Taking Advance Directives Seriously

Prospective Autonomy and Decisions near the End of Life

Robert S. Olick

GEORGETOWN UNIVERSITY PRESS/Washington, D.C.

Georgetown University Press, Wasington, D.C.
© 2001 by Georgetown University Press. All rights reserved.
Printed in the United States of America
10 9 8 7 6 5 4 3 2 1   2001
This volume is printed on acid-free offset book paper.

Library of Congress Cataloging-in-Publication Data

Olick, Robert S.
   Taking advance directives seriously : prospective autonomy and decisions near the end of life / Robert S. Olick
      p. cm.
   Includes bibliographical references and index.
   ISBN 0-87840-868-1 (cloth : alk. paper)
   1. Right to die—Law and legislation—United States. 2. Terminally ill—legal status, laws, etc.—United States. 3. Informed consent (Medical law)—United States. I. Title.

KF3827.E87 O43   2001
344.73' 04197—dc21   2001023260

*To my wife, Sally,
and to my parents, Selma and Arthur*

Contents

PREFACE TO THE PAPERBACK EDITION	ix
ACKNOWLEDGMENTS	xi
INTRODUCTION	xiii

CHAPTER ONE:	THE PLACE OF PROSPECTIVE AUTONOMY IN DECIDING FOR INCOMPETENT PATIENTS	1
	Introduction	1
	The *Quinlan* Legacy	2
	The Trial Court	3
	The New Jersey Supreme Court's Decision	4
	The Right to Refuse Treatment	4
	The Substituted Judgment Standard	5
	Guidelines for Decision Making	7
	Emergence of a Judicial Consensus	9
	The Right to Refuse Treatment	9
	Equating the Rights of Competent and Incompetent Patients	13
	Substituted Judgment and the Evidentiary Standard	14
	Process and Review	18
	Cruzan Case	18
	The Assisted Suicide Cases	20
	Legislatures Respond: The Proliferation of Advance Directive Laws	21
	An Overview of State Statutes	21

	The Patient Self-Determination Act	25
	Should Advance Directives Always Be Followed?	26
	Conclusion	29
	Notes	31
CHAPTER TWO:	**THE ETHICAL FOUNDATIONS OF PROSPECTIVE AUTONOMY**	45
	Introduction	45
	Autonomy, Integrity, and Our Critical Interests	47
	The Autonomous Pursuit of Interests	47
	Critical Interests, Character, and Integrity	50
	The Pursuit of Death with Dignity and Respect for Autonomy	53
	The Pursuit of Death with Dignity	53
	Respect for Autonomy	55
	Experiential and Surviving Interests	57
	The Current Interests Alternative	57
	Surviving Interests and Harm	59
	Respect for Persons	62
	Posthumous Harm and Interests that Survive Death	63
	Testamentary Wills	65
	Death Rituals (Funerals and Burial)	67
	Conclusion	68
	Notes	68
CHAPTER THREE:	**PROSPECTIVE DECISIONAL AUTONOMY**	77
	Introduction	77
	Autonomy as Intentionality: Action Willed in Accordance with a Plan	81
	Autonomy as Integrity: The Idea of Reflective Acceptance	85

Intentionality, Integrity, and
  Respect for Autonomy 88
    The Problem of Infinite Regress 88
    Respecting the Treatment Choices of
      Ordinary Persons 90
    Opening the Gates to Physician Paternalism 91
Case Scenario: A Recent Conversion 93
What Makes an Advance Directive Effective? 97
  Instructions for Future Care (The Living Will) 98
    An Outcome-Oriented Understanding
      (The Common Sense View) 99
    Putting a Premium on Specificity
      (The Reactionary View) 103
  Appointing a Proxy 107
  Summary: Effective Advance Directives 110
Conclusion 111
Notes 112

CHAPTER FOUR: THE PROBLEM OF PERSONAL IDENTITY 127

Introduction 127
The Argument from Personal Identity 130
  Statement of the Argument 130
  Psychological Continuity and Personal Identity 131
  How Strong Must Psychological
    Connectedness/Continuity Be? 133
Moral Objections to the Discontinuity Thesis 136
  A Paradigm Scenario 136
  On the Unity of a Life 139
  The Newly Dead 142
  Treatment of New Persons:
    Surviving Interests and Obligations 145
  Treating New Persons as Persons 147
  Permanently Unconscious Nonpersons 149
Conclusion 151
Notes 151

CHAPTER FIVE: RESPECTING ADVANCE DIRECTIVES: PUTTING THEORY INTO PRACTICE — 161

Introduction — 161
Toward an Ethic of Judgment — 163
Challenging an Advance Directive:
  Process and Procedure — 167
    Changing Incentives, Changing Behavior — 167
    Substantive Grounds for Overriding
      an Advance Directive — 170
      Hopeless Ambiguity — 170
      Radical Change in Circumstances — 172
      The Rebel Proxy — 174
    Process and Review — 176
      The Burden of Persuasion:
        Who Should Take the Next Step? — 176
      Mandating Accountability:
        Ethics Committees and Courts — 178
    Some Objections and Responses — 181
Case Scenarios at the Edges — 185
  Scenario One: An Ambiguous
    Instruction Directive? — 185
  Scenario Two: Apparent Inconsistency in the
    Patient's Wishes — 188
    Specificity of Prior Statements — 189
    The Ethics Committee's Role — 189
    Handling Family Discord — 190
    Contemporaneous Expressions
      in Favor of Life — 190
  Scenario Three: The Proxy Who Can't Let Go — 194
Conclusion — 197
Notes — 198

CONCLUSION — 211

INDEX — 217

Preface to the Paperback Edition

When my journey into the field of bioethics began in the mid-1980s, the right to refuse life-sustaining treatment was still mired in controversy. As a participant in, advocate for, and observer of the emergence of the contemporary consensus surrounding the rights of patients and families to shape the dying process, I have often been struck by the various ways in which the status of "consensus" has been achieved while lively debate and disagreement persist. The preeminence of autonomy in the care of incompetent dying patients has become a cornerstone of the bioethical landscape, yet the moral authority of advance directives, the standing of close and caring family members to make surrogate decisions, and the proper role of law and policy in facilitating, limiting, and regulating end-of-life decisions,
 main contested terrain. Ethics consultants and committees continue to grapple with end-of-life dilemmas more than any other issue.

This book is about rethinking, enriching, and fortifying the case for patient and family control in the face of significant challenges to the nature, scope, and importance of autonomy in the care of incompetent dying patients. In large measure, this project has been motivated by a deep disquiet that a quarter century after *Quinlan*, dying patients' wishes often do not direct care near the end of life, even when patients' intentions and plans have previously been put to writing in a health care proxy, living will, or both. While this book is predominantly conceptual in its structure and content, its ultimate target is very pragmatic: Taking advance directives seriously where it matters most—at the bedside of dying patients.

ACKNOWLEDGMENTS

The ideas and arguments in this book have taken form over a period of approximately 15 years. The original manuscript was submitted as my doctoral dissertation. I have since revised and updated the text to reflect some new developments, especially in law; to refine the arguments; and, I hope, to improve the writing. I am deeply indebted to Robert Veatch for his insight and stewardship, as well as for the many conversations and comments on draft chapters that helped hone the arguments and identify the limits of various positions. Many thanks are due as well to Tom Beauchamp, for his support and guidance and for his teachings in the classroom that were part of my introduction to bioethics; and to Mark Lance, for his careful reading and suggestions, especially on the topic of personal identity. Gratitude and appreciation are due to Hans-Martin Sass and to the Volkswagen Foundation, whose generous support made possible the luxury of a two-year hiatus from professional duties and a return to the relatively unfettered pursuits that are the privilege of student life.

Over the years I have benefited from the insights and generosity of numerous individuals. I want to mention three in particular. Norman Cantor has graciously given of his time and thoughts and provided valuable comments at various stages of my progress. Robert Weir has been especially supportive of this project in a variety of ways. Our innumerable hallway consults and his specific comments on several near-final chapters have improved the thought and the writing. Long before I discovered the discipline of bioethics, Jerome Balmuth of Colgate University opened my mind to the wonders of philosophy. His teachings remain with me to this day.

Many of the ideas in this book took flight a decade and more ago in countless discussions with staff, in commission meetings, and in various other communications during my tenure with the New Jersey Bioethics Commission. The reader will no doubt notice more references to that state's advance directives law than to any other. It was a rare honor to serve the commission and the people of New Jersey, and I have been enriched by the experience in untold ways. No mention of the bioethics commission would be complete without acknowledging the abiding friendship and colleagueship I formed there with the commission's chair, Paul Armstrong, to whom I am indebted beyond words.

INTRODUCTION

Approximately 2.3 million Americans die each year.[1] Of these deaths, approximately 1.7 million (more than two-thirds) are among persons 65 years of age and older,[2] for whom chronic conditions constitute five of the six leading causes of death.[3] Of the more than 1.3 million people who die in a hospital setting each year (more than half of all U.S. deaths annually), nearly 70 percent die after a decision to forego life-sustaining treatment has been made.[4] In the large majority of cases, by the time illness and disease have progressed to the point that a decision not to provide life-sustaining medical intervention is considered seriously, illness and disease also have robbed the patient of the mental faculties required to make the difficult decision to forego aggressive measures on his or her own behalf. On a daily basis, families and health care professionals are called upon to ask and answer the questions: How are decisions to terminate treatment to be made on behalf of incompetent patients? What ethical and legal principles and rules should guide us in deciding for others?

In the 25 years since the New Jersey Supreme Court's seminal opinion in the case of Karen Ann Quinlan, an ethical, legal, and societal consensus about forgoing life-sustaining treatment has emerged. In the exercise of autonomy, seriously ill patients—competent and incompetent—have the right to refuse treatment, including life-sustaining treatment, and health care professionals and families have correlative obligations to respect treatment refusals. For competent patients, autonomy and self-determination find expression in the ethical and legal doctrine of informed consent, which encompasses the right to refuse unwanted life-sustaining medical interventions when such patients are seriously ill and dying. This same principle has been extended to decision making for incompetent patients, on the premise that the right of self-determination in matters of medical treatment should not be lost or impaired when one is no longer able to personally exercise that right. In deciding for an incompetent patient, family members, physicians, and others who are responsible for the patient's care should look first and foremost to the patient's statements, values, and wishes as expressed when the patient was competent.

The strength of the principle of respect for autonomy in medical ethics lies in its priority status when the patient's wishes conflict with his or her best interests. An autonomous refusal of treatment effectively shields the patient from unwanted interventions that others—in particular, physicians—believe would promote the patient's good. Autonomy also functions as a sword: The exercise of autonomy asserts that the locus of power and authority in the physician-patient relationship (at least for this decision) rests with the patient. In short, the consensus accords respect for (prospective) autonomy reigning status in health care decisions. Only if the patient's prior expressions fail to provide a basis for decision—such as when the patient has never been competent (in which case speaking about prior autonomous expressions makes no sense)—should decisions be made in accordance with the alternative "best interests of the patient" standard.

Respecting the incompetent patient's prior autonomous wishes requires decision makers to engage in an act of recalling and reconstructing prior expressions to determine what the patient would want in the current circumstances—a task that often can prove difficult. The quest for responses to this dilemma and the value we attach to dying on our own terms has led to widespread acceptance of *advance directives* in the medical, legal, and academic communities and throughout society. Over the past quarter-century, all 50 states and the District of Columbia have enacted legislation recognizing the right to plan ahead for important decisions near the end of life at a time of future decisional incapacity by executing an advance directive. Advance directives, which are rooted in the *principle of prospective autonomy,* have come to be regarded as the preferred and legally recognized mechanism for assuring that one's own wishes and values count when treatment decisions must be made. Indeed, advance directives symbolize the right of prospective autonomy.

This is a useful point at which to offer more precise definitions of the terms *advance directive* and *prospective autonomy*. For the most part, in this book I use the term *advance directive* in its generic and most widely understood sense to refer to a *written* document that gives direction and guidance for health care decisions at a time of future incompetence (decisional incapacity). An advance directive may designate another person to make health care decisions on the patient's behalf (a *proxy directive* or *durable power of attorney for health care*); state the individual's wishes and instructions for health care (a *living will* or *instruction directive*); or both (a *combined directive*). Where appropriate, I use the more specific terms *proxy directive, instruction directive* (or *living will*), and *combined directive* to distinguish these three approaches to advance care planning. Emphasis on a written document mirrors the current state of the law, but it should not be taken as a limitation of the principle of respect for prospective autonomy that figures so prominently in this book. To the contrary, prior oral expressions play an important role in the interpretation of written directives and (as we will soon see) have been center stage in the many court cases that have recognized family members' authority to exercise "substituted judgment" that is based on prior oral expressions by incompetent patients.

The term *prospective autonomy* also appears throughout this text, often in conjunction or interchangeably with *advance directive*. Prospective autonomy (or future-oriented autonomy)—as opposed to contemporary autonomy or simply autonomy—means having a view *now* toward what will happen in the *future*. The core meaning of the term, which I develop in various ways in this book, is the idea of making plans and taking actions today that are intended to bring about a state of affairs sometime down the road. An essential feature of prospective autonomy in the context of end-of-life decisions is that choices about care are intended to take effect when one is no longer able to decide for oneself. A prospectively autonomous advance directive expresses in writing a personal plan for the dying process that is intended to control the course of care at a time of future decisional incapacity.

By far the most common purpose of advance directives is to refuse unwanted life-sustaining treatments and to choose a more natural dying process. This familiar usage and the potential conflict between patient autonomy and others' (especially physicians') contrary views of the patient's good set the stage for much of the discussion. When patients write "protreatment" directives (a choice that may well become more prevalent in the face of growing concerns about utilization of health care resources, the high cost of dying, and the spread of managed care), autonomy asserts an opposite claim. Controversy abounds when the family's affirmative request is for treatment that is not recommended—or even is opposed—by the physician. The argument for respecting advance directives presented here might well be applied to claim equal respect for pro-treatment directives. Meaningful analysis of this problem cannot proceed, however, without serious attention to issues such as the nature and limits of a right to health care and whether any such right extends to treatment that others judge to be "inappropriate" or "futile." Each of these inquiries, in turn, is fruitfully pursued only within the larger framework of a theory of social justice, or at least a social ethic of terminal care—topics that are well beyond the scope of this book.

Despite their featured place in strategies for decision making in behalf of incompetent patients, advance directives to refuse treatment have fallen far short of widely shared expectations. Most of us do not write advance directives; over the years, an estimated 5–20 percent of us have actually done so (most observers would put the figure closer to 20 percent today). More frequent use of directives can be found among specific populations, such as elderly persons, seriously ill persons, and persons living with HIV/AIDS.[5]

The lessons of experience and more rigorous empirical studies point to a range of now-familiar practical difficulties that are endemic to advance directives and advance care planning. Physicians, patients, and families often are ill-informed about their respective rights and obligations and the options available to them (advance directives, hospice, home care) or fail to communicate effectively, if at all. For those who take this step, written documents cannot escape the limitations of human foresight or the inflexibility of the "four corners" of the document. Advance directives are still a relatively new kid on the block; physicians and other health care professionals often receive them through the lens of a medical culture that remains wedded to the Hippocratic commitment "to benefit the patient according to the physician's ability and judgment."[6] In many quarters, longevity of life is identified with quality of life, and death is considered the ultimate failure. The leading national study of end-of-life care, the Study to Understand Prognoses and Preferences for Outcomes and Risks of Treatments (SUPPORT), sounds a disquieting alarm—aptly captured by the headlines of two of our nation's leading newspapers following release of the study's initial findings: "Doctors Often Fail to Heed Wishes of Dying Patient"[7] and "Patients' Wishes Often Ignored."[8] Advance directives have yet to win the battle for respect in clinical practice.

These realities fuel an ongoing debate about the moral and legal weight of advance directives in terminating life-sustaining treatment for incompetent patients. A growing number of people question the core premise that autonomy-based rights and interests apply equally for incompetent patients. Some people contend that autonomy-based interests that inform advance directives cease to be meaningful when patients can no longer appreciate whether those interests are honored or disregarded. Theoretical and empirical work has begun to challenge the generally accepted premise that advance directives are effective expressions of autonomy that are worthy of respect. Raising questions about the personal identity of incompetent patients, some writers posit that severely demented and comatose individuals are no longer the same persons they once were and that a prior directive authored by *someone else* has no moral authority to direct treatment decisions. These challenges collectively counter that, rather than accord autonomy a privileged place in treatment decision making, we should give priority to now-incompetent patients' current best interests—perhaps disregarding altogether prior directives.

The place of prospective autonomy and advance directives in deciding for incompetent patients remains unsettled. Disagreement persists about the nature and limits of prospective autonomy and about the strength of the obligation to respect advance directives in the care of dying patients.

The ongoing controversy signals the need for a new generation of debate. It shows as well the need for new, more discriminating guidelines for addressing ethical issues in the care of the dying.

This book is an argument about *why* and *how* advance directives should be taken seriously. My central task is to develop a theory of prospective autonomy that recasts and reaffirms our commitment to prospective autonomy and advance directives and defends the consensus against these challenges. Another objective is to clarify widespread confusion about the moral and legal weight of advance directives. Following the path of theory into the world of practice, I offer a prescription for emendations in law, policy, and practice that are designed to give advance directives the full measure of respect they deserve in the care of dying persons. I use cases and examples throughout to illustrate the meaning of core concepts and ideas and to demonstrate their application to decision making with advance directives.

The analysis and argument proceed in the following manner. Chapter one sets forth the foundations and central tenets of the ethical and legal consensus that ascribes priority status to the autonomy-based right to refuse life-sustaining treatment. This account, which is presented largely through the eyes of the law, is intended for the most part to be descriptive of key points that have come to shape the current landscape and that inform the analysis of subsequent chapters.

Building on this foundation, chapter two turns to the ethical foundations of prospective autonomy. I develop a *theory of prospective autonomy* that is grounded in an *integrity view of autonomous persons*. This account locates the profound importance of societal commitment to the right to die on our own terms in life's commitments to a set of concerns, projects, and core values to which we ascribe critical priority and that are closely linked to who we are. To appreciate the meaning of our interests in *personal dignity* and *family welfare* is to understand what is at stake when those interests are furthered or frustrated, honored or ignored, and reveals the profound importance of respect for autonomous advance directives. Chapter two considers and rejects the *current interests alternative*, which would have us cast advance directives aside as meaningless in favor of promoting the patient's current best interests.

The distinction between autonomous persons and autonomous actions sets the stage for chapter three. Extending the account of prospective autonomy to compass a theory of *prospective decisional autonomy*, the analysis turns to what making future-oriented choices and plans means. I present, compare, and contrast an intentionality model and an integrity (authenticity) model of autonomous actions (decisions), concluding that advance directives are best understood as intentional plans. The latter part of the chapter turns to the question of what makes an advance directive an effective exercise of prospective autonomy that gives persons who are responsible for the patient's care sufficient guidance to make treatment decisions in accordance with the patient's intent.

The *argument from personal identity* is the subject of chapter four. I first present the position that loss of psychological connectedness and continuity with the past that is the fate of severely demented and comatose persons strips prior directives of their moral authority because the now-incompetent patient and the author of the directive are *no longer the same person*. The heart of my critical response is that the logical and moral implications of regarding incompetent patients as *new persons* and *nonpersons* (the permanently unconscious) and authors of prior directives as former, *no longer existing persons* would lead us down a morally perilous path.

Chapter five turns to the practical implications of the developed theory and to the *duty to respect advance directives*. Expanding on the conclusions of chapter three, the discussion first espouses an *ethic of judgment* to characterize the broad discretion that is the special province of proxies and families in the task of interpreting and implementing advance directives. Two positions form the core of the analysis and of the emendations of policy and practice for which I argue. The first, suggested by chapter three, is that there are *three, and only three,* grounds on which an advance directive may *justifiably be overridden*. The second is that we should reverse the medical culture that places the onus on proxies and families to advocate the patient's wishes in the face of conflict. The time has come for law, policy, and practice to articulate specific and narrow grounds for justifiably overriding advance directives and to *place the burden of persuasion squarely with those who would challenge a directive's authority*. No less is required to give true voice to the place of prospective autonomy and advance directives at the bedside of dying patients and their families.

NOTES

1. National Data Bank, U.S. Department of Commerce, Economics and Statistics Administration, Bureau of the Census, *Statistical Abstract of the United States 1999*, 119th ed. (Washington, D.C.: U.S.G.P.O., 1999), 99; *MMWR—Morbidity & Mortality Weekly Report* 48, no. 30 (August 6, 1999): 664–68. This figure represents the number of registered deaths in the United States in 1997.
2. *Statistical Abstract 1999*, 102.
3. Federal Interagency Forum on Aging Related Statistics, *Older Americans 2000: Key Indicators of Well-Being* (Washington, D.C.: Federal Interagency Forum, 2000), 23, 24. The six leading causes of death for persons age 65 or older are heart disease, cancer, stroke, chronic obstructive pulmonary diseases, pneumonia and influenza, and diabetes.
4. This frequently stated number appears in the following sources: *amicus* brief of the American Hospital Association in *Cruzan v. Director, Missouri Dept. of Health*, No. 88-1503, filed 1 September 1989, 3; Thomas J. Prendergast, "Withholding or Withdrawal of Life-Sustaining Therapy," *Hospital Practice (Office Edi-*

tion) 35, no. 6 (June 15, 2000): 91–92, 95–100, 102; Charis Conn and Lewis H. Lapham, eds., *The Harper's Index Book* (New York: Franklin Square Press, 2000), 160 (citing Neil Wenger, UCLA School of Medicine).
5. John La Puma, David Orentlicher, and Robert J. Moss, "Advance Directives on Admission: Clinical Implications and Analysis of the Patient Self-Determination Act of 1990," *Journal of the American Medical Association* 266, no. 3 (July 17, 1991): 402–12 (summarizing prior studies); Joanne Lynn and Joan Teno, "After the Patient Self-Determination Act: The Need for Empirical Research on Formal Advance Directives," *Hastings Center Report* (January-February 1993): 20–21; Joan Teno et al., "The Use of Formal Advance Directives among Patients with HIV-Related Disease," *Journal of General Internal Medicine* 5 (1990): 490–94.
6. Robert M. Veatch, *A Theory of Medical Ethics* (New York: Basic Books, 1981), 10.
7. *New York Times*, November 22, 1995, 1.
8. *Washington Post*, November 22, 1995, 1.

Chapter One

THE PLACE OF PROSPECTIVE AUTONOMY IN DECIDING FOR INCOMPETENT PATIENTS

> We have no doubt, in these unhappy circumstances, that if Karen were herself miraculously lucid for an interval (not altering the existing prognosis of the condition to which she could soon return) and perceptive of her irreversible condition, she could effectively decide upon discontinuance of the life-support apparatus, even if it meant the prospect of natural death.
>
> Chief Justice Richard J. Hughes,
> New Jersey Supreme Court,
> *In re Quinlan* (1976)[1]

> The primary and most reliable indication of [a national] consensus is . . . the pattern of enacted laws.
>
> Chief Justice William Rehnquist,
> U.S. Supreme Court,
> *Washington v. Glucksberg* (1997)[2]

INTRODUCTION

In this chapter I describe the consensus regarding withholding and withdrawing of life support for incompetent patients as it has developed in law. This is a familiar starting point and perhaps a more familiar context for decisions near the end of life. The "right to die" is readily identified with the names and legal battles of Karen Ann Quinlan, Joseph Saikewicz, Claire Conroy, William Bartling, Nancy Cruzan, and others—people we know for the way they died, and for their families' courageous love, much more than for the way they lived. In the field of death and dying, law and morality are closely intertwined and have been mutually influential and reinforcing in carving out the place of autonomy in end-of-life decisions. Both, in turn, have shaped and been shaped by shared societal values. Although the issue of which field has had the greater influence on the other is a matter of some speculation, clearly the marriage of law and bioethics is to be credited with the reigning conceptual framework. [3] The principle of autonomy emerged from the embryonic stages of the bioethics movement and continues to be the idea with which bioethics is most closely identified. The current status of prospective autonomy and advance directives as integral to strategies for decisions near the end of life owes its greatest debt to its instantiation and legitimation in law. In this chapter I describe the consensus through the eyes of the law; succeeding chapters may be regarded in part as a philosophical analysis of the law and policy consensus.[4]

Taking law as a starting point, this chapter frames the issues predominantly in the "rights" language of the law. The idea of rights is especially well-suited to discussion of the place of autonomy in deciding for incompetent patients. The language of rights, particularly legal rights, underscores the dual sense of autonomy as both sword and shield in the physician-patient-family relationship. To assert a right of autonomy is to declare a claim of respect for autonomous decisions; to have a right means that others have certain obligations (the correlativity theory of rights), including the duty not to interfere with the exercise of autonomous choice. Failure to live up to those obligations is a violation of the right of respect for patient autonomy. In this way, rights empower patients with decisional authority and protect patients from the intrusions of others. Law and bioethics have embraced the concept of rights as an essential tool for redefinition of the physician-patient relationship.[5] Moreover, the notion of rights is not only a foundation of the consensus; it is deeply embedded in the fabric of how we understand patient autonomy to make treatment decisions—especially decisions to refuse life support. In sum, in making decisions near the end of life, autonomy and rights go hand in hand.[6]

The law's commitment to the autonomy-based right to refuse treatment begins with *Quinlan*, the case that has been called "the *Brown v. Board of Education* of the right-to-die movement."[7]

THE *QUINLAN* LEGACY

On September 10, 1975, Joseph and Julia Quinlan instituted legal proceedings in a New Jersey courthouse seeking permission to direct removal of the respirator that was sustaining the life of their 21-year-old daughter Karen Ann in a persistent vegetative state (PVS). Approximately six months earlier, Karen had been rushed to the emergency room of Newton Memorial Hospital after suffering cardiac arrest and falling into a coma.[8] Soon thereafter, Karen was transferred to St. Claire's Hospital, a larger and better-equipped facility known to the Quinlans. PVS is a condition in which all cognitive functions of the brain have been lost, resulting in complete unawareness of self and the environment. When PVS is properly diagnosed, there is virtually no hope of recovery to a cognitive sapient state.[9]

After much private and public agonizing, the Quinlans decided that Karen should "be free from the tyranny of the machine thought to be sustaining her life past the point at which she would have wanted to live."[10] In keeping with the treating physician's initial suggestion, they requested that the respirator be removed, allowing her to die. The hospital's initial response was to agree to honor their request. The Quinlans were asked to sign a consent and release form directing the physician to "discontinue all extraordinary measures, including the use of a respirator" and releasing the physician and the hospital from liability.[11] Shortly thereafter, however, the attending physician and the hospital changed their minds and refused to comply with the parents' request—setting the stage for the landmark litigation to follow.

The Trial Court

The Quinlans' petition to the court sought to have Mr. Quinlan appointed as his daughter's legal guardian, with "express power of authorizing the discontinuance of all extraordinary means of sustaining the vital processes of his daughter."[12] Karen's right to refuse treatment was premised on a number of grounds, most significantly the constitutional right of privacy. The petition was opposed by the hospital, the physicians, state and local authorities, and the guardian *ad litem* appointed by the court to represent Karen's best interests. In essence, these parties collectively countered that there is no constitutional right to die; that there is a compelling state interest in favor of preserving human life; and that to remove the respirator would be "homicide and an act of euthanasia." The physicians argued that whether the respirator should be removed was a judgment within the exclusive province of the medical profession and that such action would be contrary to accepted norms of medical practice, which required aggressive efforts to sustain life. Furthermore, a decision to terminate the respirator would impermissibly demand assessment of Karen's quality of life and would set a precedent allowing "quality of life standards to serve as future guidelines."[13]

Judge Robert Muir rejected the arguments made on behalf of the Quinlans and adopted the positions advanced by the medical profession and the state. In siding with the medical profession, the judge ruled that "[t]here *is* a duty to continue the life-assisting apparatus if, within the treating physician's opinion, it should be done."[14] The Quinlans' petition was denied. Striking an extra blow at the family, the court refused to appoint Joseph Quinlan as Karen's guardian and chose instead to continue the authority of the court-appointed attorney as guardian of the person. (The Quinlans' reaction to the trial court's ruling is described in their book *Karen Ann*.)[15] Judge Muir's ruling was soon followed by an expedited appeal to the New Jersey Supreme Court.

The New Jersey Supreme Court's Decision

The Right to Refuse Treatment

In the first judicial ruling of its kind, the New Jersey Supreme Court held that Karen Quinlan, an incompetent patient in a PVS, had the right to refuse the respirator that artificially sustained her life and appointed her father as the legal guardian with authority to exercise this right on his daughter's behalf. Reversing the ruling below, the New Jersey Supreme Court held that a patient has a fundamental constitutional right to refuse life-sustaining treatment, grounded in the right of privacy under the federal and state constitutions.[16] Finding the legal underpinnings for the right of privacy in the U.S. Supreme Court's decisions in the area of procreation,[17] the *Quinlan* court held that "this right is broad enough to encompass a patient's decision to decline medical treatment under certain circumstances."[18] The court also held that the right of privacy protected by the New Jersey state constitution encompasses the right to refuse life-sustaining treatment.[19]

The constitutional right to refuse treatment, like other constitutional rights, is not absolute; it must be balanced against certain countervailing state (societal) interests. To determine whether Ms. Quinlan's privacy right could be exercised in this case, the court went on to balance these competing interests. At issue in *Quinlan* were the state's interests in preserving life, in preventing suicide, and in safeguarding the integrity of the medical profession.[20] In an oft-quoted passage, the New Jersey Supreme Court held that "the State's interest *contra* weakens and the individual's right to privacy grows as the degree of bodily invasion increases and the prognosis dims."[21] The state's interest in preserving the life of a vegetative patient with no hope of recovery must be subordinated to the contrary assertion of the patient's right to refuse unwanted life support. Furthermore, rejection of life support in these circumstances is an exercise of self-determination, not an act of purposeful self-destruction that defines suicide.[22] Nor did removal of the respirator in accordance with the family's request offend principles of medical ethics. The Court's strongly worded conclusion was that "no external compelling interest of the State could compel Karen to endure the unendurable, only to vegetate a few measurable months with no realistic possibility of returning to any semblance of cognitive or sapient life."[23]

Quinlan's assessment of professional medical ethics is especially instructive because it set the tone for the ascendance of the patient's personal judgment over the physician's medical judgment in end-of-life decisions. Initially, Chief Justice Hughes' opinion rejected the premise that the decision about whether to terminate treatment rests within the exclusive province of the medical profession. To the contrary, "the interests of the patient, as seen by her surrogate, the guardian, must be evaluated by the court as predominant, even in the face of an opinion *contra* by the present attending physicians."[24] The law has a special responsibility to respond to individuals' dilemmas "in the face of modern technological marvels presenting questions hitherto unthought of."[25] The New Jersey Supreme Court flatly rejected the lower court's finding that the law, and society as a whole, should play no role in treatment decisions because "[t]he morality and conscience of our society places the responsibility in the hands of the physician."[26] Instead, such decisions "must, in the ultimate, be responsive not only to the concepts of medicine but also to the common moral judgment of the community at large."[27]

A clear message of *Quinlan* is that ultimate decisional authority rests with the patient and family, not with the physician. Individuals and society are not bound by prevailing standards of medical practice; the consensus of members of a professional organization, such as the American Medical Association, must yield to more foundational principles of medical ethics found in the legal and moral rules of the larger society that medicine serves.[28]

Notably, however, rather than reject outright, as irrelevant, the prevailing medical standards of the time, the court went to some length to reconcile those standards with the family's refusal of the respirator. Sensitive to the court's responsibility to respect (if not embrace) established medical standards, Chief Justice Hughes discussed at length whether the "internal consistency and rationality" of such standards would constitute sufficient reason not to honor the family's request. The opinion noted that physicians "have sometimes refused to treat the hopeless and dying as if they were curable" and that "many [physicians] have refused to inflict an undesired prolongation of the process of dying on a patient in irreversible condition when it is clear that such 'therapy' offers neither human nor humane benefit."[29] In other words, although no evidence was adduced that the Quinlans' position found consensus support in the medical profession, there also were no consistent and rational medical standards opposed to removal of the respirator in these circumstances.[30]

The Substituted Judgment Standard

Having clothed the personal right to refuse unwanted treatment in constitutional protections and having found that this right could be exercised in the circumstances before it, the New Jersey Supreme Court readily concluded that this right is not lost through deprivation of the ability to decide for oneself. To the contrary, this right survives incompetency and may be exercised by another person on the patient's behalf. Another frequently quoted passage from the opinion states that if a decision to forego life-sustaining treatment is

> a valuable incident of [Karen's] right of privacy, as we believe it to be, then it should not be discarded solely on the basis that her condition prevents her conscious exercise of the choice. The only practical way to prevent destruction of the right is to permit the guardian and family of Karen to render their best judgment, subject to the qualifications hereinafter stated, as to whether she would exercise it in these circumstances.[31]

Thus, the court had little trouble extending the right to refuse treatment to an incompetent patient who would never regain consciousness. It then turned to the procedural mechanism by which Karen's right of self-determination could be protected. The approach was to appoint Mr. Quinlan as guardian and to grant to the family authority to act as their daughter's proxy and to seek to determine what Karen's own wishes would be in these circumstances.

Although deciding *who* should exercise the incompetent patient's right in this case was straightforward,[32] deciding *how* such decisions should be made—that is, by what substantive standard—was more challenging. The Quinlans were authorized to use their "best judgment" to effectuate Karen's interests and wishes. This standard has come to be known as the "substituted judgment" test.

In the literal sense, substituted judgment means that the decision maker is substituted for the decisionally incapable patient and "dons the mental mantle of the incompetent," charged with responsibility to make the decision the patient would make for herself if she were competent to do so.[33] More realistically, substituted judgment most often involves a mix of subjective and objective factors in the decisional process.

Karen's family knew that she had made prior statements expressing a "distaste for continuance of life by extraordinary medical procedures"[34] in similar circumstances and that a continued vegetative existence would offend her personal values. As a legal matter, however, scant evidence was presented about what Karen would actually choose for herself. Stating that "we cannot discern her supposed choice based on the testimony of her previous conversations with friends," the court discounted this evidence as "without sufficient probative weight."[35] At the same time, in exercising their "best judgment" on behalf of their daughter, the Quinlans also were authorized to use their own judgment of what would be best for Karen; in other words, they also were empowered to employ a best interests standard. As I discuss further below, this mix of subjective and objective factors has long been part of the legal doctrine of substituted judgment developed in other contexts.

Nonetheless, substituted judgment is widely and properly viewed as an autonomy-based doctrine because it gives the patient's previously expressed wishes and values priority ranking in deciding for incompetent patients. A surrogate's primary task is to ascertain and effectuate what the patient would want; best-interest assessments are supplementary and should be patient-centered and made from the patient's point of view to the extent possible. *Quinlan*'s recognition of an incompetent patient's autonomy-based right to refuse treatment, together with the court's practical approach of looking to close family to reconstruct the patient's prior expressions and values, planted the seeds for rapid evolution of the principle of prospective autonomy in end-of-life decisions.

Guidelines for Decision Making

One further aspect of the *Quinlan* case is important to the consensus that subsequently emerged. The case also is notable for its introduction of institutional ethics committees as participants in end-of-life decisions. In its order for declaratory relief, the court set forth the process to be followed in this and future cases in which termination of life support for a permanently unconscious patient is considered:

> Upon the concurrence of the guardian and family of Karen, should the responsible attending physicians conclude that there is no reasonable possibility of Karen's ever emerging from her present comatose condition to a cognitive, sapient state and that the life-support apparatus now being administered to Karen should be discontinued, they shall consult with the hospital "Ethics Committee" or like body of the institution in which Karen is then hospitalized. If that consultative body agrees that there is no reasonable possibility of Karen's ever emerging from her present comatose condition to a cognitive, sapient state, the present life-support system may be withdrawn and said action shall be without any civil or criminal liability therefor on the part of any participant, whether guardian, physician, hospital, or others.[36]

The rationale for mandating the additional procedural step of consulting a hospital ethics committee was multifaceted. Of immediate concern was resolution of the case at hand. Recognizing that some time had passed since Karen's medical condition had been confirmed and that her parents might well choose different physicians to care for their daughter following the conclusion of the case, the committee's prognosis confirmation function was designed to foster post-judgment resolution of the treatment issue. The much more significant impact of the ethics committee's role, however, came from the intent to craft a decision-making process for future cases that would alleviate the perceived need to involve the courts in resolving similar treatment dilemmas. Here the court seized on the idea of an ethics committee as "a way to free physicians, in the pursuit of their healing vocation, from possible contamination by self-interest or self-protection concerns which would inhibit their independent medical judgments for the well-being of their dying patients."[37] Going one step further, *Quinlan* established a grant of judicial immunity from civil and criminal liability for future cases in which the so-called "Quinlan procedures" are followed. The hoped-for consequence of this approach was to facilitate resolution of similar future treatment dilemmas without court intervention. The court also was concerned, of course, with assuring accurate diagnosis of PVS for future patients.

Quinlan's deployment of ethics committees has engendered confusion and criticism among some otherwise strong supporters. The confusion stems from the fact that the court used the term "ethics committee" but assigned to the committee a prognosis confirmation function. This confusion might be explained by the posture of the case at hand; that is, the court had already resolved the legal and ethical issues, leaving for the committee only the question of confirming prognosis. As the decision subsequently was interpreted by New Jersey hospitals, other courts, and the New Jersey Supreme Court itself, the *Quinlan* procedure mandates prognosis confirmation for PVS patients by a "prognosis committee" composed of physicians (or by qualified physicians in the absence of a committee). It does not mandate review of the ethical issues by a multidisciplinary ethics committee.

Nonetheless, in the aftermath of *Quinlan*, with the proliferation of ethics committees there also has been confusion about the functions of such ethics committees and of prognosis committees.[38] Early critical commentary on this aspect of the opinion also suggested that this part of the *Quinlan* approach cedes back to the medical profession some of the family's authority.[39] Although these concerns are valid, they have proven to be largely theoretical. In fact, ethics committees have come to be regarded as empowering to patients and families facing conflict with physicians; the more common complaint has come from physicians who see ethics committees as an intrusion on their traditional prerogatives. The important point here is not concerns about ethics committees themselves (a question to which I return in chapter five). It is *Quinlan's* salutary and lasting effect—namely, the evolution of a local institutional process that allows private decisions to be made privately, away from the public glare of the courtroom in the vast majority of instances.

EMERGENCE OF A JUDICIAL CONSENSUS

The landmark *Quinlan* case brought unprecedented media coverage; the name Karen Ann Quinlan quickly became known nationally and internationally.[40] In strictly legal terms, *Quinlan* was binding precedent only in the state of New Jersey. The reasoning in *Quinlan* soon began to take hold as persuasive authority across the country, however. With rare exceptions, court after court has followed the core approach of *Quinlan*, holding that incompetent patients retain the right to refuse unwanted life support and that family members may exercise this right on the patient's behalf under the rubric of substituted judgment. Subsequent cases have added to this foundation the best interests standard, which authorizes forgoing of life support when such a decision would serve the best interests of the patient. This objective test applies when there is little or no evidence to satisfy the subjective standard of what the patient would choose.

Thus, the judicial consensus holds that a decision to forego life support for an incompetent patient may be made in accordance with the patient's previously expressed wishes or, in appropriate cases, in accordance with the patient's best interests.[41] Significantly, judges have rarely authorized forgoing of life support solely on the grounds that such a decision would serve the patient's interests and have strained to find at least some justification for this decision in the patient's prior expressions. Current law offers little guidance about when continued treatment of an incompetent adult patient would be contrary to the patient's objective interests.

The Right to Refuse Treatment

Since *Quinlan*, a patient's right to refuse life-sustaining treatment has become a well-established seam in the fabric of patients' rights in health care. In recognizing this right, courts in several states also have embraced the constitutional right of privacy.[42] More often, courts have preferred not to address the constitutional question and have recognized the common-law basis of the right to refuse treatment.[43] The common law has long recognized the individual's right to control one's own body and to be free from nonconsensual bodily invasions. In matters of medical treatment, the right to make choices about one's own health care is protected by the doctrine of informed consent. In essence, the law of informed consent requires that physicians obtain consent from patients prior to performing a treatment or procedure; this requirement is designed to ensure that patients receive information about their medical condition and the risks, benefits, and burdens of treatment options necessary to reach an informed decision.[44] The right to refuse treatment is the logical corollary of the right to consent to treatment.

Thus, the common law right of self-determination encompasses the right to accept or to refuse medical treatment, including life-sustaining treatment. Whether this right is grounded in common law or constitutional law, courts uniformly have recognized a patient's right to refuse life-sustaining treatment as a fundamental tenet of respect for patient autonomy and self-determination.[45]

Courts across the country also have uniformly held that the right to refuse life support is not absolute; it must be balanced against potentially countervailing state interests in preserving life, preventing suicide, safeguarding the integrity of the medical profession, and protecting innocent third parties. The most significant of these state interests is the preservation of life—understood to embrace "an interest in preserving the life of the particular patient, and an interest in preserving the sanctity of all life."[46] Although the state interest in preventing suicide has been identified as a distinct concern, it is encompassed within the state interest in preserving life.[47]

Courts have consistently ruled that society's indirect and abstract interest in preserving life must yield to the individual's much stronger, direct and personal claim to control over the course of his or her own life. Judicial decisions also have uniformly found that a patient's refusal of life support is not suicide—that is, it is not an act of direct and purposeful self-destruction motivated by an intent to die. Where the termination of life support allows the underlying disease or condition to take its course, the patient's death is primarily a result of the underlying disease or condition, not of a self-inflicted injury. Furthermore, respecting the patient's refusal of life support respects the patient's intent—not to die but to refuse medical intervention and to choose a personally preferred dying process.[48]

In a few instances, protecting innocent third parties from harm has been held to justify requiring competent adults to undergo medical procedures. The interests of others have not been found sufficient ground, however, to override an incompetent dying patient's refusal of treatment.[49]

With respect to the state's interest in maintaining the integrity of the medical profession, courts have asked the same question posed in *Quinlan*—namely, whether the patient's refusal of life-sustaining treatment is consonant with existing norms of medical ethics promulgated by the profession. Looking to well-established medical authorities—including official policy statements from the American Medical Association and state-level professional and regulatory bodies (such as state professional licensing boards)—for guidance, judge after judge has found that medical authorities strongly support the physician's professional obligation to respect a patient's right to self-determination, including refusal of life support. The medical profession also acknowledges that when the patient is incompetent this right may be exercised on the patient's behalf by a family member, health care representative, or legally appointed guardian.[50] The contention that decisions to terminate life support belong exclusively to the medical profession—which so occupied the *Quinlan* court—has rarely received serious consideration since. The issue has been fully recast as one of assessing whether the patient's refusal is outside the bounds of accepted professional norms, and the consistent answer to this query has been that it is not.

In sum, the incompetent patient's right to refuse life support has consistently prevailed over these four countervailing state interests, as has the family's authority to exercise this right on behalf of loved ones. Nevertheless, although the consensus stands on firm ground here, controversy persists. A small but significant number of courts have reached a contrary result, refusing to sanction a family member's authority to direct that life support be withheld or withdrawn. The consistent theme of this group of cases (discussed further below) has been that the patient's surrogate (most often a spouse) has not shown by clear and convincing evidence that forgoing of life support is grounded in the patient's own wishes. Most notably, the Missouri Supreme Court's ruling that the family of Nancy Beth Cruzan failed to present clear and convincing evidence that she would refuse life support rather than be sustained indefinitely in a PVS thrust the issue (and the family's tragedy) once again into the national spotlight—this time before the U.S. Supreme Court. Judicial departures from the mainstream through embrace of this more demanding evidentiary standard appear to be motivated in part by a different weighting of the value of life, not by rejection of the right to refuse treatment—which the U.S. Supreme Court in fact affirmed as a constitutional right in *Cruzan*. They may be influenced as well by a less hospitable disposition toward the role of close family attending a dying loved one. (I discuss *Cruzan* and the evidentiary standard governing termination of treatment for incompetent patients further below.)

Most reported cases have involved incompetent patients who were either terminally ill or in a PVS. As a general matter, life support may be foregone on behalf of an incompetent patient if the patient is in one of these two conditions or categories. Few cases have squarely reached the issue of forgoing life support for an incompetent patient suffering from a nonterminal, progressive, and irreversible illness, such as early stages of Alzheimer's dementia. Among those that have, several have involved patients in what has been called a "minimally conscious state"—that is, these patients were substantially cognitively impaired and had extremely limited capacity for interaction, but they were not clinically in PVS.[51]

Courts in California (severe brain damage following a motor vehicle accident),[52] Michigan (same),[53] and Wisconsin (Alzheimer's dementia)[54] have all ruled against a family member's petition for authorization to direct that life support be foregone. Each held that evidence of the patient's wishes was not clear and convincing. The California court ruled, however, that a feeding tube could be withdrawn if doing so were in the best interests of the patient (relying on that state's conservatorship statute). In a confused opinion, the Wisconsin court rejected the idea that termination of life support for a non-PVS patient is ever in the patient's (objective?) best interests but went on to hold that if there is "a clear statement of [the patient's] desires in these circumstances, then it is in the best interests of [the patient] to honor those wishes."

These cases and future developments at the edges of the consensus warrant more extensive analysis. At present, it is fair to say that refusal of treatment in such cases cannot be counted under the umbrella of the judicial consensus (nor can these circumstances be uncontroversially counted in the ethical consensus). Clearly, however, the competent patient's right of refusal is not expressly bounded by the nature of his or her medical condition and prognosis.[55] Arguably, the same may be said of the rights of incompetent patients in light of the frequent pronouncement that individuals do not lose these important rights on loss of competence. As these cases "the other way" themselves suggest, there is good reason to believe that courts would similarly reject such limits for incompetent patients, at least where there is credible evidence of the patient's treatment refusal.[56] In future cases, the irreversibility of the patient's medical condition will continue to be a central factor in balancing the right to refuse treatment with competing principles.[57]

Is the patient's right to refuse life-sustaining treatment dependent on or limited by the nature of the *medical treatment* in question? The consistent answer to this question has been no. Of particular concern has been whether artificially provided fluids and nutrition constitute medical treatment that a patient is entitled to refuse on the same basis as other forms of treatment, such as a respirator. This issue was first addressed by the New Jersey Supreme Court in *In re Conroy*, which involved a request to withdraw a nasogastric feeding tube from an 84-year-old woman with serious and irreversible physical and mental impairments and a life expectancy of one year or less. In *In re Conroy*, the court held that "artificial feedings such as nasogastric tubes, gastrostomies, and intravenous infusions . . . are medical procedures."[58] Although the symbolic meaning of providing fluids and nutrition to a patient should not be ignored, analytically, artificially provided fluids and nutrition is equivalent to artificial breathing by means of a respirator. "Both prolong life through artificial means when the body is no longer able to perform a vital bodily function on its own."[59] Therefore, "[a] competent patient has the right to decline any medical treatment, including artificial feeding, and should retain that right when and if he becomes incompetent."[60] Courts nationally have reached the same conclusion and have drawn no distinction between artificially provided fluids and nutrition and other forms of life-sustaining treatment.[61]

Equating the Rights of Competent and Incompetent Patients

The validity in principle of equating the rights of incompetent patients with those of competent patients has been readily accepted. This position rests on three interrelated yet distinct ideas: self-determination, best interests, and equality. Most familiar is that self-determination remains an important value "even when [the patient] is no longer able to assert that right or to appreciate its effectuation."[62] Respect for self-determination honors the intrinsic human worth of persons. To disregard the patient's prior wishes is to violate the patient's intrinsic worth, even if the patient is not aware that his or her prior wishes are being ignored. To hold otherwise would be to "permit obliteration of an incompetent's panoply of rights merely because the patient could no longer sense the violation of those rights."[63] This straightforward statement of prospective autonomy has well-established analogues elsewhere in the law. For example, the law respects a person's testamentary dispositions and estate plans even though the testator will never know whether his or her bequests have been carried out.[64] Ignoring the decedent's chosen means for distributing personal assets would offend his or her dignity.

Effectuating the patient's wishes often promotes patient well-being as well. Individuals ordinarily are the best judges of their own interests. If continued treatment and a prolonged dying process is not always in the interests of competent patients, it cannot always be in the interests of incompetent patients. As the court in *Superintendent of Belchertown State School v. Saikewicz* stated, "[t]he 'best interests' of an incompetent person are not necessarily served by imposing on such persons results not mandated as to competent persons similarly situated."[65] Once the view that continued treatment is always in the patient's interest is rejected, upholding the right of self-determination complements the law's responsibility to protect the interests of incompetent and vulnerable patients as they themselves have defined them.

Equating the rights of incompetent patients with those of competent patients also embraces the law's long-standing commitment to equality and to protection of disabled and vulnerable persons from discrimination and abuse. The value of human dignity and worth extends to all persons equally, not just to competent and healthy persons. To conclude otherwise would be "to downgrade the status of the incompetent person"[66] and would do violence to incompetent patients' interests in self-determination and well-being. As law professors George Annas and Leonard Glantz have stated, "Courts could probably come to no other conclusion without seriously undermining the rights of the weakest members of society: the mentally incompetent who are unable to protect their own interests."[67]

To be sure, this position has its critics. Some find the idea of self-determination incompatible with incompetence. For some, autonomy requires a competent contemporaneous choice; treating the incompetent patient as if he or she were competent is absurd. Others also challenge the notion that prior expressions are the appropriate measure of the incompetent patient's current interests.[68] I return to these objections at length in developing the ethical argument for prospective autonomy in chapter two. The point to be made here is that the prevailing legal paradigm holds that respect for autonomy and self-determination provides the primary justification for terminating life support for competent and incompetent patients alike. The difference is that prospective autonomy must be implemented in a different manner.[69]

Substituted Judgment and the Evidentiary Standard

Like-minded courts have implemented prospective autonomy by adopting the substituted judgment standard. Time and again a surrogate decision maker—most often a close and caring family member—has been charged with responsibility to "don the mental mantle of the incompetent"[70] with the goal of ascertaining and effectuating what the patient would want under the circumstances. Through the mechanism of substituted judgment, the autonomy rights of incompetent patients are honored on a par with those of competent patients.

In applying substituted judgment to deciding for incompetent patients, courts have essentially borrowed from a long history of legal precedent. The substituted judgment doctrine has its origins in the area of estate administration and can be traced as far back as the early 1800s in English law and the mid-1800s in American law. At that time, the doctrine was employed to determine whether a now-incompetent person would have made a gift to someone to whom an obligation of support was not otherwise owed.[71] More recent foundations are found in the health care arena. For example, in the well-known case *Strunk v. Strunk*, the court authorized removal of a kidney from an incompetent adult "donor" for transplantation into his brother on the grounds that both parties would benefit and that the donor would consent to the procedure if he were competent.[72] Thus, the historical antecedents of substituted judgment reveal some mixed strains. Under the guise of self-determination, substituted judgment also has been used to protect the individual's best interests and to achieve altruistic goals of protecting the interests of others. Although its application in deciding for incompetent patients vindicates choosing as the patient would, as illustrated by *Quinlan*, courts also have admitted under the same rubric a place for third-party judgments of what is best for the patient. This is one reason some commentators have referred to the substituted judgment doctrine as a "legal fiction." Another is the challenge of reconstructing the past (to some an "imaginative exercise") to satisfy the substantive standard of fidelity to the patient's previously expressed wishes.[73]

In fact, the substantive standard of choosing as the patient would has been the most controverted and troublesome aspect in life-and-death litigation. The primary reason is that implementing this standard and determining whether to authorize the surrogate to direct forgoing of life support can become a thorny evidentiary question. Couched against the law's time-honored presumption in favor of life, the burden of proof that the patient would refuse life support rests with the surrogate. In each case, courts have received testimony from family, friends, and sometimes religious advisors attesting to the patient's prior statements, preferences, and values—the same process that occurs informally when such decisions are contemplated within the private confines of the physician-patient-family relationship.

Courts repeatedly have struggled with the "probative value" (reliability) of the evidence presented, weighing factors such as specificity, consistency, remoteness in time, and thoughtfulness of prior statements and actions.[74] In doing so, courts have articulated several legal standards that the evidence must satisfy to meet the burden of proof and overcome the presumption in favor of continued treatment. The most prevalent standard employed is proof by "a preponderance of the evidence."[75] The most stringent rule is that there must be "clear and convincing evidence" of the patient's refusal of treatment.

Although most courts have adopted some version of the "preponderance of the evidence" test, as of the year 2001, judicial opinions in at least eight states have embraced the clear and convincing evidence standard.[76] This test demands that proof be sufficiently clear to convince the court that the patient would refuse life support and choose death under the circumstances. An alternative formulation requires that there be "proof sufficient to persuade the trier of fact that the patient held a firm and settled commitment to the termination of life supports under the circumstances like those presented."[77] At least two states provide by statute that courts should adopt a clear and convincing standard when asked to resolve disputes—perhaps suggesting, together with judicial rulings the same way, a strong minority trend in this direction.[78]

The evidentiary problem that is endemic to substituted judgment has been the subject of much scholarly debate. The contrasting positions of law professors Nancy Rhoden and Rebecca Dresser are illustrative. Each observes that in refusal-of-treatment cases, the result reached—termination of life support—is rarely justified by the court's reasoning. Evidence of the patient's wishes often fails to satisfy the articulated evidentiary standard justifying the conclusion that honoring the request to terminate life support honors patient self-determination. As the late professor Rhoden has stated,

"[C]ourts require a higher quantum of justification than is typically available, and are led to write opinions that misleadingly imply that such a justification is possible."[79] She argues further that the underlying rationale at work is deference to families as the appropriate decision makers and the often implicit acknowledgment that in fact substituted judgment promotes the dual values of respecting patient self-determination and promoting patient well-being. The theoretical implication is the "notion that acting upon a patient's unexpressed but probable desires can be equated with implementing the patient's right of choice."[80] Rhoden contends that the law should seek to remedy its conceptual inconsistency by straightforwardly recognizing a presumption in favor of family authority, placing the burden of proof to overcome this presumption on those who oppose discontinuing life support.

In contrast, Dresser points to the inherent weakness of the substituted judgment approach as reason to abandon it altogether. She argues that these conceptual infirmities mask courts' hidden resistance to taking responsibility for quality-of-life judgments that are involved in deciding when the patient should be allowed to die.[81] According to Dresser, the law should abandon substituted judgment in favor of an outright best interests analysis for incompetent patients. A supporter of prospective autonomy, Rhoden believes that advance directives offer clear proof of the patient's wishes and should be obeyed. For Dresser, advance directives suffer from essentially the same faults as substituted judgment and should be considered "nearly irrelevant."[82]

The evidentiary problem continues to plague the courts, whose posture in deciding individual cases is by necessity one of looking backward. The same dilemma also continues to plague decisions at the bedside. Clearly a state's legal standard has a significant impact on patient care decisions. The more stringent "clear and convincing evidence" rule (the New York rule) can have a chilling effect on respect for patients' previously expressed wishes and the authority of families to decide. Holding families to a less rigorous standard, such as having some trustworthy evidence (the New Jersey rule), induces greater deference to the special role of loving family members. The practical effect of the two approaches is significant and can be seen in the respective climates of these two states.[83]

In practice, moreover, attaching a legal label to the degree of certainty required to warrant termination of life support does little to help family members and physicians decide when to take comfort in the belief that this choice is what the patient would want. "Clear and convincing" is an empty concept that must be filled in by the patient's prior expressions and values and appropriate inferences to the medical circumstances. The clear and convincing standard suggests that family members and physicians must believe that the patient would refuse life support with a bit more certainty but offers little guidance to those who must daily weigh and balance what is known of the patient's prior expressions.

People widely believe that a written advance directive resolves this evidentiary problem. Yet health care professionals frequently complain that patients' living wills are vague, ambiguous, and unhelpful. Bridging the gap between these two views is one of the important themes of this book. Legal sources offer limited insights into the judiciary's stance here, but judges appear to lean toward the former, more widely held understanding. Judicial opinions point to the living will as the "best evidence" of the patient's wishes[84] or state that it is "evidence of the most persuasive quality."[85] These pronouncements suggest that a written document would satisfy the applicable evidentiary standard, including the clear and convincing standard.

Among the very few reported cases that actually have involved advance directives, at least three support this interpretation. In *John F. Kennedy Hosp. v. Bludworth*, the high court of Florida declared that a comatose terminally ill patient's surrogate can implement an advance directive refusing continued life support without the need for court approval, finding that "a so-called 'living will' or 'mercy will' [is] persuasive evidence of [the] incompetent person's intention and it should be given great weight."[86] A 1990 Georgia opinion, *Zodin v. Manor Healthcare Corp.*, ordered—virtually without discussion—that the living will of a terminally ill, chronically vegetative patient refusing life-sustaining procedures in the event of terminal illness be honored.[87] *Saunders v. State*,[88] decided under New York law, characterized a living will as "evidence of the most persuasive quality" and a "clear and convincing demonstration" that the patient would refuse treatment if terminally ill. Another New York case, however, reached a seemingly opposite conclusion. *Evans v. Bellevue Hosp.*[89] recognized an AIDS patient's proxy appointment but found his living will ambiguous and refused to authorize termination of life support. The *Evans* decision (which I discuss in chapter five) also rested on the fact that the patient's toxoplasmosis could be treated, restoring the patient to competence at least for a period of time.

Perhaps more revealing of the judiciary's stance towards advance directives is the 1993 report of the Coordinating Council on Life-Sustaining Medical Treatment Decision Making by the Courts. In a survey of 384 state trial judges nationally, although only 1 percent of judges indicated that they had actually heard a case in which an advance directive was at issue, 82 percent believed "that a properly executed document representing the patient's wishes should be dispositive where the patient is not currently competent to express such wishes."[90] This finding is consistent with the prevailing view that a written document stands as a convincing and reliable statement of the patient's wishes. The law has further contributed to this understanding through its legitimation of advance directives in statutory law. Before turning to these enactments, however, we must complete the judicial picture.[91]

Process and Review

Overall, the response to *Quinlan's* deployment of ethics committees has been far less uniform. Several states mirror the *Quinlan* procedure for PVS patients.[92] Other courts encourage, but do not require, resort to ethics committees in their broader, more familiar role.[93] Massachusetts decisions insist that ethics committees are no substitute for judicial review to resolve disputes (but do not require routine recourse to the courts);[94] Illinois case law calls for judicial review if the treatment at issue is artificially provided fluids and nutrition.[95]

Nonetheless, there is broad acceptance of *Quinlan's* underlying objective. Decisions near the end of life should be made privately, with resort to a local review process to resolve disagreements where necessary. Courts should not be involved in life-sustaining treatment decisions except in unusual circumstances.[96] Against this legal backdrop, ethics committees have emerged to play an important dispute resolution role in hospitals across the country. The ethics committee "movement" received a major shot in the arm in the early 1990s when the Joint Commission on Accreditation of Healthcare Organizations (JCAHO) mandated that all facilities it accredits establish and maintain "a mechanism for the consideration of ethical issues arising in the care of patients . . ."[97]—a quasi-legal mandate that has been widely interpreted to mean an ethics committee. Though hospitals rarely have been legally required to establish ethics committees,[98] most hospitals across the nation have done so; those that have not typically rely on one or more ethics consultants.[99]

The *Cruzan* Case

Cruzan v. Director, Missouri Dept. of Health[100] is the only case addressing refusal of life support to reach the U.S. Supreme Court. The bare facts of *Cruzan* are similar to those of *Quinlan*. In summary, a young Missouri woman, Nancy Beth Cruzan, fell into a PVS following an automobile accident. After several agonizing years, her parents sought to discontinue the feeding tube sustaining her in this condition. The hospital's refusal to comply with their request led to extended litigation through the Missouri courts to the U.S. Supreme Court.

Initially, the trial court joined the chorus of judicial voices in support of the family's right to decide and appointed Joseph and Joyce Cruzan as co-guardians of their daughter, with authority to direct discontinuance of the feeding tube. The Missouri Supreme Court disagreed, however.

Adopting a vitalist posture toward the state's interests, Missouri's highest court rejected the asserted right to refuse treatment, finding that "[t]he state's concern with the sanctity of life rests on the principle that life is precious and worthy of preservation without regard to its quality."[101] Swimming against the tide, the court also refused to equate the rights of competent patients with those of incompetent patients, stating that "it is logically inconsistent" to claim that "personal autonomy can be exercised by another absent the most rigid of formalities."[102] In a further attack on the foundations of prospective autonomy, the opinion contends that "it is definitionally impossible for a person to make an informed decision—either to consent or to refuse—under hypothetical circumstances."[103] Even assuming that Nancy's wishes could be implemented by her family, her prior statements, in the court's view, failed to satisfy the standard of being "clear and convincing, inherently reliable evidence."[104]

When the U.S. Supreme Court granted *certiorari* and accepted the Missouri Supreme Court's decision for review, many observers perceived a substantial threat to the consensus support for patients' rights that had developed over more than a decade of litigation in state courts. What appeared to be an aberrational (and perhaps ideologically and politically motivated)[105] Missouri decision might be stretched far beyond Missouri's borders when subjected to scrutiny by a U.S. Supreme Court that was widely regarded as increasingly conservative, particularly on the question of the constitutional right of privacy.

This perceived threat to the consensus proved to be largely unfounded. The U.S. Supreme Court in *Cruzan* reaffirmed that the right to refuse treatment is protected by the federal constitution. Writing for the majority, Chief Justice Rehnquist states that "[t]he liberty interest in refusing unwanted medical treatment may be inferred from our prior decisions."[106] The Court goes on to state that "for purposes of this case, we assume that the United States Constitution would grant a competent person a constitutionally protected right to refuse lifesaving hydration and nutrition."[107] Taking the majority and concurring opinions together, eight of the nine justices (excluding Justice Scalia) agreed that the right to refuse life-sustaining treatment, including artificially provided fluids and nutrition, enjoys constitutional protections. This position is most forcefully stated in Justice O'Connor's concurrence: "The liberty guaranteed by the Due Process Clause must protect, if it protects anything, an individual's deeply personal decision to reject medical treatment, including the artificial delivery of food and water."[108]

The Court also held, however, that it is constitutionally permissible—though not constitutionally required—for a state to impose appropriate procedural guidelines for making end-of-life decisions on behalf of incompetent patients.[109] It thus upheld Missouri's clear and convincing evidence standard of proof, as well as the Missouri high court's finding that the evidence of Nancy's wishes did not meet this test. Ultimately, the Cruzans were forced to return to a Missouri trial court for another hearing at which new (though limited) evidence of their daughter's wishes was presented. Finally, the Cruzans got the relief they had long requested—authority to direct removal of the feeding tube.

Cruzan disappoints in its deliberate avoidance of constitutional privacy concerns and most importantly in its failure to grant the Cruzan family and Nancy relief from their prolonged tragedy. Patients' rights advocates would prefer that the opinion had not left room for state law to demand the higher clear and convincing standard for the exercise of prospective autonomy—a legal rule that in practice can have a chilling effect on respect for patients' wishes. The salutary impact of *Cruzan* for the foreseeable future, however, is to further cement the prospective autonomy consensus. Justice O'Connor's concurrence even suggests that implementing the decisions of a duly appointed health care agent "may well be constitutionally required."[110] From another vantage point, *Cruzan*'s most enduring legacy may be that it engrained in the collective consciousness the inherent evidentiary problems that arise when family members and physicians are called upon to choose as the now-incompetent patient would choose if he or she were able.

The Assisted Suicide Cases

End-of-life issues came before the Supreme Court again in 1997, in the assisted suicide cases. In stark contrast to the climate seven years earlier, few observers feared a narrowing of the patients' rights consensus (beyond the usual scholarly speculation, perhaps, about the potential implications of a well- or poorly reasoned opinion). Instead, the national spotlight turned to the issue of whether rights of treatment refusal would be expanded to include more active assistance in the dying process. The specific question at stake was whether competent, terminally ill patients have a constitutionally protected right to request—and physicians the freedom to write—prescriptions for drugs to be self-administered by the patient with the intention of inducing a peaceful death (what some people refer to as physician aid-in-dying).

The cases originated out of the states of Washington and New York, each brought by a group of physicians who treat terminally ill patients. In Washington, the physicians were joined by Compassion in Dying, a nonprofit organization that advocates patient rights—including the right to assisted suicide. Each case presented a constitutional challenge to that state's law prohibiting physician-assisted suicide and criminalizing the practice. In essence, the Washington proceeding contended that the same principles on which the right to refuse treatment is based should, as a matter of substantive due process, be extended to compass a right to choose the time and manner of one's own death. The New York proceeding rested on equal protection grounds; the plaintiffs argued that allowing terminally ill patients who are dependent on life support to choose death by refusing treatment while denying the same choice to similarly situated terminally ill patients who are *not* dependent on life support is unfair. Following rulings in the federal district courts, the Ninth and Second Circuit Courts of Appeal (for Washington and New York, respectively) agreed, striking down the statutory prohibitions in each state.[111] The stage was set for the Attorneys General of Washington and New York to bring the issue before the U.S. Supreme Court.

Chief Justice William Rehnquist again authored the opinion, this time for a unanimous Supreme Court. The rulings in *Washington v. Glucksberg*[112] and *Vacco v. Quill*[113] rejected the due process and equal protection arguments, overruled the Ninth and Second Circuits, and strongly affirmed the state's prerogative to legislate a blanket prohibition of assisted suicide. At the heart of the Court's reasoning is the clear message that refusal of life support and assistance in suicide are factually and legally distinct.[114] Acutely aware that proponents of physician-assisted suicide, as well as the Ninth and Second Circuits, relied heavily on the Court's prior ruling in *Cruzan*, the opinion went to some lengths to distinguish the *Cruzan* precedent. After reciting its prior holding that the right to refuse unwanted medical treatment enjoys constitutional protection, the opinion in *Glucksberg* states that "the decision to commit suicide with the assistance of another . . . [is] widely and reasonably regarded as quite distinct."[115] Echoing this passage, the opinion in *Vacco* asserts that "the distinction between assisting suicide and withdrawing life-sustaining treatment, a distinction widely recognized and endorsed in the medical profession and in our legal traditions, is both important and logical; it is certainly rational."[116] The Court's considered efforts to delimit the boundaries of the extant consensus and to situate its own *Cruzan* ruling in that body of jurisprudence also once again reaffirmed and cemented the right to refuse life-sustaining treatment.

LEGISLATURES RESPOND: THE PROLIFERATION OF ADVANCE DIRECTIVE LAWS

An Overview of State Statutes

Concurrent with the judiciary's involvement in resolving refusal-of-treatment cases, state legislatures began to grapple with end-of-life decisions. In many cases, the issues first played out in a poignant and public courtroom drama that contributed to heightened public demand for the right to control one's own dying process and stimulated an otherwise reticent state legislature to action. Legislative activity focused on the root problem in deciding for incompetent patients: How can we know what the patient would choose? The answer was to allow competent individuals to put their wishes in writing to govern future post-competence health care. The written advance directive is widely regarded as resolving the courts' evidentiary dilemma.[117]

The first advance directive law was enacted by California in 1976, several months after the *Quinlan* decision. The California "Natural Death Act" (advance directive statutes often have been styled as "Natural Death Acts" or "Death With Dignity Acts") established a statutory right to direct in a written living will the withholding or withdrawal of life support in the event of terminal illness. The statute's legislative findings acknowledge that the capacity of modern medical technology to artificially prolong life may "violate patient dignity and cause unnecessary pain and suffering." The stated purpose of the law is "recognition of the dignity and privacy that a person has a right to expect" and to "protect individual autonomy."[118]

Sounding a similar chord, by mid-1990 a total of 43 states had enacted some form of advance directive legislation. In the post-*Cruzan* period, the remaining 7 states adopted laws, and several states amended existing laws. All 50 states and the District of Columbia now have laws that recognize the right of citizens to author a durable power of attorney for health care (proxy), a living will, or both. The vast majority of states have statutorily recognized both approaches. A handful of states (Massachusetts, Michigan, and New York) give statutory warrant only to the health care proxy. Alaska is the sole state that recognizes only the living will.[119]

The common theme and animating principle of advance directive laws is their embrace of the principle of prospective autonomy. Like the judiciary, legislatures readily accepted the validity of extending competent patients' rights of self-determination to incompetent patients. Operative statutory language typically states that a proxy is authorized "to make any and all health care decisions on the [incompetent patient's] behalf that the [competent patient] could make," including decisions about life-sustaining treatment.[120]

A look at selected statutory preambles further exemplifies this fundamental rationale. The Colorado statute "affirms the traditional right to accept or reject medical or surgical treatment . . . and creates a procedure by which a competent adult may make such decisions in advance, before he becomes unconscious or otherwise incompetent to do so."[121] The express purpose of the Alabama law is to assure "that the rights of individuals may be respected even after they are no longer able to participate actively in decisions about themselves" by recognizing "the right of a competent adult person to make a written declaration instructing his or her physician to provide, withhold or withdraw life-sustaining treatment."[122] All state laws accept the core premise that the right of self-determination should not be lost with loss of competence and that competent (written) expressions have a legitimate role in shaping post-competence treatment.

In contrast to the court decisions, however, legislation—particularly in the pre-*Cruzan* era—has been marked by substantive and procedural limitations on the scope of permissible patient choice. Many of the early statutes limited the patient's right to refuse treatment to circumstances of a terminal condition, excluding from the coverage of the statute permanent unconsciousness or other serious, irreversible, life-threatening conditions. The term "terminal condition" has been variously defined. A common early definition was that a "qualified patient" was one for whom, in the judgment of one or more physicians, illness will cause death within a "short time," regardless of medical intervention. Another familiar formulation is that life support would serve "only to prolong the dying process." These and other legislative phrases effectively circumscribe the patient's right to determine the course of the dying process.

Mirroring the judicial consensus, today virtually every state expressly authorizes the use of advance directives to refuse life support when a patient is terminally ill *or* permanently unconscious. Narrow definitions of terminal illness have been broadened, are interpreted more flexibly (does the treatment sustain life or prolong the dying process?), or are simply ignored in practice. Only a handful of states, however, have given clear voice to patients' rights when the patient is suffering from a progressive, debilitating, and ultimately fatal illness or disease (such as Alzheimer's dementia) that does not qualify as "terminal" even on more generous understandings of the term (e.g., a prognosis of one year of life or less remaining). New Jersey law states that life-sustaining treatment may be withheld or withdrawn pursuant to a directive "when the patient has a serious irreversible illness or condition" that is not terminal and "the likely risks and burdens of the medical intervention . . . are reasonably judged to outweigh the likely benefits to the patient. . . ."[123] Florida provides that advance directives apply when the patient has a "terminal condition, has an end-stage condition, or is in a persistent vegetative state."[124] Under the Oregon statute, life-sustaining procedures may be forgone for patients who are neither in a terminal condition nor permanently unconscious if such treatment would "not benefit the [patient's] medical condition and would cause permanent and severe pain; or . . . the person has a progressive illness that will be fatal and is in an advanced stage."[125]

In many parts of the country, the symbolic and cultural significance of providing basic sustenance, combined with the mistaken belief that discontinuing artificial fluids and nutrition for PVS patients causes death by starvation and dehydration, made the feeding tube issue the most contentious issue in the advance directives debate.[126] One outcome of the controversy was that several early statutes excluded artificially provided fluids and nutrition from the range of life-sustaining procedures that could be refused in an advance directive; others imposed procedural hurdles, such as requiring a specific statement refusing feeding tubes. This reasoning has been resoundingly rejected by the courts, which have held uniformly that all medical interventions count as medical treatments that the patient has the right to refuse. Since *Cruzan*, many of these laws have been amended. Some states have eliminated restrictions on the removal of feeding tubes, thereby expanding the scope of patients' rights. Others maintain some special conditions for the exercise of the right to refuse, such as requiring that refusal of artificially provided fluids and nutrition be reasonably and specifically known[127] or proved by clear and convincing evidence.[128] Ohio imposes the unusual and extremely burdensome requirement that withholding or withdrawal of nutrition or hydration must be ordered by a probate court on the basis of clear and convincing evidence of the patient's wishes.[129]

Statutory limitations on the right to refuse treatment, past and present, are an important piece of the overall legal landscape.[130] Arguably, lawmakers' actions are justified by reference to other competing principles—in particular, society's interests in the preservation of life and the protection of patient well-being. Like judges, lawmakers balanced autonomy against countervailing state interests. Although the record of legislative reasoning is far less accessible than the rationale of judicial opinions (many legislatures keep no record of floor debates, and statutes often contain little justifying explanation, requiring reliance on media accounts of legislative debates), the public policy arena clearly has given greater voice to the state's interest in preserving life. Charged with the responsibilities of crafting comprehensive policy, lawmakers have been understandably concerned (especially in the first decade after *Quinlan*) with protecting the most vulnerable people in society—such as elderly and institutionalized persons—from abuse. Moreover, legislatures, like courts, have been extremely reluctant to make what appear to be quality-of-life judgments. Unfortunately, in many cases state legislatures have been moved by less laudable political pressures, including the more conservative voices of some religious groups and right-to-life advocates. (Another significant limitation in several advance directive laws is suspension of a woman's directive in the event of pregnancy.) Legislatures historically have erred much more than the judiciary in the direction of a vitalist posture.

A good argument can be made that as a matter of law, these statutory restrictions are nevertheless largely hortatory.[131] Most state statutes expressly preserve patients' common law and constitutional rights, stating that the statute is intended as cumulative, not limiting, of rights that have been or may be recognized by the courts or under the Constitution.[132] Moreover, statutory law in any event cannot preempt constitutional rights.

There can be a large gap, however, between the niceties of legal interpretation and the daily practice of medicine. Statutory limitations on the right to refuse treatment through an advance directive often are taken literally by health care professionals and (sadly) attorneys who advise them. Too often, health care professionals believe the myth that anything the law does not expressly permit it therefore prohibits.[133] Moreover, health care professionals often believe that statutory law is more important than case law and are more familiar with statutes addressing an area of medical practice than with individual cases. Collectively, these factors can create a climate of reluctance (if not hostility) to honor more expansive instruments.

Nevertheless, these "letter of the law" limitations (which are unjustifiable) pale in comparison to the law's pervasive message. In stamping the law's imprimatur on advance directives, legislative enactments nationwide announce that prospective autonomy is a cherished value and the exercise of this right through issuance of an advance directive is entitled to respect. Advance directive laws have affirmed and established the autonomy-based rights of incompetent patients to refuse unwanted life-sustaining interventions. *In principle*, patients and family members now have decisional authority at the bedside.

The Patient Self-Determination Act

On the heals of *Cruzan*, Congress entered the termination-of-treatment arena by enacting the Patient Self-Determination Act (PSDA) in 1990.[134] One of the moving forces behind the PSDA was Senator John Danforth of Missouri (Nancy Cruzan's home state), who together with Senator Daniel Patrick Moynihan of New York was a primary sponsor of the bill. The goal of the PSDA was to promote greater knowledge and use of advance directives, as well as to foster respect for these documents. Beyond the Act's clear commitment to patient autonomy, other factors underlying Congressional interest in this area included the belief that more widespread use of advance directives would reduce the amount and the cost of aggressive end-of-life treatment for terminally ill and dying patients.[135]

The federal law is largely procedural; it defers to the laws of the 50 states, as well as Constitutional law, as the source of individuals' substantive rights. Under the PSDA, on admission to a health care facility (or coming under the care of a provider), all persons are to be asked whether they have or wish to receive information on advance directives for health care. The patient's "advance directive status" is to be documented in the medical record. All persons are to be provided on admission with a state-approved, written description of their rights to execute advance directives. The PSDA also imposes on health care facilities obligations to provide for staff and community education and to maintain written policies and procedures with respect to advance directives and the facility's obligations under their state's law.

The tenor of the PSDA is to encourage individuals to take responsibility for their health care futures. The law does not require individuals to execute an advance directive, and it prohibits health care providers and insurers from engaging in practices that are intended to coerce the use of advance directives—such as by making care or coverage conditional on execution of an advance directive document. The PSDA applies to all health care institutions and provider organizations that receive federal Medicare and Medicaid funds. The law is notably silent about the role of physicians in the advance directive dialogue. In the words of one commentator, the PSDA targets the "right church, wrong pew."[136]

Thus, the PSDA is designed to foster greater communication about advance directives, increase the frequency with which individuals use these documents, and secure respect for patients' advance directives. Although the PSDA defers to state law on substantive issues, such as the circumstances in which life support may be refused, the federal law fully embraces the principle of prospective autonomy and cements its embodiment in law nationally.[137]

SHOULD ADVANCE DIRECTIVES ALWAYS BE FOLLOWED?

Despite uniform endorsement of prospective autonomy and advance directives, the issue of whether directives must always be followed or sometimes may be overridden—and, if so, on what grounds—remain open questions.[138] The query shifts our attention from individual rights to the correlative obligations of others. It occupies substantial attention in subsequent chapters of this book (particularly chapter five). My immediate purpose here is to sketch the bare parameters of the legal context and to highlight the pervasive confusion in clinical practice.

Legal and ethical commentary are replete with references to advance directives as "legally binding" (or simply "binding") documents. Yet there is much ambiguity at work in the use of this term. What does it mean to call an advance directive binding? At a minimum, to say that a document is binding is to assert that once it becomes operative (that is, when the patient has been determined to be incompetent and the directive is known to those responsible for the patient's care), others are placed under certain obligations. What of the nature and extent of obligations imposed by advance directives, however?

Generally, there are at least three senses in which advance directives are regarded as binding. First, a properly executed (that is, signed and witnessed) and competently issued advance directive establishes a presumption that it should be followed. It imposes on others—proxy, family, physicians, nurses, institutions—a *prima facie* duty to follow the directive. This duty may be overcome and a directive overridden (set aside and not followed) in some cases, but only for good reasons; moreover, the burden of justification lies with those who would override the directive. Second, advance directives impose absolute duties and must be strictly followed in all cases. There is no room for discretion—at least, not without the risk of adverse consequences such as exposure to legal liability. A third understanding measures the strength of physicians' obligations by whether the directive is enforceable. When conjoined with the presumptive sense of the term, enforceability means that penalties apply for unjustified noncompliance. The view that directives are absolutely binding holds that no justification outweighs the transgression of noncompliance. References to directives as legally binding (or simply as binding) variously suggest each of these meanings and most often vacillate between suggesting that advance directives are presumptively or absolutely binding. Scant attention is paid to the question of enforceability.

The state of affairs in clinical practice reveals considerable confusion. Many physicians believe that there is a (near) absolute legal duty to follow an advance directive with little or no room for interpretation or discretion. Occasional moral qualms to the contrary are secondary to the law's command and take a back seat to the belief that adherence to the written document is the best way to avoid legal entanglements. The law's strong suggestion that a written statement satisfies the applicable evidentiary standard for termination of treatment and the law's preoccupation with rights in an excessively litigious society have been powerful forces in shaping this understanding. On the other hand, recent studies have found that many physicians feel little or no obligation to honor an advance directive and are inclined to do so only when the directive is consistent with their own judgment about what is best for the patient.[139] Many physicians continue to resist advance directives, clinging to the old ethic that subordinates patient autonomy to the physician's judgment about the patient's good. Another respected study reveals that many physicians have continued treatment contrary to the patient's wishes *and* in violation of the physician's personal conscience.[140] Thus, the daily practice of medicine appears to reveal several contradictory "norms" of behavior.

Extant law is palpably ambivalent about the legal weight of advance directives and has failed to articulate a consistent message to guide clinicians. Numerous advance directive statutes provide for the imposition of penalties against physicians for *willful* failure to follow the terms of an advance directive; some authorize quasi-legal disciplinary proceedings. Yet these provisions are little known, have rarely been invoked, and have never been subjected to judicial scrutiny. Although the judiciary appears to view advance directives as dispositive, neither courts nor legislatures have attributed to such documents traditional contract notions of breach and remedy. To date, cases seeking monetary damages against a physician or hospital for failure to honor a patient's refusal of treatment near the end of life (none of which have involved an advance directive) are few in number and show mixed results. Decisions validating claims of battery (an unauthorized intrusion upon the body)—the initial basis for development of the legal doctrine of informed consent—also have severely limited monetary recovery to "nominal damages."[141]

In sum, the law has yet to develop the teeth of enforceability. It has not lived up to the maxim that for every right there is a remedy, and it has given clinicians reason to believe that there is little or no price to pay for disregarding a patient's directive. The same is true of the law's response to family members who resist following a patient's directive. (I discuss cases seeking monetary damages and legal enforcement of advance directives in chapter five.)

There is another, more subtle, measure of the law's commitment that takes the form of structuring affirmative incentives for compliance with established rights. Numerous state laws shield physicians from legal liability when they abide by a directive *in good faith*, and several courts, as in *Quinlan*, have carved out a sphere of judicial immunity for physicians who follow the patient's wishes in accordance with a court-prescribed process. These grants of immunity can provide powerful incentives for compliance—sometimes at the expense of more considered judgment. In contrast, some states permit physicians to exercise discretion to disregard advance directives by granting legal protection for the provision of life support in good faith even when the patient's directive refuses it.[142] Some states give physicians an easy out: allowing physicians who choose to aggressively sustain life to place the burden of responsibility for arranging a transfer of care with the patient and family. Protections afforded health care institutions follow a similar path. (Curiously, far fewer advance directive laws address the legal status of family compliance/noncompliance with a directive.)

Overall, the predominant message is that there is little to fear from the heavy hand of the law. Willful disregard (neglect) of patients' wishes may subject physicians and hospitals to civil liability or professional discipline. Short of willful or intentional disregard, however, good faith behavior enjoys a safe harbor from legal entanglements. This assessment likely is true as well of the potentially large gap between these two standards, leaving a huge harbor of safe conduct. Presumably, a physician would find it a relatively easy task to justify overriding a directive on the "good faith" belief that the terms of the directive were ambiguous and that continuing life support served the patient's interests. Conversely, proving that the physician did *not* act in good faith (not quite the same as showing bad faith or willful neglect) probably would pose a considerable challenge.[143]

The popular understanding among the lay public is that advance directives should be strictly followed and that physicians have legal obligations to do so. This perception generally has been considered uniform. Experience shows that patients and families are shocked and outraged at the suggestion that an advance directive will not be followed according to its terms. On the other hand, some studies suggest that growing numbers of patients believe that some degree of flexibility and discretion is appropriate.[144]

The divide between public and professional perceptions is further illustrated by the example of advance directive policy at the New York University Medical Center in place in the mid-1990s, not long after enactment of New York's health care proxy law and the PSDA. Following New York law, standard language on the health care proxy form typically states that the author intends the directive to be "legally binding." Hospital policy, however, provides that evidence of the patient's wishes must be "clear and convincing" (the evidentiary standard required by New York courts) and calls for institutional ethics committee review in cases of disagreement. Should the patient be confident that his or her previously stated wishes will be honored?

Clearly there is no consensus on the legal and moral weight to be accorded to advance directives in individual cases. The reigning confusion cries out for articulation of clear guidelines to govern when advance directives must be followed and when they may justifiably be overridden. The position that advance directives are presumptively (*prima facie*) binding is essentially correct but incomplete. The critical issues are the weight to be given to that presumption and, conversely, the justification required to override it. The approach for which I argue demands a coherent understanding of the concept of prospective decisional autonomy (the subject of chapter three) and a set of practical and narrow rules for whether and how advance directives may justifiably be overridden (the subject of chapter five).

CONCLUSION

Concerning the nature of the judicial process, Justice Benjamin Cardozo eloquently wrote, "The sordid controversies of litigants are the stuff out of which great and shining truths will ultimately be shaped. The accidental and the transitory will yield the essential and the permanent."[145] Such has been the history of the right to refuse treatment. In fashioning a legal consensus, the courts indeed have been cognizant of these interrelated responsibilities. They have looked to the past for the facts required to resolve the accidental, transitory, and tragic dilemmas before them. They also have cast an eye to the future, setting forth precedent and guidance for the difficult decisions that many other patients and families, and those caring for them, were yet to face. The resulting consensus—embodied as well in advance directive laws, the bioethics literature, official policy statements of various professional groups, and public and professional values—can be summarized by reference to seven principles. These principles form the pillars of the widely accepted framework for deciding to forgo life-sustaining treatment in behalf of incompetent patients. In many respects, they may be said to be a part of the legacy of Karen Ann Quinlan and her family.[146]

1. Competent patients have an autonomy-based right, recognized under Constitutional and common law, to refuse treatment, including life-sustaining treatment. Life-sustaining treatment includes artificially provided nutrition and hydration.

2. Incompetent patients have the same panoply of rights as competent patients, although the manner in which those rights are exercised is different.

3. No right is absolute, but instances in which a patient's right to refuse life support is outweighed by societal interests are rare.

4. Withholding and withdrawal of treatment from a terminally ill or permanently unconscious patient allows a natural dying process to take its course. It does not constitute killing or assisted suicide.

5. In making decisions for incompetent patients, surrogate decision makers should seek first and foremost to follow a subjective standard of implementing the patient's wishes. When this test proves inadequate, a best interests standard may be applied.

6. In ascertaining an incompetent patient's wishes, the proxy, family, and physician should rely on a patient's advance directive if one has been issued.

7. A local process of review in the clinical setting should be employed to facilitate resolution of disagreements. Recourse to the courts should be rare.

These seven principles arise at various places in subsequent chapters of this book. My primary concern, however, is with the principles that constitute the dominant reasoning in support of the autonomy-based rights of incompetent patients—namely, the conjoint premises that incompetent patients have the same rights as competent patients (point 2); that those responsible for the patient's care should give top priority to ascertaining and applying the patient's previously expressed wishes (point 5); and that decision makers should rely on the patient's advance directive (point 6). Each of these points raises questions and reaches conclusions about the nature and strength of the principle of prospective autonomy and about the correlative obligations of others.

In chapter two I present a deeper argument for the moral foundations of the principle of prospective autonomy and why we ought to value, exercise, and protect the right to plan ahead for our health care futures. The arguments in chapter two develop a stronger moral grounding for the current consensus and critique the opposing position that decision making for incompetent patients ought instead to prioritize the patient's current best interests.

NOTES

1. *In re Quinlan*, 70 N.J. 10, 355 A.2d 647, 663, *cert. denied sub nom. Garger v. New Jersey*, 429 U.S. 922 (1976).
2. *Washington v. Glucksberg*, 521 U.S. 702, 710 (quoting *Stanford v. Kentucky*, 492 U.S. 361, 373 (1989)).
3. George Annas believes that the law's dedication to individual rights and attentiveness to redressing the arbitrary use of power under the rubric of patients' rights has made "American law, not philosophy or medicine, . . . primarily responsible for the agenda, development and current state of American bioethics." George J. Annas, *Standard of Care: The Law of American Bioethics* (New York: Oxford University Press, 1993), 3. Others contend that "[r]eciprocally, bioethics has shaped the law." Alexander Morgan Capron and Vicki Michel, "Law and Bioethics," *Loyola of Los Angeles Law Review* 27, no. 1 (1993): 32.
4. In charting the landscape of the consensus, the work of numerous bodies and individuals can be chronicled, together with numerous significant events, all of which have influenced general societal acceptance of prospective autonomy and advance directives and their embrace in law, policy, morality, and medicine. Among them are The Belmont Report of the National Commission for the Protection of Human Subjects (1978), which gave the principle of autonomy (along with those of beneficence and justice) philosophical and policy rigor and credibility; the writings of Henry Beecher that exposed abuses in human subjects research; and the reports of the President's Commission for the Study of Ethical Problems in Medicine and Biomedical and Behavioral Research on *Making Health Care Decisions* (1981) and *Deciding to Forgo Life-Sustaining Treatment* (1983). The Hastings Center, through Robert Veatch and the Working Group on Death and Dying, and the Kennedy Institute of Ethics, in the person of Richard McCormick, played important consultative roles in the *Quinlan* case. Much is missing from this list, including the fine scholarship of many pioneers in the nascent field of bioethics. A retrospective look at watershed work in the field of bioethics over the past 25 years appears in a collection of short essays on "The Birth of Bioethics," *Hastings Center Report* 23, no. 6 (November-December 1993): S1–S16. For an account of the origins and history of bioethics from one of the field's pioneers, see Albert R. Jonsen, *The Birth of Bioethics* (New York: Oxford University Press, 1998). Jonsen identifies the years 1947–1987 as the period when bioethics emerged as a distinct discipline.
5. "Legal commentators suggested—and most bioethicists embraced—redefinition of [the physician-patient relationship] in terms of rights." Capron and Michel, "Law and Bioethics," 36.

6. "The law's rights discourse has seemed delightfully suited to that engine of bioethical thought, the doctrine of autonomy." Carl E. Schneider, "Bioethics in the Language of the Law," *Hastings Center Report* 24, no. 4 (July-August 1994): 18.
7. Peter G. Filene, *In the Arms of Others: A Cultural History of the Right-to-Die in America* (Chicago: Ivan R. Dee, 1998), 73.
8. The precise cause of Karen's coma has long been a matter of some speculation. Initially the attending physician suspected a combination of alcohol and tranquilizers. A toxicology screen performed within hours of admission to the hospital, however, failed to detect any sign of drugs or medication above normal therapeutic levels, leaving room for doubt in this diagnosis. See Joseph and Julia Quinlan, with Phyllis Battelle, *Karen Ann: The Quinlans Tell Their Story* (New York: Doubleday & Co., 1977). Reported results of a 10-year anatomical study of Karen's brain confirm that she suffered a cardiopulmonary arrest "after accidentally ingesting a combination of prescription sedatives and alcohol." The autopsy findings also revealed an unusual and uncommon abnormality of the thalamus that was believed to have been a significant factor in the fate that befell Karen. Hannah C. Kinney et al., "Neuropathological Findings in the Brain of Karen Ann Quinlan," *New England Journal of Medicine* 330, no. 21 (May 26, 1994): 1469–75.
9. In PVS, some portion of the brainstem remains intact, sustaining some autonomic functions—often including respiration. Patients in this condition often are described as awake but not aware. There have been some isolated reports of modest recovery from diagnosed PVS, but such cases are extremely rare. For analysis of the clinical aspects of PVS, see Multi-Society Task Force on PVS, "Medical Aspects of the Persistent Vegetative State," *New England Journal of Medicine* 330, no. 21 (May 26, 1994): 1499–1508. PVS patients are not legally dead. Current law in all 50 states and the District of Columbia defines "brain death" as the irreversible loss of all functions of the entire brain, including the brain stem. Hence, for PVS patients the legal and clinical issue is termination of treatment for a living patient, not removal of life support from a dead patient. Some philosophers—most notably Robert Veatch and Daniel Wikler—contend that patients who have suffered so-called "higher brain death," like the PVS patient, are dead in a morally relevant sense. I touch on this question from a different and limited perspective in chapter four, where I consider the position that PVS patients are "nonpersons."
10. Paul W. Armstrong and B.D. Colen, "From Quinlan to Jobes: The Courts and the PVS Patient," *Hastings Center Report* 18, no. 1 (February/March 1988): 38.
11. The consent and release read as follows:

    We authorize and direct Doctor Morse to discontinue all extraordinary measures, including the use of a respirator, for our daughter Karen Quinlan. We acknowledge that the above named physician has thoroughly discussed the above with us and that the consequences have been fully explained to us. Therefore, we hereby RELEASE from any and all liability the above named physician, associates and assistants of his choice, Saint Claire's Hospital and its agents and employees.

    In re Quinlan, 137 N.J. Super. 227, 250 (1975).
12. Ibid. at 236 (quoting the initial pleading in the case).
13. Ibid. at 251.
14. Ibid. at 259 (emphasis in original).

15. Quinlan, *Karen Ann*.
16. *Quinlan*, 70 N.J. 10 at 41–42.
17. Ibid. at 39–40 (citing *Eisenstadt v. Baird*, 405 U.S. 438 (1972); *Stanley v. Georgia*, 394 U.S. 557 (1969); *Griswold v. Connecticut*, 381 U.S. 479 (1965)).
18. Ibid.
19. Ibid.
20. The physician defendants actually framed their argument somewhat differently, asserting "the right of the physician to administer medical treatment according to his best judgment." 70 N.J. at 40. This more narrow contention actually is a claim to respect for the conscience of the individual physician, rather than one concerning the medical profession and its standards of practice as a whole.
21. 70 N.J. at 41.
22. Ibid. at 42.
23. Ibid. at 39.
24. Ibid. at 40.
25. Ibid. at 44.
26. 137 N.J. Super. at 259.
27. 70 N.J. at 44. In another passage, the court states that "the overwhelming majority" of citizens would concur in the decision to remove the respirator for a patient in PVS. This point was intended to support the view that the Quinlans' decision also was consistent with prevailing societal values and that the court's ruling did not offend those values. This passage subsequently has fueled growing debate about whether societal values offer sufficient justification for a public policy that would favor withholding or withdrawing life support in "hopeless" situations, perhaps even in the face of affirmative requests for such treatment.
28. The leading work propounding this view in a systematic fashion is Robert M. Veatch, *A Theory of Medical Ethics* (New York: Basic Books, 1981).
29. 70 N.J. at 45–47.
30. Discussing *Quinlan's* approach to the role of the physician and prevailing medical standards, Veatch notes that at the time *Quinlan* was decided, stopping a respirator for a patient in Karen's condition clearly was not contrary to prevailing professional practice. Robert M. Veatch, *Death, Dying and the Biological Revolution: Our Last Quest for Responsibility*, rev. ed. (New Haven, Conn.: Yale University Press, 1989), 119–21. Curiously, in reaching this conclusion, the *Quinlan* court also found that the physicians' initial decision not to withdraw life support was consistent with the "then existing medical standards and practices" (70 N.J. at 45). This apparent contradiction seems to suggest that medical standards had changed between 1975 and 1976. A more plausible interpretation is that the physicians' refusal was justified (or at least reasonable) because at the time there was no medical consensus either way and that prior to 1976 the law had not yet embraced the patient's right to refuse life-sustaining treatment, leaving physicians in uncharted legal waters when faced with such a request. The court's concern for the role of law in shaping medical practice is evident from its efforts to craft a decision-making process for this and future cases that would allow physicians to honor requests to terminate treatment without fear of legal liability. I discuss a central feature of this

process—the ethics committee—elsewhere in this chapter and at greater length in chapter five.
31. 70 N.J. at 41.
32. The law has long deferred to a private sphere of family decision making in a range of areas and has presumed that next-of-kin ordinarily are best-suited to serve as guardian for an incompetent loved one. Throughout the *Quinlan* litigation, the New Jersey courts had shown great solicitude for the Quinlans' tragedy and their love for their daughter.
33. Tom L. Beauchamp and James F. Childress, *Principles of Biomedical Ethics*, 4th ed. (New York: Oxford University Press, 1994), 171 (quoting *Superintendent of Belchertown State School v. Saikewicz*, 370 N.E.2d 417 (Mass. 1977)).
34. 70 N.J. at 21.
35. Ibid. at 41. The New Jersey Supreme Court later overruled its evidentiary ruling that such conversations are not probative and allowed all such evidence of the patient's wishes to be admitted. *In re Conroy*, 98 N.J. 321, 486 A.2d 1209, 1230 (1985).
36. 70 N.J. at 54.
37. Ibid. at 49. Here the court adopted the suggestion of pediatrician Karen Teel, whose law review article the year before, "The Physician's Dilemma: A Doctor's View: What the Law Should Be," *Baylor Law Review* 27, no. 1 (Winter 1975): 6–9, had argued that a mechanism like an ethics committee could serve the laudable purpose of diffusing responsibility for difficult decisions, thereby freeing physicians from excessive concerns for legal liability in the practice of medicine. Interestingly, this idea was not presented by any of the parties to the case; it was introduced *sua sponte* by the court on the basis of its own research. (Personal communication with Paul W. Armstrong, counsel to the Quinlan family.)
38. Veatch, *Death, Dying, and the Biological Revolution*, 123.
39. Norman L. Cantor, "Quinlan, Privacy, and the Handling of Incompetent Dying Patients," *Rutgers Law Review* 30, no. 2 (Winter 1977): 253 ("The New Jersey Supreme Court significantly circumscribed the prerogatives of an incompetent patient's guardian by injecting a hospital ethics committee, with ostensible veto power, into the decisionmaking process."). Veatch, *Death, Dying and the Biological Revolution*, 122–23, notes that a close reading of this passage of *Quinlan* suggests a return to the physician of authority to decide whether life support should be discontinued. Clearly the court misspoke here, but this lapse should not be interpreted in any way to undermine the clear message of *Quinlan*.
40. The media's overwhelming interest in Karen's story is partially chronicled in the Quinlans' book, including some of the indicia of the international impact of the Quinlan case. A small illustration of the intense media scrutiny here and abroad is the fact that a picture of Karen, taken on her high school graduation, appeared on the covers of both *Newsweek* and the French magazine *Paris Match* in 1975–76.
41. Though these substantive standards are stated and analyzed as separate tests, they also may be regarded as involving "a continuum of subjective and objective information about the patient that will support a reliable decision." Stewart G. Pollock, "Life and Death Decisions: Who Makes Them and by What Standards?" *Rutgers Law Review* 41, no. 2 (Winter 1989): 518. In other words, as evidence of what the patient would want becomes weaker, other objective measures of the patient's interests (such as whether continued treatment will

be painful) take on greater significance; the standard begins to shade into a best interests analysis.
42. See, e.g., *Gray v. Romeo*, 697 F.Supp. 580 (D.R.I. 1988); *Rasmussen v. Fleming*, 154 Ariz. 207, 741 P.2d 674 (1987); *Corbett v. D' Allesandro*, 487 So. 2d 368 (Fla. App.), rev. denied, 492 So. 2d 1331 (Fla. 1986).
43. See, e.g., *Conservatorship of Drabick*, 200 Cal. App. 3d 185, 245 Cal. Rptr. 840 (Ct. App. 1988); *In re Estate of Longeway*, 133 Ill.2d 33, 549 N.E.2d 292 (1989); *In re Gardner*, 534 A.2d 947 (Me. 1987); *Matter of Westchester County Medical Center (O'Connor)*, 72 N.Y.2d 517, 534 N.Y.S.2d 886, 531 N.E.2d 607 (1988).
44. For comprehensive analysis of the law of informed consent, see Paul S. Appelbaum, Charles W. Lidz, and Alan Meisel, *Informed Consent: Legal Theory and Clinical Practice* (New York: Oxford University Press, 1987).
45. The New Jersey Supreme Court's 1985 *Conroy* opinion rested its decision regarding the right to refuse life support on the common-law right of self-determination, leaving some question about the court's commitment to the constitutional basis of the right. *Conroy* did not, however, reject the constitutional basis of the right. 98 N.J. 321, 348, 486 A.2d 1209 (1985); Pollock, "Life and Death Decisions," 530–31 ("Without rejecting the constitutional right, the court shifted the basis of its decision to the common-law right of self-determination in *Conroy*."). The *Farrell* opinion, rendered two years after *Conroy*, resolves any doubt in this regard under New Jersey law by reaffirming the constitutional right of privacy as a fundamental right to be protected against unwanted interventions and invasions of bodily integrity. In *Farrell* the court states: "While we held that a patient's right to refuse medical treatment even at the risk of personal injury or death is primarily protected by the common law, we recognized that it is also protected by the federal and state constitutional right of privacy." 108 N.J. 335, 348, 529 A.2d 404 (1987) (citing *Conroy*, 98 N.J. at 348; *Quinlan*, 70 N.J. at 38–42). New Jersey's continuing commitment to patients' rights to refuse unwanted treatment near the end of life is summarized in the 1987 *Peter* decision: "All patients, competent or incompetent, with some limited cognitive ability or in a persistent vegetative state, terminally ill or not terminally ill, are entitled to choose whether or not they want life-sustaining medical treatment." *In re Peter*, 108 N.J. 365, 372, 529 A.2d 419 (1987).
46. *Farrell*, 108 N.J. at 349; *Conroy*, 98 N.J. at 349.
47. *Conroy*, 98 N.J. at 350; see *Farrell*, 108 N.J. at 349–50 (quoting *Conroy*).
48. *Conroy*, 98 N.J. at 350–51; *Farrell*, 108 N.J. at 350; *Bartling v. Superior Court of Los Angeles County*, 163 Cal. App. 3d 186, 209 Cal. Rptr. 220, 225–26 (Ct. App. 1984); *Gardner*, 534 A.2d at 955–56.
49. Competent adults have been compelled to accept medical treatment to protect the public health: *Jacobson v. Massachusetts*, 197 U.S. 11 (1905) (enforcing compulsory smallpox vaccination law); to protect the patient's minor children against emotional and financial abandonment: *Application of President & Directors of Georgetown College*, 331 F.2d 1000, 1008 (D.C. Cir.), cert. denied, 377 U.S. 978 (1964) (ordering a blood transfusion for a mother because of her "responsibility to the community to care for her infant"); and to protect the life of an unborn child: *Raleigh Fitkin-Paul Morgan Memorial Hosp. v. Anderson*, 42 N.J. 421, cert. denied, 377 U.S. 985 (1964) (interests of an unborn infant were sufficiently compelling to order a life-saving blood transfusion for a pregnant woman). In the latter two circumstances, the interest in protecting minor children was most compelling where the parent's prospect for recovery was good and the

parent's death would have put the child's security or life at risk. Scenarios in which the interests of others would put an incompetent patient's refusal of treatment to the test are extremely rare. One such scenario would be proposed imposition of treatment on a terminally ill woman in the late stages of pregnancy for the benefit of a viable fetus.

50. The AMA position can be found in American Medical Association Council on Ethical and Judicial Affairs, *Code of Medical Ethics: Current Opinions with Annotations*, 1998–99 ed. (Chicago: American Medical Association, 1999), sec. 2.20. The commentary to this section includes an annotated listing of the many court decisions in which this section of the AMA Code has been cited in the court's opinion. Of relevance to the historical context and the *Quinlan* court's view of the then-prevailing medical ethic, recognition of the patient's right to refuse treatment and corresponding professional obligations did not appear in the AMA Code until 1980.

51. Lawrence J. Nelson and Ronald E. Cranford, "Michael Martin and Robert Wendland: Beyond the Vegetative State," *Journal of Contemporary Health Law and Policy* 15 (Spring 1999): 427–53 (using this term).

52. *Conservatorship of Wendland*, 78 Cal.App.4th 517, 93 Cal.Rptr.2d 550 (Ct.App. 2000). Rose Wendland has brought an appeal of the decision to the California Supreme Court.

53. *In re Martin*, 450 Mich. 204, 538 N.W.2d 399 (1995).

54. *Guardianship of Edna M.F. (Spahn)*, 210 Wis.2d 557, 563 N.W.2d 485 (1997).

55. Some courts have upheld a competent patient's right to refuse life-sustaining treatment when he or she is suffering from an irreversible and debilitating condition but is not terminally ill. See *Bouvia v. Super. Ct. of Los Angeles County*, 179 Cal. App. 3d 1127, 225 Cal. Rptr. 297 (Ct. App. 1986) (patient with severe cerebral palsy and quadriplegia had a right to refuse artificially provided fluids and nutrition); *Bartling* (patient with lung cancer and chronic respiratory failure had right to refuse a respirator); *State v. McAfee*, 385 S.E.2d 651 (Ga.1989) (patient with quadriplegia had right to refuse a respirator); *In re Culham*, No. 87-340537-AZ, slip op. (Cir. Ct. Mich., Dec. 15, 1987) (patient with nonterminal amyotrophic lateral sclerosis [ALS] had a right to refuse a respirator). This is not to say that treatment refusals by competent patients will *always* be upheld by the law. One issue on the horizon involves a competent patient's refusal of life-sustaining treatment when the patient is not terminally ill and the proposed treatment offers substantial benefit of recovery from the underlying illness or disease process. Cases upholding the right to refuse treatment under these circumstances usually have involved patients whose refusal was grounded in religious beliefs. See, e.g., *In re Osborne*, 294 A.2d 372 (D.C. 1972) (upholding the right of a Jehovah's Witness to refuse a blood transfusion); *In re Boyd*, 403 A.2d 744 (D.C. 1979) (upholding the right of a Christian Scientist to refuse medication).

56. Two early Massachusetts cases applying the substituted judgment test appear to support this proposition, but neither makes clear whether the patients were considered to be terminally ill. *Matter of Spring*, 380 Mass. 629, 405 N.E.2d 115 (1980) (end-stage kidney disease); *Matter of Hier*, 18 Mass.App.Ct. 200, 464 N.E2d 959 (1984) (92-year-old woman with severe mental illness in need of a gastrostomy tube).

57. See *Superintendent of Belchertown State School v. Saikewicz*, 370 N.E.2d 417, 425-26 (Mass. 1977): "[T]here is a substantial distinction in the State's insistence that

human life be saved where the affliction is curable as opposed to the State interest where, as here, the issue is not whether, but when, for how long and at what cost to the individual [his] life may be briefly extended."

58. 98 N.J. at 373.
59. Ibid.
60. Ibid. at 374. *Accord* Peter, 108 N.J. at 382; *Jobes*, 108 N.J. at 427.
61. See, e.g., *Rasmussen; Drabick; Corbett; McConnell v. Beverly Enterprises-Connecticut, Inc.*, 209 Conn. 692, 553 A.2d 596 (1989); *Brophy v. New England Sinai Hosp.*, 398 Mass. 417, 497 N.E.2d 626 (1986). This position is reaffirmed by the U.S. Supreme Court in *Cruzan*, which I discuss separately.
62. *Conroy*, 486 A.2d at 1229 (citing *John F. Kennedy Mem. Hosp., Inc. v. Bludworth*, 452 So.2d 921, 924 (Fla. 1984)).
63. Cantor, "Quinlan, Privacy, and the Handling of Incompetent Dying Patients," 252 (quoted in *Conroy*, 486 A.2d at 1229).
64. *Conroy*, 486 A. 2d at 1229 (quoting Cantor, "Quinlan, Privacy, and the Handling of Incompetent Dying Patients," 259).
65. 370 N.E.2d at 428.
66. Ibid.
67. George J. Annas and Leonard H. Glantz, "The Rights of Elderly Patients to Refuse Life-Sustaining Treatment," *Milbank Quarterly* 64 (Supp. 2) (1986): 104.
68. Rebecca S. Dresser and John A. Robertson, "Quality of Life and Non-Treatment Decisions for Incompetent Patients: A Critique of the Orthodox Approach," *Law, Medicine & Health Care* 17, no. 3 (Fall 1989): 234–44.
69. Nancy Rhoden, "Litigating Life and Death," *Harvard Law Review* 102, no. 2 (1988): 384.
70. This oft-quoted language, which often is attributed to *Saikewicz*, can be traced to *In re Carson*, 39 Misc.2d 544, 545, 241 N.Y.S.2d 288, 289 (N.Y.Sup.Ct. 1962).
71. Histories of the substituted judgment doctrine appear in John A. Robertson, "Organ Donations by Incompetents and the Substituted Judgment Doctrine," *Columbia Law Review* 76, no. 1 (1976): 48–78; and Louise Harmon, "Falling Off the Vine: Legal Fictions and the Doctrine of Substituted Judgment," *Yale Law Journal* 100, no. 1 (1990): 1–71.
72. 445 S.W.2d 145 (Ky.Ct.App. 1969). See also *Hart v. Brown*, 289 A.2d 386 (Conn. Super. Ct. 1972) (applying substituted judgment to authorize parents of seven-year-old identical twins to consent to a kidney transplant from one to the other).
73. Harmon, "Falling off the Vine."
74. See, e.g., *Conroy*, 486 A.2d at 1230.
75. See, e.g., *Gray; Brophy*. Other courts have stated that surrogates must have "some trustworthy evidence" of the patient's wishes (*Jobes*).
76. *In re Westchester County Med. Ctr. (O'Connor)*, 72 N.Y.2d 517, 531 N.E.2d 607 (1988); *Mack v. Mack*, 618 A.2d 744 (Md. 1993); *Martin; Gardner; In re Estate of Longeway*, 133 Ill.2d 33, 549 N.E.2d 292 (1989); *In re Tavel*, 661 A.2d 1061 (Del. 1995); *Guardianship of Edna M.F. (Spahn). Cruzan v. Director, Missouri Dept. of Health*, 497 U.S. 261 (1990), upheld the constitutionality of Missouri's clear and convincing evidence standard. For further analysis of the evidentiary standards

applied in termination of treatment cases, see Alan Meisel, *The Right to Die* (New York: John Wiley & Sons, 1989), sections 10.21–10.27.
77. *Eichner v. Dillon*, 52 N.Y.2d 363, 420 N.E.2d 64, 72, *cert. denied*, 454 U.S. 858 (1981). See also *O'Connor* (quoting *Eichner*).
78. *Conn. Gen. Stat.* §19a-580c (1999); *Md. Code Ann.—Est & Trusts* §13-712(b) (Michie's Supp. 2000).
79. Rhoden, "Litigating Life and Death," 390.
80. Ibid., 384.
81. Rebecca Dresser, "Life, Death, and Incompetent Patients: Conceptual Infirmities and Hidden Values in the Law," *Arizona Law Review* 28, no. 3 (1986): 373–405.
82. Ibid.; Rebecca Dresser, "Confronting the 'Near Irrelevance' of Advance Directives," *Journal of Clinical Ethics* 5, no. 1 (Spring 1994): 55–56.
83. This issue sometimes is illustrated from the podium by posing the question, "If you were in a serious car accident on the George Washington Bridge and did not have an advance directive, would you rather be taken to a hospital in New York or New Jersey?" The hypothetical also illustrates that patients' rights often are matters of state law and are not always portable across state lines.
84. *Peter*, 108 N.J. at 426.
85. *Saunders v. State*, 129 Misc.2d 45, 492 N.Y.S.2d 510, 517 (1985).
86. 452 So.2d 921, 926 (Fla. 1984).
87. *Zodin v. Manor Healthcare Corp.*, No. 9010821007, Slip op. (Sup.Ct.Ga., Cobb Cty. Nov. 21, 1990). The Georgia court upheld an advance directive issued in Texas.
88. 492 N.Y.S.2d at 517.
89. *New York Law Journal* (July 28, 1987), 11.
90. Coordinating Council on Life-Sustaining Medical Treatment Decision Making by the Courts, *Guidelines for State Court Decision Making in Life-Sustaining Medical Treatment Cases* (St. Paul, Minn.: West Publishing, 1993), 13–14. Summarizing the survey findings, the *Guidelines* go on to state (p. 15) that "the results of this survey suggested that few differences arose among responding judges over the weight to be given advance directives and that they considered them dispositive."
91. Meisel apparently concludes otherwise, stating that "courts generally agree that an advance directive must be proved by clear and convincing evidence." Meisel, *The Right to Die*, section 10.27. It may be fair to say that this question is unsettled because it has rarely been squarely addressed. Nevertheless, in addition to the indicia of the judiciary's stance I discuss, there is no reason to think that courts that have not adopted the clear and convincing evidence standard for surrogate decision making by families in the absence of a directive would hold a written advance directive to a higher standard.
92. *DeGrella v. Elston*, 858 S.W.2d 698 (Ky. 1993); *In re Colyer*, 99 Wash.2d 114, 660 P.2d 738 (1983); *Guardianship of L.W.*, 167 Wis.2d 53, 482 N.W.2d 60 (1992) (prognosis confirmation by two independent neurologists required).
93. *In re Lawrance*, 579 N.E.2d 32 (Ind. 1991); *In re Barry*, 445 So.2d 365 (Fla.Dist.Ct.App. 1984); *In re Hamlin*, 102 Wash. 2d 810, 689 P.2d 1373 (1984); *In re Torres*, 357 N.W.2d 332 (Minn. 1984).

94. *Saikewicz.* See also the later decision of the Supreme Judicial Court in *Guardianship of Doe,* 411 Mass. 512, 583 N.E.2d 1263 (1992).
95. *In re Estate of Greenspan,* 137 Ill.2d 1, 558 N.E.2d 1194 (1990); *Longeway.*
96. See, e.g., *Rasmussen; Lawrance; In re Morrison,* 206 Cal. App. 3d 304, 253 Cal. Rptr. 530 (1988); *In re Browning,* 543 So.2d 258 (Fla. Dist. Ct. 1989), *aff'd* 568 So. 2d 4 (Fla. 1990). For an overview of procedural mechanisms for review and insightful analysis of the mediation function of ethics committees, see Dianne Hoffmann, "Mediating Life and Death Decisions," *Arizona Law Review* 36, no. 4 (Winter 1994): 821–77.
97. Joint Commission on Accreditation of Healthcare Organizations, *1994 Accreditation Manual for Hospitals, Vol. I, Standards* (Oakbrook Terrace, Ill.: Joint Commission, 1994), RI.1.1.6.1.
98. Only the state of Maryland has enacted legislation to require creation of institutional ethics committees (called "patient care review committees"). *Md. Code Ann., Health—Gen.* §§19-370, *et seq.* (Michie 1996). *Haw. Rev. Stat.* §663-1.7 (Michie 1993) establishes legal immunities for consultation with an ethics committee. Regulations issued by New Jersey's Department of Health, originally adopted in the aftermath of the state's advance directives legislation, require establishment of ethics committees in all hospitals and establishment of ethics committees or similar mechanisms at other facilities and agencies. *N.J. Admin. Code* title 8, §43G-5.1; 8:42-6.3 (1999). The stated purpose of the ethics committee is to resolve conflicts. Regulations issued by the Texas Department of Mental Health and Mental Retardation require all facilities under its jurisdiction to establish an ethics committee to be available for consultation with regard to decisions about life-sustaining treatment. *Tex. Admin. Code* title 25, §405.60 (1999). I discuss the Maryland statute further in chapter five.
99. Ethics committees are less prevalent in nursing homes, although a large number of long-term-care facilities have established a committee, share a committee with an affiliated hospital, or participate in a network that offers access to committee consultation.
100. 497 U.S. 261 (1990).
101. *Cruzan by Cruzan v. Harmon,* 760 S.W.2d 408, 419 (Mo. S.Ct., *en banc* 1988).
102. Ibid. at 425.
103. Ibid. at 417.
104. Ibid. at 411, 425.
105. After the *Cruzan* appeal had been filed in the Missouri Supreme Court, a vacancy occurred on the five-member panel assigned to hear the case. The newly assigned judge was known to be a right-to-life advocate. The panel ruled against the Cruzan family by a three-to-two vote.
106. 497 U.S. at 278. In contrast to most state courts, a five-member majority of the U.S. Supreme Court carefully avoided addressing the right of privacy, choosing instead to articulate the right to refuse treatment as a protected liberty interest. Justice Brennan, speaking for four members of the Court in his minority opinion, embraced these established privacy principles. This constitutional distinction between the liberty and privacy interests is of no concern to the current status of patients' rights to refuse life support. It is of some significance, however, to constitutional scholars who recognize that calling refusal of treatment a liberty interest rather than a fundamental privacy right implicitly lowers the burden of justification required of states that restrict this right, should

such restrictions be subjected to constitutional scrutiny. This point is made by John A. Robertson, "Cruzan and the Constitutional Status of Nontreatment Decisions for Incompetent Patients," *Georgia Law Review* 25, no. 5 (Summer 1991): 1174.
107. 497 U.S. at 279.
108. Ibid. at 289.
109. Ibid. at 282, 284.
110. Ibid. at 289. Justices Brennan, Blackmun, Marshall, and Stevens, in dissent, seemed to agree with Justice O'Connor on this point (497 U.S. at 302). Thus, this view garnered a majority of the members of the Court when the opinion was issued. Of this group, only Justices O'Connor and Stevens sit on the current Court.
111. *Compassion in Dying v. Washington*, 79 F.3d 790 (9th Cir. 1996) (rehearing *en banc*); *Vacco v. Quill*, 80 F.3d 716 (2d Cir. 1996).
112. 521 U.S. 702 (1997).
113. Ibid., 793.
114. Although the Supreme Court held that there is no constitutional barrier to state laws banning assisted suicide, the Court also was unanimous in its judgment that the debate about physician-assisted suicide can and should continue in the laboratory of the states. In the words of the Court: "Throughout the Nation, Americans are engaged in an earnest and profound debate about the morality, legality, and practicality of physician-assisted suicide. Our holding permits this debate to continue, as it should, in a democratic society." Ibid., 735. Bans on assisted suicide have been challenged on constitutional grounds in state courts on at least two occasions. The Florida case of *Krischer v. McIver*, 697 So.2d 97 (Fla. 1997), and the California case of *Donaldson v. Lundgren*, 2 Cal.App.4th 1614, 4 Cal.Rptr.2d 59 (1992), both held that state constitutional privacy protections did not include a right to physician-assisted suicide. More than 40 states prohibit physician-assisted suicide and make it a crime to assist another person in committing suicide. Only the state of Oregon has legalized the practice, under limited conditions; this initiative began at the ballot box with a statewide referendum in 1994. *Or. Rev. Stat.*, §§127.800, et seq. (Supp. 1998). Similar ballot measures have failed in Washington (1991) and California (1993). On April 30, 1997—two months prior to the Supreme Court decisions—the Federal Assisted Suicide Funding Restriction Act of 1997 was enacted to prohibit federal funding for physician-assisted suicide. Pub. L. 105-12, 111 Stat. 23 (codified at 42 *U.S.C.A.* §§ 14401, et seq. (West, pamphlet, 2000)).
115. 521 U.S. 725.
116. Ibid., 800–801.
117. In most instances, a combination of factors moved state legislatures to address these issues. Each state no doubt has its own unique story, which includes a role for the courts, public opinion, interest group politics, the personal concerns of individual legislators, and (in New Jersey and New York) bioethics study commissions. The role of the courts should not be underestimated. Beyond the effects of bringing the plights of patients and families before the media spotlight, many cases evidence a form of judicial activism. Several courts have expressly called on their state legislatures to act as the appropriate body to craft a comprehensive approach to end-of-life decision making. See, e.g., *Rasmussen*; *Jobes*; *Torres*; *Colyer*.

118. The language quoted is from the legislative findings and declaration of California's 1991 revision and repeal of the original Natural Death Act. *Cal. Health & Safety Code* §§7185, *et seq.* (West Supp. 1996). For discussion of the original California Natural Death Act and proposed amendments thereto, see Sherri Schaeffer, "Death with Dignity: Proposed Amendments to the California Natural Death Act," *San Diego Law Review* 25, no. 4 (1988): 781–828.
119. Choice in Dying maintains a current national map, available at its website, <www.choices.org> (visited 14 August 2000).
120. *N.Y. Public Health Law* §2982 (Consol.1997).
121. *Col. Rev. Stat. Ann.* §15-18-102 (West 1997).
122. *Ala. Code* §22-8A-2 (Michie 1997).
123. *N.J. Stat. Ann.* §26:2H-67 (West 1996). The full text of this provision states that life support may be withheld or withdrawn when the patient is neither terminally ill nor permanently unconscious and "when the patient has a serious irreversible illness or condition, and the likely risks and burdens associated with the medical intervention to be withheld or withdrawn may reasonably be judged to outweigh the likely benefits to the patient from such intervention, or imposition of the medical intervention on an unwilling patient would be inhumane." The rationale is discussed in New Jersey Commission on Legal and Ethical Problems in the Delivery of Health Care, *The New Jersey Advance Directives for Health Care and Declaration of Death Acts: Statutes, Commentaries and Analyses* (Princeton, N.J.: New Jersey Commission, 1991), 54–55.
124. *Fla. Stat. Ann.* §765.302 (West Supp. 1999).
125. *Or. Rev. Stat.* §127.531 (Supp. 1999). Oregon's approach here actually is a bit more demanding. The full text of the statutory form asks the author to make an election about feeding tubes "[I]f I have a progressive illness that will be fatal and is in an advanced stage, and I am consistently and permanently unable to communicate by any means, swallow food and water safely, care for myself and recognize my family and other people, and it is very unlikely that my condition will substantially improve."
126. An excellent collection of essays on the topic is Joann Lynn, ed., *By No Extraordinary Means: The Choice to Forgo Life-Sustaining Food and Water* (Bloomington: Indiana University Press, 1986).
127. *N.Y. Public Health Law* §2982 (Consol.1997). This requirement is commonly interpreted to mean that the patient's refusal of artificial nutrition and hydration must be expressly stated in writing and documents in use in New York invariably contain a specific place to make this choice.
128. *Neb. Rev. Stat.* §30-3418 (Michie 1995) (the attorney-in-fact—the proxy—must have express authority or establish the patient's refusal by clear and convincing evidence); *Okla. Stat. Ann.* §3080.4 (West 1997) (to overcome the presumption in favor of treatment, the attending physician or a court must find, by clear and convincing evidence, that the patient when competent made an informed decision to refuse nutrition and hydration); *Ala. Code* §22-8A-11 (Michie 1997) (applies to a surrogate's decision for a PVS patient).
129. *Ohio Rev. Code Ann.* §2133.09 (Baldwin 1994).
130. The first generation of state laws are collected in Society for the Right to Die, *Handbook of Living Will Laws* (New York: Society for the Right to Die, 1987). For a critique of pre-*Cruzan* advance directive laws, see George J. Alexander, "Time

for a New Law on Health Care Advance Directives," *Hastings Law Journal* 42, no. 3 (March 1991): 755–78.
131. A persuasive argument that the familiar statutory restrictions on patients' rights are unjustified appears in Norman L. Cantor, *Advance Directives and the Pursuit of Death with Dignity* (Bloomington: Indiana University Press, 1993).
132. More than half of the states included provisions of this nature in their laws as of the mid-1980s. See Gregory Gelfand, "Living Will Statutes: The First Decade," *Wisconsin Law Review 1987*: 784, n. 202 (compiling statutes). More recent enactments commonly have done the same.
133. Alan Meisel, "Legal Myths About Terminating Life Support," *Archives of Internal Medicine* 151 (August 1991): 1497.
134. P.L. No. 101-508, codified at 42 U.S.C.A. §1395cc (West 1992). The Patient Self-Determination Act took effect December 1, 1991.
135. Edward J. Larson and Thomas A. Eaton, "The Limits of Advance Directives: A History and Assessment of the Patient Self-Determination Act," *Wake Forest Law Review* 32 (Summer 1997): 249–93; George J. Annas and Frances H. Miller, "The Empire of Death: How Culture and Economics Affect Informed Consent in the U.S., the U.K., and Japan," *American Journal of Law & Medicine* 20, no. 4 (1994): 367–68 ("Congress had both cost containment and autonomy objectives in mind when it passed the Patient Self-Determination Act.").
136. Claire C. Obade, "The Patient Self-Determination Act: Right Church, Wrong Pew," *Journal of Clinical Ethics* 1, no. 4 (Winter 1990): 320–22.
137. The most comprehensive account of the PSDA and its meaning for hospitals, health care professionals, and patients is Lawrence P. Ulrich, *The Patient Self-Determination Act: Meeting the Challenges of Patient Care* (Washington, D.C.: Georgetown University Press, 1999). The PSDA's predominantly procedural posture was dictated in large measure by dual concerns about the potentially controversial nature of the issues and the proper role of the federal government (questions of "federalism"). Elizabeth Leibold McCloskey, "The Patient Self-Determination Act," *Kennedy Institute of Ethics Journal* 1, no. 2 (June 1991): 163–69, offers an inside look at the politics of the PSDA's origins and path through Congress. An early practical guide to implementing the PSDA is Concern for Dying, *Advance Directive Protocols and the Patient Self-Determination Act: A Resource Manual for the Development of Institutional Protocols* (New York: Concern for Dying, undated).
138. Dan W. Brock, "Good Decisionmaking for Incompetent Patients," *Hastings Center Report* 24, no. 6 (November-December 1994): S10.
139. See The SUPPORT Principal Investigators, "A Controlled Trial to Improve Care for Seriously Ill Hospitalized Patients," *Journal of the American Medical Association* 274, no. 20 (November 22/29, 1995): 1591–98; David Orentlicher, "The Illusion of Patient Choice in End-of-Life Decisions," *Journal of the American Medical Association* 267, no. 15 (April 15, 1992): 2101–04 (summarizing pre-SUPPORT empirical studies).
140. Mildred Z. Solomon et al., "Decisions near the End of Life: Professional Views on Life-Sustaining Treatments," *American Journal of Public Health* 83, no. 1 (January 1993): 14–23. The authors conclude that disagreement with and misunderstanding of ethical and legal guidelines are major factors that explain this pattern of physician behavior.

141. The most pertinent cases are *Estate of Leach v. Shapiro*, 13 Ohio App.3d 393, 469 N.E.2d 1047 (1984); *Anderson v. St. Francis-St. George Hosp., Inc.*, 77 Ohio St. 3d 82, 671 N.E.2d 225 (1996); and *Osgood v. Genesys Regional Medical Center*, slip op., no. 94-26731-NH (Mich.Cir.Ct., Genesee Cty., Mar. 7, 1997).

142. *Md. Code Ann., Health—Gen.* §5-609 (Michie 1996); *Or. Rev. Stat* § 127.555 (Supp. 1998); *Va. Code Ann.* §54.1-2988 (Michie 1998); *Iowa Code Ann.* §144B.12 (West 1997). The Maryland, Oregon, and Virginia laws extend the immunity to claims that are based on lack of consent or authorization. The Iowa and Virginia laws may be the most egregious. Iowa law states that "[n]otwithstanding a contrary health care decision of an attorney in fact, the health care provider is not subject to criminal prosecution, civil liability, or professional disciplinary action for failing to withhold or withdraw health care necessary to keep the principal alive." The next sentence makes a transfer of care the responsibility of the attorney in fact (the proxy). Virginia allows the physician to refuse compliance if the physician believes the treatment to be "medically or ethically inappropriate." *Va. Code Ann.* §54.1-2990 (Michie Supp. 1998).

143. In future litigation, patients' rights advocates can point to Justice O'Connor's assertion in *Cruzan* that honoring a proxy's decisions "may well be constitutionally required" to support a claim for violation of the constitutional right to refuse treatment.

144. Ashwini Sehgal et al., "How Strictly Do Dialysis Patients Want Their Advance Directives Followed?" *Journal of the American Medical Association* 267, no. 1 (January 1, 1992): 59–63.

145. Benjamin N. Cardozo, *The Nature of the Judicial Process* (New Haven, Conn.: Yale University Press, 1921), 35.

146. Although I cast the consensus in slightly different terms, the summary here is consistent with that given by Alan Meisel in "The Legal Consensus about Forgoing Life-Sustaining Treatment: Its Status and Its Prospects," *Kennedy Institute of Ethics Journal* 2, no. 4 (December 1992): 315. See also Allen E. Buchanan and Dan W. Brock, *Deciding for Others: The Ethics of Surrogate Decision Making* (Cambridge: Cambridge University Press, 1989), 90: "The dominant tendency, both in recent legal doctrine and in the bioethics literature, has been to view the rights of incompetent individuals as an extension of the rights of competent individuals, through arrangements by which these rights are exercised for the incompetent by others."

Chapter Two

THE ETHICAL FOUNDATIONS OF PROSPECTIVE AUTONOMY

[W]e not only have, in common with all sensate creatures, experiential interests in the quality of our future experiences but also critical interests in the character and value of our lives as a whole. These critical interests are connected . . . to our convictions about the intrinsic value—the sanctity or inviolability—of our own lives. . . . A person's right to be treated with dignity . . . is the right that others acknowledge his genuine critical interests.

Law professor Ronald Dworkin, 1993[1]

The most appropriate method is to adopt a variation of the "best interests" standard and to ask whether treatment will advance the current and future welfare of the patient. This approach requires a systematic evaluation of the incompetent patient's personal contemporaneous interests, rather than the interests competent persons might have in those situations. . . . The important question is whether patients who cannot experience the richness of normal life still have experiences that make continued existence from their own perspective better than no life at all.

Law professors Rebecca Dresser and John Robertson, 1989[2]

INTRODUCTION

In the account of the prevailing consensus (chapter one), we saw that the dominant approach to the place of prospective autonomy in end-of-life decisions has been to regard the rights of incompetent patients as an extension of rights to self-determination and privacy that belong to competent patients. The goal of this chapter is to present and defend a deeper claim about the importance of the principle of prospective autonomy—namely, that future-oriented actions and decisions are integral to the life of autonomous persons, no less concerning the way we die than the way we live. The consensus presupposes this view—implicit in the banner of "death with dignity" under which the battle for these rights has been fought—but fails to articulate the more fundamental roots of prospective autonomy in the moral life. Nor does it adequately explain the connections between autonomy and dignity. These failings are at least partially attributable to the fact that the predominant framework obscures the reality that advance directives are grounded in the rights, interests, and concerns that autonomous individuals have with respect to their health care futures. These rights and interests are not derivative of those of competent persons (patients); they are future-oriented rights and interests *of* competent persons.

In the long history of social and political philosophy, discussions of autonomy have taken many forms. The term *autonomy*—derived from the Greek *auto* (self) and *nomos* (rule)—has been used to express the ideas of self-rule, self-determination, independence, freedom of choice, privacy, and responsibility for one's actions. In different contexts, autonomy refers to the capacity for self-governance; the actual exercise of choice; an ideal of character, integrity, and authorship; and sovereign authority, particularly with regard to individual freedom from external constraints of others such as the state or institutions.[3] In the vast literature on the concept of autonomy, contemporary and historical, the notion of autonomy as involving current, contemporary capacities, choices, and actions predominates. Comparatively little attention has been devoted to our concern here—the concept of future-oriented autonomy. Although the foregoing list of terms and descriptions remains relevant, their meaning and significance take on different contours within the realm of prospective autonomy and in the context of decisions near the end of life.

In this chapter I articulate an understanding of prospective autonomy that is grounded in a model of autonomy as integrity. I argue that the deeper importance of prospective autonomy in the moral life generally and in control over the dying process in particular springs from the idea of the autonomous life as one of commitments to critical concerns, projects, and core values. The main point of the argument is that we have *critical interests* (borrowing Ronald Dworkin's term) in pursuing the commitments and projects that matter most to us—those that define a good life—in a way that is consistent with our core values. Living a life of integrity—loosely speaking, a life that is "in character" and in keeping with the projects and values that are identity-conferring because of the importance we attach to them—matters in important ways. Our interests in personal dignity and familial welfare that are at stake in how we die are critical to integrity not only for their own sake but also because issuance of an advance directive asserts authorship over a closing chapter in the story of a person's life.[4]

The latter part of the discussion turns to the chief challenge to this view—namely, that incompetent patients' current experiential interests should command priority attention. The essential claim made by proponents of the *current interests alternative* is that the autonomy-based interests that inform advance directives are meaningless to patients who have lost the capacity to appreciate whether their wishes are honored (or dishonored). My argument rejects this critique; I show that the familial and dignity interests that are at stake in our response to advance directives survive incompetency; their validity and importance are not contingent on the patient's present experiential and cognitive abilities.

The analysis leads to the conclusion that failure to respect an autonomous advance directive is a serious harm to the patient. The concept of harm recurs often, and some brief clarification is useful here. Following the lead of Joel Feinberg's highly regarded work on the concept of harm, I intend the term *harm* to be understood in the broad sense of *setback to interests*—including a person's interests in having his or her rights respected.[5] When an autonomous advance directive is ignored, the patient's critical interests are frustrated, thwarted, or in the general sense set back, and this setback is a harm to the patient. Insofar as disregard for an autonomous directive violates the patient's rights, it may be equally apt to say that the patient has been *wronged*. Some observers may even find this characterization more appropriate, particularly if no tangible injury—added pain, suffering, monetary loss—is done to the patient when treatment is continued. I take the term *harm*, understood in this broad sense of setback to interests, to be more descriptive of what is at stake when advance directives are overridden. The point of the argument, however, does not depend on rigorous analysis of the concepts of harming and wronging.

AUTONOMY, INTEGRITY, AND OUR CRITICAL INTERESTS

The Autonomous Pursuit of Interests

Only a moment's reflection is required to appreciate that living an autonomous life is inextricably connected with the idea of having a set of concerns, desires, and *interests* that we pursue in the living of that life. At one level, daily life involves a variety of concerns—deciding what to wear to work tomorrow, what route to drive to the office, when to pick up the dry cleaning, or what to make for dinner, to name a few. These sorts of activities for which we plan and prepare, however briefly, often go unnoticed and seem trivial (unless, of course, traffic is a major headache in one's work week) when we contrast them with larger and longer-term goals such as having a successful career, raising a family, pursuing a passion for singing, dedicating oneself to a religious faith, or giving scarce time and energy to a cherished cause (human rights, a clean environment, freedom of speech). In each case—and we could develop a much longer, perhaps endless, list—we endeavor in our actions to promote or satisfy some interest. Indeed, in a meaningful way, the object and purpose of our undertaking is to promote some interest(s).

In the pursuit of our various interests, we may be said to *have a stake in the outcome*. It matters whether we get what we are after, whether things go well or badly. Clearly, however, not all interests are equally significant. A person does not pursue his or her entire constellation of interests with equal vigor. Nor are our obligations to respect and not interfere with someone else's pursuit of his or her interests of equal weight. Thus, to determine what respect is due the interests of others we need a measure of the importance of various interests to their possessor. For the purposes of the present inquiry, we need a way to construe and evaluate the moral weight of the interests of incompetent patients with advance directives.

In this task we can distinguish, as does Ronald Dworkin, our *experiential* interests from our *critical* interests. Dworkin characterizes an individual's *critical interests* as those that it makes his/her life "genuinely better to satisfy"—interests that if not satisfied would make a person worse off in a meaningful way.[6] Most of us take seriously the idea that we want to *do something* with our lives. We have what philosophers have variously called focal aims, ulterior interests, or projects.[7] For some people, these projects entail having a successful career, living a life marked by professional or personal achievement, seeing our families flourish, or being a valued member of the community. For others, it means a life marked by freedom to have numerous experiences—to travel the world, be an avid outdoorsman, or be a passionate mountain climber.[8] Although these tangible projects offer ready illustrations, we also have a set of less tangible but equally important interests that involve the *kind of person* each of us is. Most of us value dearly some number of personal qualities: honesty, kindness, compassion, generosity, toughness, shrewdness, and so on. We strive in our endeavors to cultivate and remain true to the character traits we value—often to the point at which, in an Aristotelian sense, we are habituated to certain character traits and *are* honest or compassionate. By the same token, most of us care about how others think of us (even when we reject the opinions of others as a measure of self-worth). We have an important stake in our reputation, in being thought of and remembered as kind, honest, generous, and the like.[9] Finding that others think us cold, "slick," or mean-spirited when we have committed our lives to precisely the opposite is a deeply felt injury.

Whatever our interests—and most of us pursue many of them simultaneously—what distinguishes our critical interests is that they are central to our pursuit of a good life, defined in terms of our own values and commitments. Our critical interests are directly connected to whether we view our lives as going well or badly, as successful and fulfilling or frustrating and disappointing.[10] We value these interests dearly for their own sake, as ends in themselves, and gain a level of intrinsic satisfaction not only at their attainment but in their pursuit as well.

In contrast, our *experiential* interests are interests that we choose to pursue largely because we enjoy or find satisfaction in the activity. The experience of doing things such as playing tennis, going to the theater, watching television, or cooking constitutes the primary reason for doing so. Pleasurable activities are important to living a good life, of course, and are instrumental to larger goods in life—such as good health, intellectual stimulation, and friendship. However, "the value of these experiences, judged one by one, depends precisely on the fact that we do find them pleasurable or exciting *as experiences*."[11] The primary value for us, the dominant reason for choosing some activities as opposed to others, lies in the pleasure and satisfaction of the experience itself.

We do not personally identify the many pursuits we value as experiences as constitutive of what it means to have a good life in the deeper way that we value our critical interests. If we are suddenly deprived of the ability to play tennis or go to the theater, the usual response is regret and disappointment rather than worry, depression (at least not for long) or sorrow, and we often compensate by finding some other interest that brings equal enjoyment. This is not to suggest, of course, that we do not experience our critical interests, nor that experience itself separates our critical and experiential interests. Moreover, what some people consider pleasurable activities that they "could live without," others value as critically important. The devastation felt by the baseball pitcher forced into early retirement by a rotator cuff injury or by the vocalist who loses her singing voice to throat cancer are real; such losses are less tragic, however, if they happen to someone who is not athletic or could not hold a tune in the first place.

We also can observe that the pursuit of our critical interests characteristically involves future-oriented decisions and substantial investment in the future. Few of life's most valued pursuits are achieved overnight. For most people, securing the welfare of one's family is a lifelong commitment and concern (a large inheritance or winning the lottery notwithstanding). A successful career—as musician, physician, lawyer, professor, or businessperson—is measured not by a single achievement but by a life of accomplishment. Pitching a shutout, even in the World Series, does not make one a great baseball player. (A no-hitter, however, will get your name entered in the Hall of Fame in Cooperstown.) This point is poignantly illustrated by the fact that the converse does not always hold. As the lives of public figures (especially politicians) demonstrate, a single act of dishonesty or infidelity can end a career and devastate one's reputation, tarnishing forever the image that one has spent the better part of a life cultivating. Despite many fine achievements and herculean efforts to amend the history books, the life story of former president Nixon will always have a chapter (or two) known as Watergate. In short, as compared to our experiential interests, substantial investment in our critical interests gives us all the greater stake in the outcome. When critical projects fail badly, we do not view our failure as a disappointment or a mere setback; we are more likely to see it as a serious harm with a deeper significance and, depending on the magnitude of the harm, to use terms such as *crisis* or *tragedy*.

In sum, what marks off our critical and experiential interests in a morally significant way is the personal importance we assign to various interests and the ways in which we identify ourselves with some interests more strongly than with others. We have a greater stake in the success or failure of our critical interests precisely because they are constitutive of our own view of the good life. This point is made more clear by a deeper distinguishing fact about our critical interests: Investment in our most cherished commitments is intimately connected to our values and involves a process of identification and authorship that defines who we are.

Critical Interests, Character, and Integrity

We can regard a person's constellation of interests as a sort of network in which the pursuit of one project is not only an end but also a means to another important end. As Feinberg puts it, our ultimate interests (Feinberg's term) "characteristically resemble . . . ends (not *the* end) which are also means to many other divergent ends."[12] For most of us, an autonomous life is structured around the projects to which we assign priority and the critical interests at which they aim. To be sure, a good life includes having many of our experiential interests fulfilled, but it is not merely a collection of rewarding and pleasurable experiences (at least for most of us). A *good* life has a structure and coherence that binds what we value and forms a portrait and narrative of the kind of person that each of us is.[13]

For many (though not all) people, this coherence comes from the fact that commitments to our critical interests are in various ways *identity-conferring*.[14] The things that matter most to us are those with which we identify as constitutive of our character—not just what we do but who we are. Through pursuit of our most valued projects and goals, we identify ourselves with those projects and make them *ours*. Conversely, we choose many of our projects because of the commitments we have. A life of engagement in the things we hold most dear is a process of self-identification and self-authorship.[15] Some philosophers have used the term *authenticity* to express essentially this same idea, stressing that autonomy involves a process of reflective acceptance and internalization of values and commitments that imprints a personal stamp on who we are.[16] By the same token, this process of moral agency makes each of us the author (to a significant extent) of how others identify us—of who others believe us to be.

The concept of *integrity* captures the place of structure and coherence in the moral life. To say that someone lives a life of integrity is to say that that person's life is marked by consistency of commitment and conviction over time, by a sense of wholeness that binds.[17] This wholeness comes from at least two sorts of consistency in the moral life. The first involves coherent integration of a person's core values and commitments; the second entails translation of values into action.[18] A person of integrity possesses a consistent and integrated pattern of internal commitments that in turn are reflected in the person's decisions and actions. If someone's projects and values were constantly changing and showed little temporal investment, we would be hard-pressed to describe any of these interests as critical, nor could we ascribe the label of integrity to that person's life. At the same time, we could hardly consider honesty to be an identity-conferring trait for someone who lies whenever doing so will bring personal advantage.[19]

Beyond the outward and readily observable meaning of having interests and projects (wanting a successful career, raising a family, having friends), for most people pursuing life plans in accordance with a set of core values and principles is of critical importance. In many respects these values—whatever they may be—bind a person's interest network, contributing in crucial ways to a core definition of the self. These core values anchor an internal coherence in the moral life. Most of us care about whether we are honest and trustworthy, keep our promises, are selfish or altruistic; we make substantial investments in *living up to* our ideal about the kind of person we choose to be. A person of integrity is consistently guided by a personal moral compass lodged at the center of the person's interest network. A life of integrity involves conscious reflection about one's values and commitments such that one's *significant* choices stay the course, manifesting substantial investment in personal values and commitments. (It is not necessary to integrity that every decision and action, however inconsequential, presupposes conscious reflection and selection.)

For example, we value professional success for its own sake and as a means of providing for the welfare of ourselves and our families. To most of us, however, how we achieve that success also matters. It makes a difference whether we tell the truth, keep our promises, and are respected by others. It also matters whether we are able to balance a career with things that are important to being a good spouse, child, or parent—such as spending "quality time," making the holidays special, always being kinder than necessary, and so on. The exercise of our faculties in the pursuit of our projects is closely connected to our values, especially values that we have so internalized that they constitute dispositions of character to conduct ourselves in certain ways.

Integrity itself, then, counts among our most important interests. A person's commitment to and investment in a structured and coherent life give it independent intrinsic value. There is much at stake in the quest to live a life of integrity. When commitments to important projects are frustrated, when core values are compromised, when the moral compass is off course, the setback to pursuit of a good life is deeply felt, at times tragic.[20]

Several further points about integrity are relevant to the present inquiry. We commonly think of integrity in terms of honesty, uprightness, and moral virtue. Whether someone is a good or bad person is not central to this understanding of integrity, however.[21] Integrity in the relevant sense here is personal and subjective. It involves reflection on one's own choices in relation to one's accepted values and commitments.[22] To say that someone is a person of integrity, we need not agree with or approve of the person's values, commitments, or choices. The fact that the person behaves consistently with his or her settled commitments and makes authentic choices ordinarily is sufficient warrant for this ascription.[23] Ebenezer Scrooge was no role model for our children, but he lived his life in character (until the Ghost of Christmas Past induced a character-altering change of perspective). Had Scrooge died prior to his character transformation, leaving a written request to be buried with his life's fortune, complying with his request, however distasteful, would honor his autonomy and integrity.

It also is not necessary to integrity that someone rigidly adhere to the same values always or that the person always assign the same priority to personal projects. Nor is it crucial to integrity that all of one's decisions, actions, and beliefs are consistent, that they are thoroughly in character, or that a person's character is considered fixed after a certain term of years as if to set a standard against which all future behavior is measured. It is a fact of life that we modify and change our values, priorities, and plans, and we often (though not always) do so without sacrificing our integrity.[24] Metaphorically, the internal compass may adjust direction, but it remains centered. Integrity in its fullest sense is an ideal. It is an aspiration and model of an autonomous life. It would have little practical meaning in the moral life, however, if rigid consistency of values and choices were a necessary condition for the ascription of integrity.[25]

The idea of personal integrity captures the dignity we attach to being in charge of our own lives and makes plain the intimate connection between autonomy and dignity. To have dignity is to have worth or to be worthy. To be treated with dignity is to have others act toward us in a manner that shows respect for our worth and esteem. Thus, dignity has an internal face and an external face. Dignity is closely connected with the ideas of self-worth, self-esteem, and self-respect. It also is closely connected with the way others perceive and behave toward us. When others treat us with disrespect, when they perceive us or behave toward us in a way that diminishes our worth and esteem, they treat us with *in*dignity.[26] Respect for autonomy honors the inherent value of a person's commitments to his or her critical interests. In crucial respects, an autonomous life that commands the respect of others is a life of dignity. When others violate, disregard, or impede someone's autonomy, it is an affront—an indignity. [27]

A point worth emphasizing is that ordinarily, having and pursuing interests means that having things go well is in a person's interest; flourishing of interests promotes the person's good. Others need not agree with our choices, however. The values of others and the choices they would make under the circumstances may have bearing on a person's reasoning—especially if alternative, even discordant, views come from family, friends, or colleagues—but the agreement of others is not the yardstick of integrity. Nor is it the yardstick of our obligations to respect autonomy. Taking the right of autonomy seriously must include the right to be wrong. To hold otherwise is to strike at the heart of integrity and dignity where it matters most: in the face of opposition from those who would choose otherwise *for* us.

How, then, should we understand the pursuit of death with dignity from the point of view of integrity? Do we have critical interests in how we die?

THE PURSUIT OF DEATH WITH DIGNITY AND RESPECT FOR AUTONOMY

The Pursuit of Death with Dignity

The phrase "death with dignity" asserts that there are more dignified and less dignified ways to die and that there are more and less *un*dignified ways to die. Few people would disagree with these conjoint propositions, other than those who insist that death is the ultimate indignity (perhaps confusing death with the dying process).[28] Indeed, the wide acceptance of this concept explains, in part, why the battle for patients' rights to refuse life support has been fought under the banner "death with dignity." (Recall that many advance directive statutes have been titled "Death with Dignity" acts.)

Refusal of life support and the decision to accept an earlier death when one is terminally ill or irreversibly comatose is variously motivated by the prospect of the pain and suffering of a protracted dying process; the diminished value of life when stroke, senility, or other assaults deprive us of mental capacity and the ability to interact meaningfully with others; the loss of freedom and control that is endemic to being nonambulatory, physically immobile, or, worse, helpless—all the while dependent on machines, tubes, and health care professionals for the basic functions of life; the loss of privacy in facing death in the company of strangers in a hospital or nursing home; and the interests of loved ones who must bear the emotional, psychological, and perhaps financial burdens of the "death watch" and beyond. The fact that all of these concerns are meaningfully connected to personal dignity resonates with our considered moral judgments. To die in terrible pain, dependent on the armamentarium of modern medicine while one's family watches an inexorable decline toward the inevitable, is to die with a diminished sense of worth and dignity—perhaps, to die in indignity.

Autonomy as integrity illuminates the essential connection between being in charge of one's own life and taking charge of the dying process; it offers an explanation of the deep-seated importance of putting one's personal stamp on the dying process. The shaping of one's post-competence fate asserts "the realm of inviolable sanctuary most of us sense in our own being."[29] It affirms that life structured by one's core values and moral compass does not end with terminal illness and loss of competence; it acknowledges that dying is part of life taken as a whole. In the face of a debilitating illness that degrades, dehumanizes, and challenges self-worth, choosing how we die—deciding how long we will suffer the indignity of dependence on medical technology—brings dignity to the dying process. It puts the countenance of dignity, of a life of integrity, on a crucial chapter in the patient's life.[30]

Because of the close historical association between the ideas of death with dignity and self-determination, advance directives often are narrowly identified with self-interest or, more precisely, with a self-referential understanding of dignity. This definition, however, does not fully capture the meaning of our critical interests in the dying process. We can shed further light on a person's critical interests in the dying process by loosely distinguishing our *dignity interests* and our *familial interests* and by reflecting on a person's interests in terms of his or her self-regarding and other-regarding dimensions.

The constellation of concerns we have for personal dignity, or the absence of indignity, in the dying process—including the (negative) value we attach to suffering, dependence, and mental incapacity—is at the heart of our *dignity interests*. At the center of our various *familial interests* are predominantly other-regarding concerns for the emotional, psychological, and financial welfare of loved ones.[31] These two concerns are closely connected in essential ways. It matters for the sake of our loved ones that they are at the bedside, that they are witness to our suffering, that they will suffer a prolonged and anguished vigil, and that they will remember how we die. It also matters for our own sake, however. It is in a person's own interest whether loved ones fare well or badly, whether felt obligations to family are met or breached.

Moreover, although dignity's lens is predominantly self-regarding, it also involves how others perceive us. From the point of view of dignity and integrity, whether we are remembered as having faced our last days with the countenance of dignity, committed to loved ones through a full life even in dying, is a significant part of the story of one's life. As Cantor writes, "[P]eople care mightily about the image and memories to be left during a period of decline and death. People strive to cultivate an image during a lifetime, and they don't want to see that image despoiled by a protracted demise in a gravely debilitated condition."[32] We "care mightily" about these things for our own sake and for the sake of our families.

Clearly there is an objective quality to our understanding of death with dignity that springs from shared moral judgments about human worth and dignity. At bottom, however, dignity and dying with dignity—like integrity—are highly personal and subjective. To pursue death with dignity is to shape the dying process in accordance with the importance one attaches to dignity and familial interests in one's personal value scheme. Each person must decide by reference to his or her own interests what is at stake in how dying and death unfold. The insight of the Values History—a document used to elicit personal values and preferences as an aid to writing an advance directive—is the attempt to illuminate the role of these critical interests (without using this term) in shaping the decisions committed to paper in advance directives.[33] For those of us who overcome the natural reluctance to confront our own deaths, advance directives offer the opportunity to impress a personal stamp on the end of life and to pen guidance on how the continuing story of our lives will be told.[34]

Respect for Autonomy

It should now be clear that the integrity view of autonomy provides compelling justification for the principle of respect for prospective autonomy and for advance directives. Once we recognize the inherent value of being in charge of one's own life, it follows that future-oriented decisions should remain valid and entitled to respect post-competence. The point of an advance directive is to guide others in promoting our interests for us—more strongly, to charge others with this responsibility. To respond otherwise, to renege on this charge, is to violate autonomy by denying the intrinsic importance of a person's critical interests in dignity, family, and a life of integrity compassing not only how one has lived but how one will die. Violation of autonomy by ignoring or deliberately overriding an advance directive is an affront to the integrity and dignity of the person who is and has been its author. It denies a patient's commitment to and right to authorship of a crucial chapter of a life story that still is being told. As Ronald Dworkin remarks, "Making someone die in a way that others approve, but he believes a horrifying contradiction of his life, is a devastating, odious form of tyranny."[35]

Thus, there is compelling reason to accord respect for prospective autonomy priority status over competing considerations of the patient's current expressions and interests. Dworkin makes this point emphatic by employing the concept of "precedent autonomy" to describe the lexical priority due to advance directives:

> A competent person's right to autonomy requires that his past decisions, about how he is to be treated if he becomes demented, be respected even if they do not represent, and even if they contradict, the desires he has when we respect them, provided he did not change his mind while he was still in charge of his own life. If we refused to accept precedent autonomy, and instead insisted that past decisions made when competent will not be enforced unless they represent the present wishes of the incompetent patient, we would be violating the point of autonomy on the integrity view.[36]

If we take seriously the critical interests that inform advance directives, we must grant that the previously expressed, written wishes of the competent person have precedence over the now-incompetent person's current experiential interests. Norman Cantor makes a similar claim. The author of an advance directive, Cantor asserts, "ought to be presumed to have deliberately formulated and constantly adhered to the sentiments of an advance directive. . . . [T]he signing of an advance directive ought to be presumed . . . to carry with it sufficient deliberation to make it binding," subject to rebuttal of this presumption.[37] Many supporters of advance directives (as well as of a family's substituted judgment in the absence of a written document) also find compelling reason for a strong presumption that prior treatment refusals should be honored.

The argument is powerful, but I am not yet prepared to fully embrace it. The concept of precedent autonomy suggests not only that autonomous advance directives as a rule should take precedence over competing considerations—in particular, the patient's current best interests—but that this presumption is virtually irrebuttable, perhaps absolutely binding.[38] Many people endorse this position, and I concur in its tone and tenor. The argument for precedent autonomy also suggests, however, a strong, perhaps irrebuttable, presumption that *all* advance directives in fact embody autonomous choices (are autonomous) and therefore have precedential weight in treatment decision making. This different sort of claim stems from the fact that the fundamental rationale for the principle of prospective autonomy is grounded in an understanding of *autonomous persons*. Yet by focusing on the meaning of an autonomous life, on what it means to be autonomous, the integrity view of autonomy paints an incomplete picture of the nature of *autonomous decisions*—of what it means to act autonomously in particular instances.

All advocates of respect for advance directives, including Cantor and Dworkin, would acknowledge that respect for advance directives presupposes autonomous decisions.[39] Do all advance directives, however, *ipso facto* express autonomous decisions? Is the presumption that an advance directive is entitled to respect because it embodies an autonomous choice rebuttable in particular instances? There is reason to inquire whether some, but not all, advance directives may count as autonomous and worthy of respect. An account of future-oriented autonomous decisions is needed. The task of chapter three is to take up this question and to develop a conception of *prospective decisional autonomy*.

In addition, the case for prospective autonomy must respond squarely to the competing claim that the incompetent patient's current welfare and interests should count in deciding for them, not the dignity and familial interests on which prior directives are based. As framed by critics of prospective autonomy, the "current interests" approach asserts that our critical interests do not survive (are not relevant) post-competence because (some) incompetent patients can no longer experience and appreciate these concerns and cannot be harmed by disregard of the prior interests that informed a prior directive. The preceding analysis has laid the foundation for a response to this attack, pointing to several ways that critical interests in how we die do not depend on actual experience of whether our interests are furthered or frustrated.

A stronger account of how our critical interests survive incompetency will strengthen the moral case for respect for prospective autonomy; a stronger account of how the dignity and familial interests that are central to advance directives survive incompetency will strengthen the moral case for respect for advance directives. I turn to this task in the remainder of this chapter, explaining and critiquing the current interests alternative and offering a richer account of surviving interests in how we die.

EXPERIENTIAL AND SURVIVING INTERESTS

The Current Interests Alternative

Law professors Rebecca Dresser and John Robertson flatly reject the principle of prospective autonomy in favor of a *current interests approach*. In a jointly authored article, they assert that formerly competent patients' autonomy interests do not survive incompetency because the incompetent patient "lacks interests in privacy, dignity, and other values that presuppose some conscious appreciation of those concerns." [40] Writing separately, Robertson argues that "the decision affects the incompetent patient as she now is, not as she previously was."[41] Thus, the "central question [is] how to value or respect incompetent patients as they are now."[42] Following this same path, Dresser asserts that because "incompetent patients are no longer capable of valuing their prior exercise of these [autonomy] rights . . . they can receive no present benefit from treatment decisions in accord with their former preferences."[43] Because the now incompetent patient cannot comprehend and experience violation of prior autonomous choices, there is no moral obligation to follow prior directives and no disrespect or injury involved in disregarding prior directives.[44]

Rather than looking to prior directives that aim to promote now "meaningless" interests, Dresser and Robertson argue that we should be concerned solely with the current welfare interests of the incompetent patient.[45] On their view, the current interests approach respects incompetent patients as persons because it privileges patients' interests as they now are. Notably, their critique of the consensus (which they refer to as the orthodox approach) is an objection to the place of instruction directives (living wills) in decisions for incompetent patients. They would allow proxies and family members to hold decisional authority, but they argue that the proxy should disregard the patient's prior expressions and focus instead on whether the patient has an interest in continued life.[46] In an initial effort to define the current interests of incompetent patients and to provide needed guidance to proxy and family, Dresser and Robertson make a further claim. Incompetent patients who retain some cognitive capacity for interaction with their environment have significant interests in continued life, even if in a gravely debilitated state. Patients who fit this description should continue to receive life support, unless this treatment would entail significant pain and discomfort for the patient.[47]

Other writers have questioned whether speaking about autonomy makes sense when the contemporaneous capacity for its exercise is absent, but Dresser and Robertson stand alone in their extended critical analysis of the consensus and their advocacy of the current interests alternative. Their position raises important questions about the role of incompetent patients' current interests in termination-of-treatment decisions, particularly dilemmas posed by conflicts between prior directives that refuse treatment and current experiential interests in continued life.[48] Consider the severely demented Alzheimer's patient with an advance directive that refuses feeding tubes, who has lost all interest in food and does not recognize his children but is not in tremendous pain and still appears to enjoy baseball, especially when the Yankees win. Such "hard cases" involve a morally important risk of premature death for incompetent patients who retain (perhaps significant) interests in continued life.

The inquiry to be pursued here is whether these sorts of cases present a serious challenge to the lexical ordering of principles that grounds the conceptual framework for deciding for incompetent patients. Whether best interests should trump advance directives in exceptional cases is a related but distinct issue, which I explore in chapters three and five.

The current interests alternative bears a heavy burden if we are to be persuaded to dethrone prospective autonomy in favor of a best interests approach to treatment decisions for incompetent patients. As we will see, the current interests alternative simply fails in this effort, for it rests on two fatally flawed premises. The first is the claim that incompetent patients do not have autonomy-based interests in dignity and family welfare that survive loss of mental capacity. The second claim, which is derivative of the first, is that giving priority to the patient's current interests respects the patient as a person.[49]

Surviving Interests and Harm

At the heart of the current interests account is the faulty assumption that a person's interests cease to be important and cannot be harmed, violated, or set back unless a person actually "has some conscious appreciation of those concerns." Again, the claim is that incompetence extinguishes a person's autonomy-based critical interests.

To begin we can observe that broadly equating incompetence with inability to appreciate concerns for privacy, dignity, or family welfare simply misdescribes the real experience of many incompetent patients. This description may be true of severely demented patients (though not uniformly so) and of permanently unconscious patients. However, many patients who lack the cognitive reasoning skills to make health care decisions nonetheless are aware of and responsive to being institutionalized, dependent on others for activities of daily living, and the hardship and suffering of loved ones. Many incompetent patients do experience previously feared humiliation, loss of self-esteem, and indignity. Many are aware of having chosen a proxy (or at least hold the expectation that a spouse or child is in charge) and may be aware of having issued specific instructions for their care, even if they cannot now understand what they had written. Thus, as a descriptive account the current interests alternative sweeps too broadly.[50]

More important, the factual observation that some incompetent patients clearly do lack the present ability to be concerned about respect for their prior autonomous choices should not be confused with the normative claim that autonomy-based interests therefore should be subordinate to the patient's best interests. To see how this position presents a radical challenge to the moral life, we need only look to a sample of the array of social practices in which we act on important interests in future events with an understanding that future setbacks to those interests are (serious) harms regardless of whether we later come to know how things turned out. When a testator's bequests are not honored, we view this as a harm to the testator (and, in the ordinary case, to beneficiaries) although the testator cannot know posthumously what has happened. To discontinue life support for an Orthodox Jew who has suffered irreversible loss of all functions of the entire brain, including the brainstem (so-called "whole brain death"), but has made known his rejection of brain death as a valid concept of death offends the individual's deep-seated religious beliefs and inflicts a serious harm.[51] Giving a blood transfusion to a dying adult Jehovah's Witness is a violation of religious beliefs even if the patient never recovers consciousness.

The same idea is at work in our approach to organ donation. The Uniform Anatomical Gift Act, adopted in some form across the nation, provides that family members may consent to donation, absent "contrary indications" that the patient would withhold consent, presupposing that individuals have the right to control disposition of their body parts after death. Is it really the case that the donor—or, more precisely, the nondonor—who voices objection to donation is not harmed by bodily invasion to retrieve internal organs?[52]

In each of these cases (there are many others), we commonly hold that we have legitimate interests in future events and that there is a profound violation of autonomy that harms the patient, despite the patient's inability to consciously appreciate this harm.[53] What informs these and other social practices in which we honor future-oriented decisions is "social respect for the intrinsic dignity interests of persons, even when violations of those interests cannot be felt by the affected individual."[54]

Autonomy as integrity resonates with our considered moral judgments in such cases by explaining how the ends of prospective autonomy are interests (in the case of family welfare, we might also say obligations) with targets that postdate incompetence. The point of the integrity view of autonomy is that a person's future-oriented interests in dignity and family welfare are nonexperiential in significant respects—that is, their importance does not depend on a person's actual experience of whether they are satisfied or frustrated. A person's interest in dying in a dignified manner consistent with his or her own settled values is fulfilled when an advance directive is honored and harmed when it is not, even though the patient will not attain the satisfaction of knowing that his or her wishes were honored, or know the frustration and anger of having an advance directive ignored. As with the foregoing examples, the harm done when a person's directive is ignored lies in the objective fact of the person's wishes being dishonored and the blocking or thwarting of critical interests, not in the subjective cognitive experience (frustration, depression, anger, humiliation) of knowing that this thwarting of interests has occurred. The chief aim of autonomy is to bring about certain states of affairs that promote our interests; the positive mental state that comes from successful investment in a project is a secondary goal and a "welcome dividend."[55] The same holds true for the unwelcome return of negative mental states associated with unsuccessful investment in important projects.

In contrast, the current interests alternative posits an unacceptably narrow view of autonomy and autonomy-based interests in the moral life. This account fails to offer a plausible explanation for these and other social practices in which respect for prospective autonomy plays a central role. It also fails to appreciate the distinction between the fact of an interest being frustrated or thwarted and the cognitive disappointment or anger of knowing this to be so.

The paucity of the current interests approach is further revealed by the odd and disturbing claims that the logic of the argument would have us embrace. We would have to accept that our interests in family welfare are not strongly other-regarding and that our stake in the welfare of loved ones is extinguished when we cannot know whether the state of affairs toward which we have worked and planned occurs. In other words, our stake in family well-being and our substantial investments in the projects that promote this end are contingent on knowing whether our investments have paid off. We also would have to accept a spare conception of personal dignity that reduces the countenance of dignity to present experience, ignoring the ways in which dignity is related to how we are perceived by others. Even more significantly, we are called on to reject the close connections between dignity, integrity, and the importance of being in charge of one's entire life. Instead, we are asked to accept that a person's meaningful, constructive participation in the telling of his or her life story ends with serious illness and mental incapacity. In these and other ways, the current interests approach demands that we regard the incompetent patient predominantly, if not exclusively, in the present—as divorced from his or her past (including past interests, projects, and relationships). The same is true for the family, who are asked to accept responsibility as proxy but set aside intimate knowledge of a loved one—of that person's values, commitments, and wishes—in favor of narrow attention to the patient's current experiential interests in continued life.

The ultimate collective message of these claims is a severely truncated understanding of prospective autonomy that asserts that it is misguided, perhaps irrational, for autonomy to posit a stake in a state of affairs that may occur post-competence. Dresser and Robertson state that "the real offense in maintaining debilitated patients is to competent observers, whose own concepts of what constitutes dignified and respectful medical treatment for seriously compromised human beings have been violated."[56] Simply explaining away the profound importance we attach to future-oriented control of how we die by pointing to the sensibilities of those who maintain vigil at the bedside gives an empty accounting of our considered moral judgments.

There is a final tag-on argument to consider: that if incompetent patients could be returned miraculously to competence for the purpose of deciding about life support (the hypothetical construct stated, but not relied upon, in *Quinlan*), they would be concerned solely with "current and future interests as incompetent individuals, not their past preferences."[57] This speculative vision of the incompetent patient as hypothetical chooser can never truly be tested—and it is far from clear why we should assume this assertion to be true. In fact, the stronger argument is to the contrary. As Cantor argues, "There is no reason to assume that a person's values and priorities would change while the person is in a permanently incapacitated state."[58] It is far more plausible to believe that the suddenly and temporarily competent patient would take into account the same future-oriented concerns for dignity and family welfare that motivated the prior directive. It is highly unlikely that future-oriented concerns would be limited to experiential interests such as pain, pleasure, and relational capacity, as these authors suggest. Indeed, it borders on the absurd to suggest that in a suddenly lucid moment the patient will abandon forward-looking concerns for personal dignity and the welfare of loved ones.

To pursue this point a step further, the miraculously competent patient probably would want to know (as before) whether he or she will experience pain, possess relational capacity, and derive previously unanticipated enjoyment from a state of "pleasant senility." The patient also will want to know (as before) whether his or her existence on life support will involve dependence, immobility, and indignity, as well as whether his or her continued life in a seriously debilitated condition will impose severe emotional, psychological, and financial burdens on family members. In short, the more logical result of this hypothetical exercise would be enhanced understanding of one's medical condition and more informed decisions that are based on the same values embodied in a prior directive.

The point is illustrated by the case of some AIDS patients who experience fluctuating decisional capacity with temporary treatment of conditions such as toxoplasmosis that impair cognitive faculties. Experience with this group of patients reveals that they not only continue to fear the inexorable physical decline of progressive illness, they also remain acutely aware of concerns for personal indignity and the welfare of others.

Respect for Persons

If the current interests approach were correct, and prior autonomous expressions were not relevant to the care of incompetent patients (as is the case with the never-competent and with those who have not previously expressed their wishes), the principle of beneficence indeed would counsel giving priority to the patient's current welfare, as measured by the patient's experiential interests. It would be plausible to hold that doing so honors respect for persons. Once we recognize, however, that the importance of our critical interests does not depend on actual experience and that denial and thwarting of the interests an advance directive aims to protect harms the patient, the secondary argument that respect for persons demands the subjugation and disregard of prior directives collapses.

As framed by its proponents, the current interests approach also rests on a sterile and unacceptable view of the principle of respect for persons.[59] On the autonomy as integrity account, respect for prior competent choices is intrinsic to "respect for the dignity and self-realization of all human beings."[60] Honoring advance directives respects the future-oriented moral agency that is integral to an autonomous life. For persons who have made the considered effort to write advance directives, honoring those directives respects the "earned prerogative" to control the dying process and authorship of a life as a whole.[61] In stark contrast, the current interests approach denies the profound significance of moral agency and authorship of a complete life. Moreover, it denies life's continuity, radically divorcing the patient from his or her personal history, as if to say, "The life you have lived—your values, plans, and relationships—no longer matters."

Rather than treating patients as persons with historicity marked by active moral agency, the current interests approach regards incompetent patients merely as the subjects of experiences. Characterizing this approach as patient-centered (Dresser)[62] does little to rescue it from the charge that it in fact treats patients as objects.[63] By definition, an objective standard relies on decisional criteria that are external to and independent of the patient's subjective values, wishes, and character. Ignoring the patient's prior autonomous wishes treats the incompetent patient as an object and shows disrespect for the person that the patient is *and has been* over the course of a lifetime. To abridge the patient's life in this way is to degrade and dehumanize the incompetent patient.[64]

Posthumous Harm and Interests that Survive Death

We can supplement the integrity view of autonomy and better understand how our familial and dignity interests in how we die survive loss of mental capacity by briefly considering two related questions: Is posthumous harm possible? If it is, what sorts of interests survive death, so that speaking of their being set back as a harm makes sense? If frustration of our interests causes posthumous harm, it necessarily follows that we can be harmed by unknown violations of our interests while we are in a comatose or seriously debilitated, cognitively impaired condition.[65] If that is the case, proponents of a current interests approach are foreclosed from insisting that the autonomy interests embodied in advance directives no longer count—at least not on the ground that setbacks to these interests must be experienced to constitute harms. They cannot maintain (to paraphrase the cliché) that what we don't know can't harm us.

Important (critical?) interests whose ultimate fulfillment or thwarting postdates a person's death can be found in many spheres of the moral life. Consider, for example, a parent's desire to see the family business continue and thrive or the philanthropist's gift to build a new research facility, endow an academic chair, or combat global warming. When these commitments do not come to pass despite substantial investment and planning—when one's will is abrogated, when contracts and promises are broken—we commonly regard these events as harms. The fact that the events do not occur until after the person's death does not negate the harm. So too with a person's reputation. When false rumors are spread after one's death ("he was unfaithful in marriage," "he cheated on his taxes," "he embezzled funds from the company"), common sense tells us that an injury has been done. The fact that the victim of such falsehoods can never know the embarrassment or anger that he or she would feel while still alive does not lead to the opposite conclusion.

The integrity view of autonomy grounds our shared, commonsense understanding that we are indeed harmed when the interests toward which future-oriented plans aim are set back in significant ways. This understanding is equally true in the domain of decisions near the end of life. Clearly, the impact of death on loved ones is felt well beyond the patient's death. Although we may say of personal dignity interests that they are satisfied with a death shaped by a person's advance directive—and thus that they do not survive death itself—this statement is not entirely true. First, there is a close connection between dignity and commitment to family welfare. Second, dignity involves how others perceive us and how others remember us. It matters deeply that the image and memories of a lived life, including those of decline and death, survive long after we die, have great meaning to loved ones, and are part of the story of each person's life. As Feinberg writes, "The final tally book on a person's life is not closed until some time after his death."[66] To dishonor an advance directive is to deprive its author of the right and opportunity to write in the tally book that his or her life has been marked throughout by dignity and integrity, including in death. At stake in doing so is the serious harm involved in having others remember how we died as a terrible contradiction of how we lived and the legacy of life's investment.[67]

Some accepted social practices—in particular, testamentary wills, funeral arrangements, and burial—seem to be more closely related to respect for advance directives than others. Each of these practices, like advance directives, is premised on the principle of prospective autonomy and on the view that there are important surviving interests at stake in death and dying that extend beyond our capacity to know whether those interests are honored and protected or demeaned and denied. Our strong commitment to respect for prior wishes in each circumstance (correlative surviving duties) provides further evidence of how respect for prior autonomous wishes honors respect for persons.[68] The remainder of the discussion in this chapter looks more closely at these practices.

Testamentary Wills

If we so readily accept the validity of implementing a deceased person's testamentary will, why not also accept a living will (or other form of advance directive)? The analogy to testamentary wills is familiar; it has been employed by courts and commentators. Since before the founding of our nation, Anglo-American law and society have recognized the personal right to make a devise by will, disposing of and distributing one's property and assets after death. This practice is so widely accepted that it seems to be a natural thread in our cultural fabric. (This is not to say, of course, that all adults execute testamentary wills. By some estimates, more than two-thirds of all people die without one.)[69]

Beyond the fact that advance directives and testamentary wills are both concerned with decisions about death and dying, the laws, rules, and practices governing these practices share several common features. In fact, laws governing property wills have served as models for development of state legislation on advance directives. As with an advance directive, a testamentary will must be executed by a competent adult and may be modified, revoked, or completely rewritten at any time while the author is competent. In both cases, the author is presumed competent (if of legal age—usually 18), challenges to the author's competence are rare, and going back in time to adduce evidence to mount such a challenge is difficult.[70]

These surface similarities may make the analogy attractive (and account in part for the fact that most law firms consider advance directives to be part of trust and estate practice), but we need to probe more deeply to see the strengths and weaknesses of the comparison. The central conceptual point is that both practices embrace the principle of prospective autonomy. Like advance directives, testamentary wills are intended to take effect only after the author has lost the ability to change prior decisions committed to writing. Is the fact that the former control health care decisions while the person is still alive and the latter control the disposition of property after death a crucial difference? Critics of advance directives argue that it is; they contend that the patient can be harmed by respect for a prior directive, whereas the deceased cannot be harmed by dishonoring a devise of property.[71]

Of course, a living patient can be harmed in ways that a deceased person cannot, and this fact demands our moral attention. Yet this observation does not diminish our obligations to respect the critical interests that ground advance directives. This view also ignores a key feature of the analogy: the fact that respect for testamentary dispositions also is firmly rooted in much the same interests as those that are at stake in how we die. We are loath to overturn a devise not only because the testator has chosen to distribute personal property in this manner but also because we presume that most persons seek to provide for the welfare of their families in doing so. We also presume that choices about how one disposes of property and assets accumulated over a lifetime say something about that life and are a form of final personal statement about the testator's character, values, and commitments. For example, we praise charitable gifts as the acts of a generous person, whereas we label as mean-spirited the person who deliberately denies children their inheritance. Thus, dishonoring a testamentary will is an affront to our familial and dignity interests in much the same way as dishonoring an advance directive.

There is a further important distinction between the two practices that can be regarded as strengthening the case for respecting advance directives. The writing of a testamentary will is understood against the backdrop of the rules of intestate succession that constitute the default mechanism governing how property is to be distributed in the absence of a will. Intestate succession laws embrace the time-honored presumption that we care about the future welfare of our families and that we want to be remembered in this way by giving priority to the transfer of property to family members. This default approach reflects societal consensus that seeks to approximate what the deceased person would have wanted had he or she written a will.[72]

No comparable consensus about how to treat patients without advance directives exists. Assuming that substituted judgment in the absence of a written document lacks evidentiary support, the current default position is far from uniform; several approaches may be vying for consensus status. In principle, treatment may be forgone if doing so would be in the patient's best interests, but there are few guidelines and no consensus about how a best interests principle should be applied. In medical practice, the prevailing view remains that we should adhere to a presumption in favor of life, although this presumption has been eroding over time. The law also continues to embrace this presumption—though with a sense of ambivalence as termination of treatment in the best interests of incompetent patients gains wider formal acceptance. Arguably there is societal consensus around the family's authority to decide. This point cannot be pressed too far, however, and it does not get us any closer to a consensus on the content and criteria for applying a substantive best interests standard (unless we choose simply to defer to family judgment—a view that also is controversial). At most, what we can say with confidence is that if termination of treatment is warranted in accordance with the incompetent patient's best interests, this judgment must be made on a case-by-case basis.[73]

In sum, we do not have a clear picture of what will happen to us if we fail to write an advance directive. Unlike the situation with testamentary wills, there are no clear and accepted rules that make plain the consequences of not taking charge of the end of one's own life. Moreover, because the content of a best interests approach is not based on consensus about what most of us would want, we cannot say (again in contrast to testamentary wills) that the default position honors what the average person would choose, nor that it necessarily serves the patient's best interests.[74]

This point might be regarded as weakening the analogy to testamentary wills. At the same time, however, it strengthens the case for honoring advance directives because the alternative is not firmly rooted in societal consensus or in clearly articulated criteria for the patient's best interests. An advance directive seeks to bring certainty to an otherwise uncertain situation. On balance, the analogy between advance directives and testamentary wills is imperfect, chiefly because the dying patient can be harmed in ways the deceased person cannot. There is good reason, however, to consider dishonoring of advance directives to be offensive on a par with dishonoring of testamentary dispositions.

Death Rituals (Funerals and Burial)

The same fundamental points can be made about funerals and burial. Our personal stake in our death ritual has ancient roots. From time immemorial, societies have ascribed great significance to whether a person's funeral and burial is in accord with the person's religious beliefs and moral convictions. Although death rituals often are rooted in religious traditions, in contemporary times we have become more accepting of the right of individuals to tailor funerals and burials to their own personal (and perhaps idiosyncratic) values. Many of us form definite views about the kind of funeral we want and how we want to be buried. Sometimes these desires and instructions are committed to writing as part of one's testamentary will; more often, they are communicated orally to a spouse or adult child.

The assertion that disregarding the deceased's personal wishes in such matters is not only offensive but also harmful to the person's interests can hardly be disputed. To perform an autopsy on an Orthodox Jew, cremate someone who desires burial, or have an open casket for someone who has stated a preference that it be closed is highly offensive (though the last example is not on the order of the first two). It is offensive not only because it is contrary to the individual's expressed choice but because it is an affront to the deceased's critical interests. The impact on the sensibilities of family and friends, on how this ending chapter of one's life is written and remembered, and on the integrity of one's full life does serious harm to the deceased's surviving interests. Again, the fact that the deceased cannot actually experience any form of harm makes the analogy to advance directives imperfect, but our considered and time-honored deference to prospective autonomy in personal matters such as these further exemplifies the importance of respect for our prior wishes in dying and in death.

CONCLUSION

The integrity view of autonomy, which is implicit in the legal and ethical consensus, provides compelling justification for the priority status of the principle of prospective autonomy and respect for advance directives in decisions near the end of life for incompetent patients. Autonomous persons are holders of future-oriented rights to control treatment decisions. Autonomy as integrity makes plain the critical interests that are at stake in the exercise of these rights and offers a persuasive account of the basis for our considered moral judgments about the pursuit of death with dignity and the value of prospective autonomy in the moral life. Failure to honor a directive harms the patient by frustrating and injuring the patient's dignity and familial interests that survive and remain critical post-competence. The integrity view of autonomy counsels continuing commitment to the strong presumption in favor of respect for prospective autonomy and respect for advance directives.

Nevertheless, we must address a further question before the account of prospective autonomy in decisions near the end of life is complete. The conclusion that advance directives are entitled to a strong presumption of respect presupposes that they embody autonomous choices. Yet being an autonomous person does not mean that all of one's actions also are autonomous. To determine whether any particular advance directive may not be entitled to the benefit of this presumption, a further account of how we can distinguish autonomous from nonautonomous decisions—that is, how we can distinguish prospectively autonomous advance directives from those that are not—is required. This analysis is the task of the next chapter.

NOTES

1. Ronald Dworkin, *Life's Dominion: An Argument About Abortion, Euthanasia, and Individual Freedom* (New York: Alfred A. Knopf, 1993), 235–36.
2. Rebecca S. Dresser and John A. Robertson, "Quality of Life and Non-Treatment Decisions for Incompetent Patients: A Critique of the Orthodox Approach," *Law, Medicine & Health Care* 17, no. 3 (Fall 1989): 240.
3. Joel Feinberg, *Harm to Self: The Moral Limits of the Criminal Law* (New York: Oxford University Press, 1986), 27–28; Ruth R. Faden and Tom L. Beauchamp,

A History and Theory of Informed Consent (New York: Oxford University Press, 1986), 7–8.

4. The model of autonomy as integrity and the close connections between integrity and the pursuit of death with dignity I present here are indebted to the previous work of law professors Ronald Dworkin and Norman Cantor. The position I develop, however, devotes more extensive attention to several key points and strikes out in some different directions from the thought of these writers.

5. Joel Feinberg, *Harm to Others: The Moral Limits of the Criminal Law* (New York: Oxford University Press, 1984), especially chapter one.

6. Dworkin, *Life's Dominion*, 201.

7. Feinberg, *Harm to Others*, 37–45, uses the term "ulterior interests" to refer to the more ultimate goals and aspirations that we consider important and that we value for their own sake as ends. Feinberg notes that this idea mirrors C. L. Stevenson's notion of "focal aims." For Bernard Williams, our "projects" are the sets of desires and concerns we possess as individuals and that shape our character. Bernard Williams, *Moral Luck* (Cambridge: Cambridge University Press, 1981), 5.

8. For more extensive lists of the types of interests that count as critical or ulterior in persons' lives, see Dworkin, *Life's Dominion*, 200–202; Feinberg, *Harm to Others*, especially 37, 60.

9. My wife's grandfather, who died in 1995 at the age of 93, undoubtedly would have been pleased to know that friends and family remembered him as "Gentleman George."

10. Dworkin, *Life's Dominion*, 201–202.

11. Ibid., 201 (emphasis in original).

12. Feinberg, *Harm to Others*, 45.

13. Dworkin, *Life's Dominion*, 205, argues that "people think it is important" that their lives have a "structure that expresses a coherent choice" among a variety of life's experiences, achievements, and commitments. I concur with this general understanding. This is not to say, however, that a good life *must* have this sort of structure and coherence. A person's life could be filled with important achievements and personal satisfactions and be considered on most accounts a good life but also lack the kind of coherence described here.

14. This term is borrowed from Lynne McFall, "Integrity," in *Ethics and Personality: Essays in Moral Psychology*, ed. John Deigh (Chicago: University of Chicago Press, 1992), 87.

15. Gabriele Taylor, *Pride, Shame and Guilt: Emotions of Self-Assessment* (New York: Oxford University Press, 1985), 109: "[W]hat he thinks very worthwhile doing, and what he thinks very important not to do, contributes essentially to his being one sort of person rather than another."

16. Harry Frankfurt's seminal analysis of authenticity as involving second-order reflection on and acceptance of first-order desires appears in Harry G. Frankfurt, "Freedom of the Will and the Concept of a Person," *Journal of Philosophy* 68 (1971): 5–20. Extended discussion of the authenticity model of autonomy also appears in Gerald Dworkin, *The Theory and Practice of Autonomy* (Cambridge: Cambridge University Press, 1988), especially chapters one and seven. In chapter three I offer a critical analysis of an authenticity/integrity model of

autonomy as the basis for a theory of autonomous actions, exploring Frankfurt's and Gerald Dworkin's views at greater length.
17. The etymological origin of the term—*integritas*—means wholeness. *Oxford English Dictionary*, 2d ed. (Oxford: Clarendon Press, 1989).
18. McFall, "Integrity," 81, argues that the requisite coherence for an ascription of integrity involves "consistency within one's own set of principles or commitments" and "coherence between principles and actions."
19. That integrity consists of consistency of commitments and wholeness is the general and broad meaning of the term. Some philosophers draw a distinction between "personal integrity" and "moral integrity." Personal integrity refers to commitments and projects that are not governed by moral values. Moral integrity refers more narrowly to consistent adherence to moral norms. See Tom L. Beauchamp and James F. Childress, *Principles of Biomedical Ethics*, 4th ed. (New York: Oxford University Press, 1994), 471; McFall, "Integrity," 88 *ff*. Some descriptions in the foregoing account of integrity would be more strictly characterized under the rubric of personal integrity because they involve nonmoral judgments. This distinction is not necessary for the present inquiry, however, because decisions near the end of life are embedded in an inherently moral context. Consequently, I use the terms *integrity, moral integrity*, and *personal integrity* somewhat interchangeably.
20. Dworkin, *Life's Dominion*, 206, holds a similar view.
21. This common understanding is reflected in typical dictionary definitions of *integrity*. For example, the *Random House Dictionary of the English Language* (New York: Random House, 1968) defines "integrity" as "adherence to moral and ethical principles; soundness of moral character; honesty," and lists *probity* and *virtue* as synonyms. *Dishonesty* is listed as an antonym for integrity.
22. James F. Childress, "Appeals to Conscience," in *Ethics and Personality: Essays in Moral Psychology*, ed. John Deigh (Chicago: University of Chicago Press, 1992), 98, gives a similar account of remaining true to one's own values under the rubric of conscience.
23. McFall, "Integrity," 85. McFall makes the further claim that when we grant integrity to a person, "we must at least recognize [that person's commitments] as ones a reasonable person might take to be of great importance...." Whether reasonableness in this sense is a necessary condition of the idea of integrity is a tangential issue for the present inquiry. I address this point in a different way in chapters three and five, where I reject the idea that third-party (objective) judgment that a treatment refusal is *un*reasonable justifies noncompliance with the patient's choice.
24. Dworkin, *Life's Dominion*, 224: "The integrity view of autonomy does not assume that competent people have consistent values or always make consistent choices, or that they always lead structured, reflective lives."
25. We might imagine an entirely different sort of person who seems to be without firm commitments to anything and always appears to be acting "out of character." Robert Jay Lifton suggests in *The Protean Self: Human Resilience in an Age of Fragmentation* (New York: Basic Books, 1993) that many of us are in fact shape-shifters (proteans) whose essential self is regularly in a state of variation, adjustment, and transformation. Arguably, even Lifton's shape-shifters are possessed of a core self that makes transformation possible without loss of identity. I discuss a similar point with respect to autonomous actions in chapter three.

26. For insightful discussion of these and other aspects of the concept of death with dignity, see Daniel P. Sulmasy, "Death and Human Dignity," *Linacre Quarterly* (November 1994): 27–35; Leon R. Kass, "Averting One's Eyes, or Facing the Music?—On Dignity in Death," *Hastings Center Studies* 2, no. 2 (May 1974): 67–80.
27. I do not mean to suggest here that only autonomous persons have dignity or can be treated with (in)dignity. All human beings have an intrinsic worth and dignity and deserve not to be treated with indignity, regardless of their capacity for autonomy—including persons who are severely handicapped, mentally ill, or comatose.
28. See Paul Ramsey, "The Indignity of 'Death with Dignity'," *Hastings Center Studies* 2, no. 2 (May 1974): 47–62.
29. Feinberg, *Harm to Self*, 27.
30. It is tempting to say here that death is the final chapter in the story of a person's life. Because, as I argue, our critical interests—and thus the final chapter—survive beyond death, this language is best avoided.
31. Popular understanding and public education about advance directives rightly stress easing of family burdens as a reason to write advance directives but obscure the fundamental significance of concern for family welfare—especially the potential fiscal impact of treatment decisions. It is worth pausing for a moment to reflect on the place of the family's fiscal well-being. In the past, emphasis on the self-referential features of dignity, as well as concerns for the propriety of allowing monetary costs to influence decisions about life and death, have led some thinkers to deemphasize fiscal issues and even place them outside the bounds of morally licit reasons to refuse life support. See Nancy S. Jecker, "Being a Burden on Others," *Journal of Clinical Ethics* 4, no. 1 (Spring 1993): 16–20; J. F. Turner et al., "Physicians' Ethical Responsibilities under Co-Pay Insurance: Should Potential Fiscal Liability Become Part of Informed Consent?" *Journal of Clinical Ethics* 6, no. 1 (Spring 1995): 68–72. We should straightforwardly acknowledge the place of costs in attending to family welfare, particularly in an era of extreme cost-consciousness when so many Americans may find themselves uninsured or underinsured.
32. Cantor, *Advance Directives*, 30. I argue that our interests in how we are remembered in fact survive death. Consequently, we can suffer posthumous harm if our efforts to shape those memories are thwarted.
33. The Values Profile document developed by Norman Cantor does an excellent job of evoking judgments about these important concerns in preparation for drafting the specific instructions of an advance directive. An important feature of Cantor's approach is the attempt to prompt individuals to assign a relative weight (intolerable, very negative factor, unimportant) to the factors of pain and suffering, immobility, the interests of loved ones, and so on, in their choices as a guide to a health care proxy. Cantor, *Advance Directives*, Appendix D. For another version of a Values History, see P. Lambert, J. M. Gibson, and P. Nathanson, "The Values History: An Innovation in Surrogate Medical Decision-Making," *Law, Medicine & Health Care* 18 (Fall 1990): 202–12.
34. To maintain attention on the interests at stake in how we die, in subsequent discussion I periodically use the terms *familial* and *dignity interests*, rather than the broader, less descriptive, term *critical interests*. I do not intend that these interests should be thought of as entirely distinct, nor that the interests at

stake in how we die can be neatly separated as self-regarding and other-regarding.
35. Dworkin, *Life's Dominion*, 217.
36. Ronald Dworkin, "Autonomy and the Demented Self," *Milbank Quarterly* 64, supp. 2 (1986): 13. See also Dworkin, *Life's Dominion*, 228.
37. Cantor, *Advance Directives*, 30 and 28.
38. Cantor and Dworkin acknowledge that there may be some circumstances in which concerns for the patient's current interests and the pull of human compassion would justify overriding an advance directive, though neither offers a case in which this would be so. For both, however, overriding an advance directive would violate autonomy. As Dworkin, *Life's Dominion*, 229, writes, "We might have other good reasons for treating [an incompetent patient] as she now wishes, rather than as, in my imaginary case, she once asked. But still, that violates rather than respects her autonomy."
39. Cantor, *Advance Directives*, 28: "[T]he nature of the deliberation surrounding an advance directive might be a proper inquiry for any health-care agent (or other person) eventually implementing the instructions"; Dworkin, "Autonomy and the Demented Self," 14: "[A]ny appeal to a right to precedent autonomy requires evidence of an actual past decision contemplating the circumstances the patient is now in." Thus, each acknowledges this point, leaving open the possibility that in particular instances an advance directive may not be entitled to the presumption that it embodies autonomous decisions.
40. Rebecca S. Dresser and John A. Robertson, "Quality of Life and Non-Treatment Decisions for Incompetent Patients: A Critique of the Orthodox Approach," *Law, Medicine & Health Care* 17, no. 3 (Fall 1989): 241.
41. John A. Robertson, "*Cruzan* and the Constitutional Status of Nontreatment Decisions for Incompetent Patients," *Georgia Law Review* 25, no. 5 (Summer 1991): 1193.
42. Ibid., 1144.
43. Rebecca S. Dresser, "Life, Death, and Incompetent Patients: Conceptual Infirmities and Hidden Values in the Law," *Arizona Law Review* 28 (1986): 381.
44. Ibid.
45. This interpretation warrants some clarification. At times, Dresser and Robertson suggest that advance directives serve a useful purpose when they express the same treatment choice that otherwise would be based on third-party judgment regarding the patient's best interests, thereby lending further support to the contemplated treatment decision; see Rebecca Dresser, "Advance Directives: Implications for Policy," *Hastings Center Report* 24, no. 6 (November/December 1994): S2–S5. Elsewhere they suggest that advance directives should carry moral weight if they are explicit and in fact anticipate medical conditions that have come to exist; see Dresser and Robertson, "Quality of Life," 237. Clearly, however, the predominant argument is that respect for prospective autonomy and advance directives should be subordinate to a current best interests approach—that advance directives are virtually "meaningless." Robertson, "*Cruzan* and the Constitutional Status of Nontreatment Decisions," 1167 (incompetent patient's prior interests "are no longer relevant"); Rebecca Dresser, "Relitigating Life and Death," *Ohio State Law Journal* 51, no. 2 (1990): 431 (incompetent patients' past values and preferences "are now meaningless to them").

46. Dresser and Robertson, "Quality of Life," 241. This is an odd, perhaps contradictory, claim. If the incompetent patient has no experiential interests in how decisions are made, why does the patient retain interests in who makes the decisions? By admitting the validity of a proxy appointment, Dresser and Robertson seem to admit as well that some interests survive incompetence, even if harm to such interests (failure to accept the proxy's legal authority) cannot be known by the patient.

47. Dresser and Robertson, "Quality of Life," 241; see also Dresser, "Relitigating Life and Death," 429: "[T]he objective standard should permit nontreatment when the patient lacks any relational capacity . . . [but] should mandate treatment that will enable the patient capable of interacting with the environment to continue life as long as significant pain and discomfort are absent." To her credit, Dresser continues to pursue the challenge of articulating an objective best interests standard grounded in the patient's subjective experience in "Missing Persons: Legal Perceptions of Incompetent Patients," *Rutgers Law Review* 46, no. 2 (Winter 1994): 609–719. This task is extremely important if we are to develop uniform guidelines for the care and treatment of seriously ill and dying patients who have not previously expressed their treatment wishes or were never competent. It offers no reason, however, to abandon the ethical and legal priority accorded to prior autonomy and advance directives.

48. Of course, the reverse situation in which a directive affirmatively requests treatment but continued treatment appears not to serve the incompetent patient's current interests in being free of pain or communicating with others also may arise. In this regard, Dresser is consistent in her attack on prospective autonomy. She would override a vitalist's affirmative request for continued life when there is no possibility for relational capacity, on the ground that this decision is best for the patient.

49. The current interests position often is linked with another line of attack on advance directives that also is posited by Dresser and alluded to by Robertson. The claim is that by virtue of loss of psychological connectedness and continuity with the past, incompetent patients have become new persons, and the wishes of the former person who authored the advance directive have no moral authority to govern current treatment decisions. The personal identity challenge to advance directives is the subject of chapter four. For now, I emphasize that although the two positions can be complementary and mutually reinforcing (*a fortiori*, the interests of the incompetent new person are not the same interests as those of the formerly competent person the patient no longer is), they raise significantly separate and distinct questions. In this chapter I assume that the incompetent patient and the author of a prior directive are the same person; I present and defend this position in chapter four.

50. See Norman L. Cantor, "Prospective Autonomy: On the Limits of Shaping One's Postcompetence Medical Fate," *The Journal of Contemporary Health Law and Policy* 8 (1992): 31, note 55, for a similar point.

51. For further discussion of this issue, see Robert S. Olick, "Brain Death, Religious Freedom, and Public Policy: New Jersey's Landmark Legislative Initiative," *Kennedy Institute of Ethics Journal* 1, no. 4 (December 1991): 275–92; Robert M. Veatch, *Death, Dying and the Biological Revolution: Our Last Quest for Responsibility* (New Haven, Conn.: Yale University Press, 1989), especially chapter 2; David Zweibel, "Accommodating Religious Objections to Brain Death: Legal

Considerations," *Journal of Halacha and Contemporary Society* 17 (Spring 1989): 49–68.

52. In fact, an organ donor card is a form of advance directive. Is it consistent to encourage organ and tissue donation and to regard overriding the donor's gift as a harm but also to hold, as some thinkers do, that treatment refusals near the end of life are not entitled to the same respect? The parallels between advance directives and organ donation are rarely discussed but are worthy of further examination. From another vantage point, the history of organ donation and procurement may hold valuable lessons about the widespread reluctance to execute advance directives and the difficulties in implementation that they have encountered. See Arthur L. Caplan, *If I Were a Rich Man Could I Buy a Pancreas?* (Bloomington: Indiana University Press, 1992), 262–63.

53. Some writers argue that declaring the death of an Orthodox Jew on the basis of neurological criteria is justified because public policy (except in the states of New Jersey and New York) does not recognize religious objections to the contrary. Some observers also have contended that disregarding objections to neurological death is justified to save the life of another patient in need of a scarce respirator. Depending on the circumstances, a blood transfusion for a Jehovah's Witness arguably could be justified as protecting the interests of the patient's young children. These arguments, however, are appeals to justificatory grounds for violations of religious beliefs. There is no suggestion here that religious beliefs have become irrelevant or that failure to honor patients' religious beliefs does not constitute a harm.

54. Cantor, "Prospective Autonomy," 24, uses similar examples to make this same point about our common understanding of the place of prospective autonomy in the moral life.

55. This understanding of what it means for an interest to be harmed is discussed in Feinberg, *Harm to Others*, 84–85.

56. Dresser and Robertson, "Quality of Life," 238.

57. Ibid., 236.

58. Cantor, "Prospective Autonomy," 30.

59. Arguably, Dresser and Robertson misconstrue the principle of respect for persons altogether. Some bioethicists hold that respect for persons derives from the principle of respect for autonomy and therefore is not implicated when autonomy is not at issue, such as for incompetent patients who have not made prior expressions about their treatment wishes. Having rejected autonomy's legitimate place in deciding for incompetent patients, the Dresser/Robertson analysis improperly grounds respect for persons on the principle of beneficence. Thus, their argument here really is iterative and adds nothing to their modified best interests challenge to prospective autonomy. The same is true under a broader understanding of the principle of respect for persons that presses beyond the boundaries of autonomy. On this construction, respect for persons would include certain duties to incompetent patients—such as veracity, promise-keeping, confidentiality of physician-patient communications, and avoidance of killing. Robert M. Veatch, "Resolving Conflicts Among Principles: Ranking, Balancing and Specifying," *Kennedy Institute of Ethics Journal* 5, no. 3 (September 1995): 203–04. Respect for persons cannot be redefined to do the work of the principle of beneficence in justifying a modified best interests approach.

60. Cantor, "Prospective Autonomy," 25.
61. Ibid., 29: "A competent person views control over the postcompetency dying process as part of the earned prerogative to shape the subsequent images and recollections of her life."
62. Dresser, "Relitigating Life and Death," 430, contends that "the assessment itself centers on the individual patient and is in this sense highly subjective." This claim confuses a *patient-centered* approach with a *subjective* approach and equivocates on the meaning of the term *subjective*. The current interests approach is subjective in the narrow sense that it takes into account the incompetent patient's current experiences of pain, discomfort, pleasure, and contentment. This claim does little more, however, than rephrase the idea that an objective standard should be patient-centered—a feature that is commonly understood to be a component of an objective best interests analysis as articulated by numerous courts and commentators. The critical distinction between subjective and objective standards rests on whose moral point of view—whose values, wishes, and beliefs about quality of life and the benefits and burdens of life support—count in the decisional process. If the incompetent patient's advance directive does not count, a modified objective standard cannot be called subjective.
63. Cantor, "Prospective Autonomy," 28: "To ignore [prior directives] would relegate the patient to the status of an object whose fate is determined by others, rather than a human who has etched his own fate."
64. Nancy K. Rhoden, "Litigating Life and Death," *Harvard Law Review* 102, no. 2 (December 1988): 409; Nancy K. Rhoden, "The Limits of Legal Objectivity," *North Carolina Law Review* 68, no. 5 (June 1990): 864.
65. Allen E. Buchanan and Dan W. Brock, *Deciding for Others: The Ethics of Surrogate Decision Making* (Cambridge: Cambridge University Press, 1989), 163: "If interests can survive death, then *a fortiori* they can survive permanent unconsciousness, loss of personal identity, and less extensive departures from competence."
66. Feinberg, *Harm to Others*, 83.
67. The idea of causing harm to the dead may seem contrary to another commonsense notion—namely, that one must be in existence to be harmed. The concept of posthumous harm points to a deeper philosophical question: the "problem of the subject." Can there be harm without a subject to be harmed? Pressing the line of reasoning to its full logic, we are led to the paradoxical conclusion that if there is no subject to be harmed, death itself is not a harm. The even stronger commonsense revulsion at this view shows that in our common experience as well, people have interests that are not extinguished with death; their satisfaction or frustration will occur some time after death. Feinberg, *Harm to Others*, 79–83, offers a thoughtful discussion of the problem of the subject and a similar response to that given here. For critiques of Feinberg's position, see Ernest Partridge, "Posthumous Interests and Posthumous Respect," *Ethics* 91 (January 1981): 243–64; Barbara Baum Levenbook, "Harming Someone after His Death," *Ethics* 94 (April 1984): 407–19. Both authors take issue with Feinberg's argument, but both also conclude, on other grounds, that posthumous harm is possible.

I also should note that if we were to engage this philosophical puzzle further, it would be of no avail to proponents of a current interests approach. They must admit that the living patient is a subject with interests, even if only experiential ones. At best, critics of advance directives could seek to minimize the importance of the interests a directive expresses by insisting that their duration is limited and expires with the declaration of death.

68. The discussion here also is apt for other well-recognized legal mechanisms for the exercise of future-oriented rights, such as creation of trusts to be administered by and for the benefit of others after death.

69. Gerry W. Beyer, "Statutory Fill-In Will Forms—The First Decade: Theoretical Constructs," *Oregon Law Review* 72 (Winter 1993): 769 (citing numerous sources).

70. Arguably, establishing that the author of a directive was not competent at the time the directive was executed may be more difficult because testamentary wills are almost always drawn up in consultation with an attorney, whereas advance directives often are not. The latter situation should change, to some extent, as health care professionals become more involved in discussing advance directives with their patients. Ordinarily, both types of documents must be witnessed, with the witnesses affixing their signatures to the document. This requirement is largely a legal formality that asks two adults (the usual rule) to attest that the author appears to be of sound mind and free of undue influence. Although witnesses often are not privy to the dialogue that preceded execution of the document and informed the choices made therein, the practice of witnessing strengthens the presumption of the author's competence. Consequently, rebutting this presumption would entail finding someone who is more knowledgeable about the author's state of mind during the time the document was being formulated and leading up to its execution. The same is true of another ground for challenging testamentary wills and advance directives: the claim that the document was not freely and voluntarily signed and that the author was subject to coercion or undue influence.

71. Dresser and Robertson, "Quality of Life," 237.

72. This point is made by Nancy M. P. King in *Making Sense of Advance Directives*, revised ed. (Washington, D.C.: Georgetown University Press, 1996), 185: "[Intestate succession] names property dispositions according to a conventional social morality: Parents, spouse, and children are the principal beneficiaries."

73. One exception is suggested by the fact that the vast majority of people believe that if they were in a PVS (or other condition of permanent unconsciousness) they would not want to be maintained on life support. Whether public policy should reverse the presumption in favor of treatment in this or any other circumstance, however, is a much more complicated question.

74. King, *Making Sense of Advance Directives*, 150–51. Cantor argues that a consensus-based default position should be based not on objective best interests, but on a constructive preference standard. Norman L. Cantor, "Discarding Substituted Judgment and Best Interests: Toward a Constructive Preference Standard for Dying, Previously Competent Patients Without Advance Instructions," *Rutgers Law Review* 48, no. 4 (Summer 1996): 1193–1272.

Chapter Three

PROSPECTIVE DECISIONAL AUTONOMY

[T]he crucial guidance in an instruction directive goes to the criteria for an intolerable quality of life—particularly the level of debilitation which renders existence degrading to the [individual]. In other words, the substantive instructions should be result oriented, focusing on the consequences of medical intervention for the patient's status rather than the nature of the medical procedures.

Law professor Norman Cantor, 1993[1]

Preferences ascertained in advance and aimed to guide treatment decisions must ordinarily be shown to be both authentic and stable over time.

Joan Teno, Hilde Lindemann Nelson, and Joanne Lynn, from a consensus document on behalf of participants in a conference on decision making for the mentally incapacitated, 1993[2]

INTRODUCTION

The ethical and policy consensus, conjoined with the deeper moral underpinnings of the integrity view of autonomous persons, offers compelling justification for the lofty status of the principle of prospective autonomy and the position of advance directives in making treatment decisions for incompetent patients. There is an important distinction, however (generally ignored by the extensive literature on advance directives), between being autonomous and acting autonomously—between autonomous persons and autonomous actions.[3] A further account of what exercising the relevant capacities for prospectively autonomous choice means is needed.[4] The chief aim of this chapter is to develop the conceptual foundations for a coherent theory of *prospective decisional autonomy*.

Faden and Beauchamp[5] and Beauchamp and Childress[6] have persuasively analyzed autonomous action in terms of (1) intentional, (2) performed with substantial understanding, and (3) without controlling influences that determine the person's actions. These three conditions of autonomy are equally apt for advance care planning, and my analysis is indebted to their work in various ways—most importantly in the analysis of advance directives as intentional plans.

Rather than analyzing each of these three conditions of autonomy, however, my more modest and specific objective is to examine what makes an advance directive an effective exercise of prospective autonomy that therefore is entitled to priority status in particular cases of conflict with the patient's current experiential interests.[7] I attempt to answer two crucial questions: First, what model of autonomy best explains prospectively autonomous decision making with advance directives? Second, what is the nature of the core decisional process manifest in an effective and autonomous advance directive? From the answers to these queries, a picture of a core pattern of understanding necessary to issuance of an effective directive emerges. Although each of these questions has been identified in some form in the bioethics literature, scholarly commentary generally has failed to offer serious and sustained normative analysis of the concept of prospectively autonomous choice. I hope that the analysis in this chapter will contribute to a more constructive and theoretically sound dialogue.[8]

As a preliminary matter, the operative background assumption of the discussion is that the author of an advance directive is called upon to make anticipatory judgments about a potentially wide range of future medical circumstances that *might* materialize. The exercise of prospective autonomy characteristically involves what some philosophers and decision theorists refer to as *judgment under uncertainty*.[9] These background conditions direct our attention to the most common and paradigmatic practice with advance directives. They also provide a prism for the most significant and interesting concerns for which a theory of prospective decisional autonomy must account—and thereby sharpen the analysis.

Of course, placing the discussion within these confines also oversimplifies the practice of advance care planning. With increasing frequency, advance directives are issued (or revised) following hospital admission or specific diagnosis of illness. Sometimes the document is tailored to a diagnosed illness or disease with a predictable clinical course (the "disease-specific" directive); in this context, it may very closely approximate the exercise of contemporaneous autonomy. More patients are discussing advance care planning with their physicians, affording opportunity for more informed decisions. In reality, the extent to which advance directives are written remotely in time from their actual use or in the face of an uncertain future can vary considerably. These concerns arise at several points, but (as will become clear) they require no emendation of the basic theory I develop.[10]

Different views of autonomy essentially are metaphors that place the concept within a given lens, calling on us to regard autonomy *as* self-determination, integrity, intentionality, rational deliberation, expression of a preference, and so on.[11] Two models of prospectively autonomous action are suggested by the analysis of autonomous persons: an integrity model and an intentionality model. Each seeks to explain what it means for a person to assert authorship over his or her health care future, shaping future treatment decisions in terms of critical values, commitments, and interests.

In the first part of this chapter I argue that *intentionality* captures the essential features of planning, identification, and authorship involved in future-oriented treatment decisions and that advance directives are best understood as intentional plans. In the next section I present the integrity model, arguing that the most plausible construction of what distinguishes an *integrity* (*authenticity*) view of actions from the intentionality model is the further condition of identification as the author and agent of an action at a deeper level of the self. Applied to advance care planning, the integrity view would require that the author of a directive reflectively accept prospective treatment decisions as consistent with his or her settled values, commitments, and critical interests.

The analysis goes on to critically compare the two approaches, offering several reasons to prefer the intentionality model as a paradigm for advance care planning. The thrust of the argument is that the intentionality paradigm resonates more closely with commonsense experience and would honor many ordinary health care decisions. On the other hand, the integrity view of actions would narrowly constrict the range of patients' choices that are entitled to respect and open the door to paternalistic disregard for patients' treatment refusals on grounds that they are nonautonomous. Comparison of the two models is further sharpened by a case analysis. In the main, the analysis is limited to critical comparison of these two theories; I do not claim to establish that intentionality offers the *only* adequate explanation of prospective decisional autonomy—although an alternative model would carry a heavy burden of justification.

The latter part of the discussion turns to the question of effective advance care planning and attempts to establish two narrow claims. First, the core pattern of effective prospective decision making with an instruction directive should be understood as fundamentally outcome-oriented and condition-specific—meaning that it is concerned with shaping a dying process marked by possible future states of incapacity, dependence, indignity, and so on. I contrast this view with its chief rival: an approach that grafts the informed consent model onto advance directives, positing that an effective directive is treatment-specific—that is, it expressly refuses a respirator, feeding tube, surgery, and so on. I argue that this alternative position fails to appreciate the nature and limits of prospective autonomy and would unjustifiably and paternalistically render many advance directives nonautonomous. Second, an effective proxy directive appoints a trusted family member or friend to act on the patient's behalf and states the nature and limits of the proxy's authority. A proxy appointment is grounded in the bond of trust between patient and proxy; the choice of who decides often is more important than giving specific direction about what should be decided. Again, I contrast and compare this position with an alternative view—here, that the sole basis for the proxy's authority is to decide as the patient would. It is argued that this alternative account embraces an improperly narrow understanding of the nature and purpose of proxy directives.

The focus on the idea of effectiveness bears further explanation. It is a fact of life that the best of intentions—and the best laid plans—can fail to meet their objectives. This observation may be all the more true when those plans are made in anticipation of significant events that have not yet begun to unfold, as is often the case with advance directives. What truly matters is whether a directive provides sufficient guidance to those who are called upon to follow it—that is, whether it is effective. Attending to effectiveness rather than understanding seeks to bridge the temporal gap between the writing of a directive and its implementation and underscores the fact that the four corners of the advance directive document are the primary—and in some cases the only—available expression of what the patient understood and intended.

Effectiveness also sheds light on a related point about autonomy. Autonomy exists on a continuum of degrees.[12] A decision about how much autonomy is enough to justify respect for autonomous decisions essentially is a normative judgment. A prospectively autonomous decision need not be made with "full" autonomy; it is a decision marked by *sufficient* autonomy.[13] *An effective directive provides sufficient guidance to those responsible for the patient's care.* Were we to insist that all advance directives be based on full and complete understanding; that the author be possessed of complete apprehension of all relevant medical information that correctly describes a range of possible future medical conditions; that the author understand the nature of the act of issuing a directive; that the author understand the foreseeable risks, benefits, burdens, and possible outcomes of accepting or refusing a range of medical interventions; *and* that this complete understanding be perfectly expressed and fit perfectly the actual circumstances in which the directive must be used, few directives would qualify as autonomous, effective, and entitled to respect. Thus, sufficiency is a placeholder that indicates a threshold level of effectiveness that justifies the statement "the directive gives us guidance as to the appropriate course of treatment."[14]

I take an effective directive to be an autonomous directive.[15] Some critics will respond that this threshold is too low; perhaps advance directives should be "substantially" or "highly" effective. Coupled with the presumptive force of advance directives, sufficiency is an appropriate standard. The further reasons for this view emerge in the course of the discussion. The analysis in the first part of the chapter assumes this operative standard of sufficient guidance.

One conclusion of this chapter is that autonomous, effective advance directives refusing life support should be honored and should trump competing concerns for the patient's current experiential interests. Another is that some advance directives may be nonautonomous. The implications of the theory for the principle of *respect for autonomy* arise at various points. This chapter lays the groundwork for extended discussion of the obligation to honor advance directives in chapter five.[16]

AUTONOMY AS INTENTIONALITY: ACTION WILLED IN ACCORDANCE WITH A PLAN

Prospectively autonomous actions ought to be understood as intentional actions. By intentional action I mean "action *willed in accordance with a plan*, whether the act [outcome] is wanted or not."[17] Having an intention involves two primary components: the cognitive and the motivational.[18] Intentional *action* also has a third component—authorship. The concept of a plan emphasizes the cognitive component; the concept of willing stresses the motivational component. The phrase "willed in accordance with a plan" expresses a special connection between the cognitive and the motivational components and an essential causal relation between motivation, action, and result.[19] This special causal connection is the idea of authorship. To be the author of an action is to identify oneself as the causal agent behind the action.[20] Thus, a person acts intentionally when he or she acts with a state of mind in which his or her conscious will, purpose, or object is to perform a particular action and bring about a particular foreseeable result or results by that action.[21] By contrast, actions performed without a plan or conscious purpose (for example, negligent acts, such as leaving a sponge in the abdomen after surgery) are not intentional actions. Nor does the mere expression of a preference that is unconnected to a plan (even a rudimentary one) to bring about a certain result qualify as an intentional action. All other things being equal, for example, absent the controlling influence of others, an intentional action is an autonomous, self-determining action.[22]

We can understand the pursuit of critical interests and projects and the issuance of advance directives in the same way. Pursuit of our critical interests characteristically involves having and following plans of intention. The value and importance we attach to critical interests and projects—having a successful career, providing for the welfare of one's family, contributing to one's community, and so on—constitute the primary reason and motivation for making it one's conscious object and purpose to achieve these goals. (There also may be other, instrumental reasons, of course.) Doing so requires a form of means-to-end reasoning about what is required to implement and achieve these projects; the actions required for the individual to be the causal agent and author of the intended result(s); and the result (goal) itself, including reasonably foreseeable consequences of pursuing the project(s). In sum, a plan of intention is "the integration of cognitions into a blueprint for action."[23] A person's network of interests can be viewed in much the same way as involving interrelated blueprints for pursuit of various interests and projects. Ideally, the fully autonomous person has a set of blueprints integrated into a master plan. (This is not to say that all intentional plans involve the pursuit of critical interests, nor that all intentional plans are necessarily complex or involve complex processes of cognitive integration. A plan of intention can be quite minimal—for example, using liquid soap to clean the dishes.)

There is an obvious sense, of course, in which performing an action that it is my conscious object and purpose to perform makes that action mine. Intentional plans that take as their aim satisfaction of our critical interests also are identity-conferring commitments in a more significant way. To illuminate this point, we can regard formulation of a plan of intention as part of a person's *evaluational* system. In other words, intentional planning entails reasoning about a set of considerations that, when combined with assessment of the factual circumstances, provides a basis for judgments of the following form: "The thing for me to do in the circumstances, all things considered, is X." To choose a particular course of action as a means to achieve a particular goal, while rejecting alternative courses, is to assign priority to a chosen course of action and the project that is its conscious object. Assigning priority to a plan of action also entails evaluating alternatives in light of reasons, motives, values, commitments, and so on that one holds important.[24] Moreover, regarding oneself as a causal agent engaged in the pursuit of projects and commitments presupposes a view of oneself as an agent in the world—a self-perception that is constitutive of a person's evaluational system. Investment in critical projects in accordance with intentional plans makes us causal agents in their success or failure, asserts that those plans and projects are ours, and imprints a personal stamp of authorship on a chosen course of action.

In making a critical project one's conscious object, a person is characteristically aware of the values and commitments that make that project critical because they are a seam in the fabric of a person's evaluational system.

Indeed, there is a close connection between the values and commitments that provide important reasons for doing something and understanding of the goal one has consciously chosen to pursue. We can make the stronger claim that planning to become a great pianist, acquire great wealth, be an honest politician, and so on, and then proceeding to follow that plan, entails some sort of evaluation of the values and commitments that make (substantial) investment in such projects worthwhile. The same is true of advance care planning and the pursuit of death with dignity.

Intentional planning does not, however, demand that a person engage in conscious evaluation of personal values and commitments in the process of forming a plan of action. Forming and acting on an intentional plan do not require that in the deliberative process a person reflectively accept, internalize, and identify as one's own the values and commitments the person holds important. In other words, an intentional plan framed within the context of one's evaluational system ordinarily involves reasoning of the following sort: "It is important to me that my family not suffer undue emotional and financial burdens if I am terminally ill." Intentionality does not require, however, that a person make a more reflective and higher-order judgment of the following sort: "I am the kind of person who cares about easing the burdens of my dying for loved ones." As will become clear, this distinction separates the intentionality and integrity approaches.[25]

Furthermore, as with autonomy itself, this account of intentional action does not require that a person's reasons for choosing a course of action—what one's intentional plan aims at—must be reasonable. The moral worth of a person's plans and projects is not a criterion of intentionality. Some people believe that accepting an earlier death to spare family members further financial hardship is morally wrong, but this belief does not make refusal of treatment for this reason any less intentional. The person who formulates and follows a very clear, well-considered plan to commit suicide (perhaps guided by Derek Humphry's how-to book *Final Exit*) has acted intentionally. The fact that others may consider the act unreasonable does not negate the fact that it was intentional. (To make this narrow point, we can set aside the more thorny question of whether depression or other psychological forces may negate the intention to commit suicide, or the autonomy of the act.)

The argument that advance care planning with an advance directive is a particular type of intentional action is straightforward.[26] More precisely, an advance directive is a plan that comprises one or more interrelated, intentional decisions. The question of how these intentions should be described and understood, however, is a more complicated matter that is critical to the issue of respect for advance directives. In the words of J. L. Austin, "[T]here is a good deal of freedom in 'structuring' the history of someone's activities by means of words like 'intention.'"[27] To avoid the charge of arbitrariness, we should endeavor to describe what is intended from the person's own point of view, asking what state of affairs he or she intended to bring about.[28]

With this analysis in mind, we may characterize what a directive intends under a variety of act-descriptions. In broad brush, an advance directive expresses an intentional plan to assert control over the dying process; it is intended as a blueprint for treatment decisions near the end of life, as the script that guides how a crucial part of a person's continuing life story is to be told. The intention(s) of an advance directive also can be characterized by reference to the document's more concrete goal(s) and purpose(s)—the state of affairs the person seeks to bring about in the dying process. Under this description, further consideration of whether a directive is entitled to respect as autonomous, and of the closely connected question of what a person should understand to issue an effective directive, can be analyzed in terms of the following formulations of intention. The author of an instruction directive understands and intends *that* he or she not receive (or receive) life-sustaining treatment when he or she is suffering from a particular medical condition(s). A proxy directive states that its author understands and intends *that* the personally selected proxy have authority to make treatment decisions in his or her behalf. These intentional decisions meaningfully constitute the elements and goals of a directive's plan and raise interesting and challenging questions about prospective autonomy.

The importance of framing intentional act-descriptions in these ways will become clearer when we turn to the nature of an effective directive. Some of the staunchest critics of advance directives generally have failed to appreciate that intentional plans should be understood in terms of their purposes and objects; these critics have insisted mistakenly that directives must be highly specific and manifest an unrealistic degree of foresight. I confront this critique later in this chapter, where I argue that specificity sometimes may be desirable (though it is not without its own problems), but it is not a necessary condition of an intentional plan nor of an effective directive.

Thus, the integrity view of persons may embrace, without inconsistency, the concept of intentional planning to explain what pursuing critical goals and projects in the living of an autonomous life means. On the intentionality model of prospective decisional autonomy, an advance directive is an intentional plan that is shaped by a person's values, commitments, and critical interests—which are part of the person's evaluational system. The phrase "death with dignity" expresses the general purpose and objective of the plan; application of this personal conception to anticipated circumstances of serious illness and incapacity expresses the more concrete goals of the plan. In choosing and following an intentional plan, the author of a directive asserts control and authorship of his or her health care future.

Intentional planning does not require, however, that reflective acceptance of the values, commitments, and interests that shape and motivate an advance care plan must be a part of the cognitive planning process. Reflective acceptance would make an advance directive that much more compelling, but it is not a necessary condition of autonomous choice. Similarly, a life of integrity does not demand that each and every autonomous action be consistent and reflectively integrated with a core self.[29]

AUTONOMY AS INTEGRITY: THE IDEA OF REFLECTIVE ACCEPTANCE

What would an integrity view of actions mean for advance directives? The familiar plea, "but this is not what she would really want," strikes an intuitive chord and points to the conceptual query about whether autonomy demands authentic action. An integrity view of actions seeks to give concrete meaning to the inchoate notion of "acting in character." What distinguishes the integrity standard is the claim that intentionality alone is not sufficient ground to count a particular action as autonomous. Autonomy demands an added level of self-identification with a person's choices.

The most plausible way to construe this requirement is to assert that autonomy involves a *reflective acceptance* of a person's choices as consistent with his or her settled values, commitments, and projects. Some bioethical commentators appear to embrace a view of this sort. Concerned that care of the dying too often fails to meet the patient's own goals, some writers have begun to explore the connections between authenticity, stability of choices, and advance directives. They suggest (without sustained theoretical analysis) that autonomy means that preferences are "authentic and stable over time"[30] or that autonomy requires a constancy and quality of reasoning reflecting "internal consistency of individual preference matrices or 'value maps.'"[31] To understand the implications of this view for advance directives, we must expand the foregoing analysis and give more specific content to the notion of reflective acceptance.

Several influential writers—in particular, Harry Frankfurt and Gerald Dworkin—have captured the core meaning of reflective acceptance by positing a hierarchical model of the self and the cognitive process that moves the will to action.[32] Frankfurt distinguishes between a person's first-order and second-order desires, values, and commitments. A first-order desire is a desire that moves (or would move) the will to action. An effective first-order desire that does move the will to action—a first-order volition—identifies the person's will. A second-order desire is a desire to have a certain desire or to have a certain desire be one's will. Thus, having second-order desires requires a reflective evaluation and acceptance of (competing) desires of the first order. To have a second-order volition is to choose for oneself the desire that one wants to be an effective first-order desire that identifies one's will and is part of one's own self. To illustrate, the statement "I want to X" describes a first-order desire; the statement "I want to want to X" describes a second-order desire and expresses the idea of reflective acceptance of a first-order desire as the desire someone wants to be his or her will (a second-order volition).[33]

Frankfurt calls someone who has second-order volitions a person (for our purposes, an autonomous person). By contrast, one who lacks second-order volitions and acts only on volitions of the first order is what Frankfurt calls a *wanton*. Though such a person may have second-order desires, he or she is indifferent about which of two or more competing first-order desires shall become an effective desire and move the will to action.[34] The wanton is not a person of integrity because acting with integrity requires having at least some effective second-order volitions that manifest valuing some desires of the first order more than others.

Frankfurt's hierarchical theory of the will does important work in articulating a way to understand what it means for a person's actions to be his or her own. For the integrity theorist, however, a somewhat stronger account of the connection between individual actions and core values is required. Frankfurt expressly allows that "a person may be capricious and irresponsible in forming his second-order volitions and give no serious consideration to what is at stake." Frankfurt places "no essential restriction on the kind of basis, if any, upon which [second-order volitions] are formed," stating that "[s]econd-order volitions express evaluations only in the sense that they are preferences."[35] Yet someone who acts in this way—as if his or her actions are isolated events, disconnected from a conception of personal history or projects—can hardly be said to be acting with integrity. As Gabriele Taylor writes, "[N]ormally someone who formed his second-order volitions capriciously and irresponsibly would hardly be thought to be valuing anything at all."[36] Integrity, then, demands a stronger sense of second-order reflection and identification that makes reference to the person's settled values and commitments and seeks to locate that special connection of ownership between persons and their actions within the reflective self.

To warrant the ascription of integrity, a person must not only evaluate and identify as his or hers the desires, values, and attitudes that move the will to action; he or she must identify a course of action as consistent with his or her coherent values and commitments. According to Gerald Dworkin (who frames his analysis of autonomy in terms of authenticity), autonomy "is a second-order capacity to reflect critically upon one's first-order preferences and desires, and the ability to either identify with these or to change them in light of higher-order preferences and values."[37] Moreover, an autonomous person adopts an attitudinal stance toward his or her decisions, asking whether he or she "views himself [or herself] as the kind of person who wishes to be motivated in these particular ways."[38]

This sort of second-order cognitive reflection upon one's desires, values, wishes, and decisions as *mine*, and as consistent with the self, is the repository of a person's "real will" and authentic self. This second-order reflection separates autonomous from nonautonomous actions. Furthermore, the attitudinal stance that marks integrity is more than a fleeting attitude. In caring about the kind of person that he or she is, a person also is aware that the contemplated action may have implications for future behavior, that living a life of integrity involves consistency and coherence of his or her values, commitments, and projects over time. A shallowly sincere person who has superficial and short-lived second-order volitions cannot be said to act with integrity because he or she does not relate second-order volitions to core values, commitments, and self-identity.[39]

Applied to advance care planning, the posit of autonomy as integrity is that to count as autonomous, decisions about future treatment must be identified and accepted as consistent with settled values, commitments, and critical interests. Assuming an intentional plan, the integrity model insists on a further reflective acceptance that consciously connects the plan of a person's advance directive with settled values, commitments, and critical interests and identifies the plan as consistent with them. Metaphorically, the author of a directive must identify with the plan as being properly steered by his or her inner moral compass. Looking again to the purposes and goals of the directive, the decisional process underlying its issuance might be describable in its most general form as follows: "I am and want to be the kind of person for whom death with dignity means there are circumstances in which my life should not be artificially prolonged." Under a more rigorous application, the directive's author must consciously identify his or her intentional treatment plan, and its purposes to refuse life support in certain medical conditions, as consistent with settled values and commitments that he or she has accepted and internalized on higher-order reflection. Treatment choices that are not based on such higher-order reflective acceptance are not authentic, are not worthy of the ascription of integrity, and are not worthy of respect as autonomous.

Many people who write advance directives may well engage in reflection about and (re-)identification with critical values, commitments, and projects in the process of developing an advance care plan.[40] When this deeper self-study is evident, the directive presents an even more commanding case for respect. Should this self-study be a requirement of autonomous action, however? Should respect for advance directives depend on the presence or absence of such reflective acceptance? In the following section, I argue that the integrity view of actions is an inappropriate standard by which to measure whether future-oriented treatment decisions are autonomous and worthy of respect.

INTENTIONALITY, INTEGRITY, AND RESPECT FOR AUTONOMY

The Problem of Infinite Regress

The hierarchical theory of the will has met with some important objections. A fundamental conceptual problem with this model is that it logically entails an infinite regress of higher-order desires—that is, desires to have a desire. Frankfurt acknowledges this concern, stating, "There is no theoretical limit to the length of the series of desires of higher and higher orders."[41] He attempts to resolve it by asserting that decisive identification with a first-order desire is a commitment that resounds throughout the self and silences scrutiny at any higher level.[42] Without an identifiable ground for such a decisive commitment, however, a person's purportedly decisive choice must be regarded as arbitrary.

We sometimes make decisive choices after considered evaluation; at other times we make them out of fatigue, lack of interest, or shortness of time. When one of the latter circumstances exerts substantial influence, why should we assume that a decisive commitment has occurred at the second-order level? To understand why the action is authentically the person's own and not that of a wanton, we need to know its relation to all lower and relevant higher orders in the sequence of volitions. We also need to know why we should look no further than the second order.[43] Moreover, the hierarchical conception allows that a person could be a wanton with respect to higher-order desires—indifferent to which of several competing third-order desires will become effective—while making a decisive commitment to an action at a lower level. At the same time, this decisive commitment to make a second-order desire an effective first-order volition itself could be arbitrary.

In principle, by insisting on a connection between a person's choices and his or her core values (as Gerald Dworkin does), the integrity view posits a stronger ground for calling an action one's own. This modified formulation, however, nonetheless is embedded in an hierarchical conception of the will and is plagued by the same problems as Frankfurt's model. Where are we to locate a person's decisive identification of a chosen course of action as being consistent with his or her settled values, commitments, and critical interests? How are we to distinguish genuine from arbitrary self-identification as the kind of person who refuses treatment to spare loved ones further emotional and financial hardship in the final days? In sum, a hierarchical theory of autonomous action posits no authoritative ground for concluding that the requisite reflective acceptance has occurred and no authoritative ground for concluding that any particular action possesses the properties that make that action peculiarly the person's own and an act marked by integrity.[44] Absent a persuasive and comprehensive theory of the self that nonarbitrarily terminates the series of desires to have a desire—

perhaps in a totally integrated value structure (the ideal of full integrity)—this problem seems inescapable.[45]

An integrity theorist might respond that despite these thorny questions of the self, the intentionality alternative fails to account for the connection between actions and values that makes an action one's own. Absent higher-order reflection, one might argue, intentional actions are first-order volitions, based on first-order desires, values, or motives. As such, they should be considered inauthentic, nonautonomous actions—even the acts of a wanton.

We can illustrate how the foregoing account of intentional planning resists this critique with some examples from everyday life. Consider the simple actions of starting a car, buying the newspaper, and wearing a tie to work. All are actions we ordinarily consider to be ours, to be chosen and performed freely, and to be worthy of respect as autonomous. Saying, like Frankfurt's wanton, that I do not care whether or not I wear a tie to work seems exceedingly odd. It seems equally odd to say that wearing a tie to work is an autonomous action only if I reflect upon whether doing so is a good idea; upon wanting to be the kind of person who wears a tie; or, perhaps more abstractly, upon the kind of person who conforms to a dress code. In fact, I may never have engaged in such reflective evaluation of the desire to wear a tie to work. Nonetheless, wearing a tie is an action willed in accordance with a plan—at least a minimal one that includes evaluation of means to ends and a rejection of the alternative course of action (i.e., not wearing a tie). I properly identify the action as mine and can hardly be said to be indifferent about whether I wear a tie.

The point is aptly demonstrated by the vast area of law-abiding conduct. Under ordinary circumstances, actions such as stopping at red lights; paying for rather than stealing groceries; or, more generally, simply respecting the person and property of others in our daily activities are intentional actions. Yet, we often have engaged in no second-order reflection upon and identification with the motivational structure underlying such actions. Perhaps such identification has occurred at some time in one's history, but habits of obedience to law often are formed without such identification. For me to pay for my groceries, I need not reflectively evaluate whether I want to be the kind of person who pays for his groceries, the kind of person who is honest, or the kind of person who obeys the law. Nevertheless, the action is my own (as are the groceries).

These common, everyday actions exemplify the point of the theoretical account of intentional action. By identifying with and committing myself to an intentional course of action—particularly a plan in which critical interests are at stake—I assert my agency and authorship and make the plan my own. The merit of autonomy as intentionality is that it offers a compelling account of what it means for an action to be autonomous while avoiding the pitfalls of a hierarchical conception of the will—and without reliance on a more thoroughgoing theory of the self.

Respecting the Treatment Choices of Ordinary Persons

The issue of which actions and decisions would count as autonomous and worthy of respect has been called "perhaps the most important test of the adequacy of an analysis of autonomy."[46] As I have suggested, insisting on reflective acceptance as a necessary condition of autonomy would be morally perilous because it would label a wide range of ordinary actions—including most law-abiding conduct—nonautonomous. In health care, the critical issue is how each model would fix the locus of decisional authority by marking off autonomous from nonautonomous decisions. A workable concept of autonomy should establish criteria for the exercise of autonomy that ordinary patients are capable of satisfying; it should qualify as autonomous an acceptable range of health care decisions. It should not posit a largely unattainable ideal "beyond the reach of normal choosers" that effectively denies patient autonomy.[47]

Many familiar health care decisions are based primarily (in some cases solely) on consideration of the nature of one's medical condition and the treatment alternatives. Choosing from among treatment options means assigning priority to the selected course of action—an evaluative judgment that commonly involves at least rudimentary reasoning about whether a course of treatment and care will serve the patient's goals and values. Yet higher-order, attitudinal reflection about personal values often is absent from the decisional process. The average patient does not reflect upon or identify with factors such as his or her attitude toward and trust of physicians, medicine, or professional expertise; the priority of health on his or her personal list of things that make for a good life; or the more complex sociocultural motivational structure underlying these or other potentially relevant considerations. When a patient formulates and acts on an intentional plan for treatment, the patient's motivational structure is present and important, but it is not (re-)evaluated and (re-)adopted as the patient's own.

To illustrate the point: A cancer patient's informed, autonomous choice between surgery and chemotherapy—or rejection of both—requires that the patient understand the nature of his or her condition and the risks, benefits, and burdens of treatment alternatives. However, the intentional act of authorizing or refusing treatment does not demand (though it may involve) reflective identification with values or attitudes such as, "I want to be the kind of person who has a low tolerance for pain." Similarly, agreeing with the physician's advice (what some consider, *simpliciter*, a waiver of decisional authority) does not require conscious reasoning of the sort, "I am the kind of person who trusts my doctor's advice," nor deliberation about why I am a trusting person. Even a competent patient's decisions that appear to be grounded in a well-integrated self-conception in fact may fail to satisfy this test. A Jehovah's Witness who refuses a blood transfusion may never have reflectively accepted the particular Witness beliefs underlying this refusal—nor even the Witness faith itself.[48]

As these few examples show, the integrity standard would render a wide range of familiar health care decisions nonautonomous; it would respect far fewer health care consents and refusals than the intentionality approach. Compounding this theoretical difficulty, in practice the inherent uncertainties of attempting to locate and verify higher-order reflective deliberation would probably invite use and abuse of this standard as a mechanism for overriding patients' otherwise autonomous treatment choices. The practical import might well be to erect an ideal that places autonomous control out of reach for far too many patients and with respect to far too many decisions.

This concern is no less true of future-oriented treatment decisions. Making it my conscious object and purpose to refuse treatment if I am dying of cancer and in severe pain at a future time requires that I understand and evaluate relevant medical information within the framework of reasons, values, and commitments that I hold important; it does not demand a further level of reflection of the sort, "I am the kind of person who does not want to be a burden to my family," nor self-inquiry about why I feel this way. This belief is present and material in my evaluative structure without having to be the object of conscious reflective acceptance.

The posit of intentionality is that decisions to refuse treatment near the end of life are embedded in an evaluative (motivational) structure that compasses personal values and attitudes about dependence, disability, privacy, dignity, and so forth. Insisting that a person's otherwise autonomous treatment refusal is not the person's own and is not entitled to respect unless he or she poses the introspective question of the sort, "Do I really care whether aggressive treatment when I am terminally ill will be a financial burden on my family?" is counterintuitive and contrary to our considered moral judgments. Holding that the author of a directive must manifest higher-order examination of his or her underlying belief structure would require that we dishonor many advance directives that we commonly consider autonomous. In fact, the integrity view leads to the troubling conclusion that the pursuit of death with dignity shaped by one's personal values and commitments is a critical interest in the moral life—but that most of us are more likely to find those interests frustrated rather than satisfied.

Opening the Gates to Physician Paternalism

An equally significant problem for an integrity theory of autonomous actions is that it would allow paternalistic physicians (and families) wide berth to challenge treatment refusals with which they disagree. Bruce Miller, an advocate of authenticity, suggests the potential use of such a theory:

> If a refusal of treatment is a free action but there is reason to believe that it is not authentic or not the result of effective deliberation, then the physician is obliged to assist the patient to effectively deliberate and reach an authentic decision.[49]

Miller's focus is the competent patient, and his narrow point is that there is an obligation to enhance patient autonomy when there is evidence that decisions may not be sufficiently autonomous. Confined to these limits, this position is plausible and may be justified by appeal to the principle of respect for autonomy or, as Miller claims, the physician's duty of beneficence.

The point to be made here is that on an integrity (authenticity) view of actions, this proposition stands as an open invitation for paternalistic physicians to question patient decisions in search of proof of reflective acceptance. This position is evident among commentators who claim that to be autonomous, "choices expressed at one point in time must correspond reasonably well to the patient's preferences in the future."[50] The suggestion that a directive that fails to satisfy a standard of stability and authenticity is nonautonomous and is not entitled to respect underscores the potential threat to prospective autonomy.

Certainly there are some familiar indicia of a person's character and values that we commonly employ in judging that someone's choices are in character. The physician-patient relationship can be an important source of insight into the patient's core values and commitments (the authentic self), and that dialogue may reveal the patient's reflectively accepted values, commitments, and life plans, as well as their connection to important health care choices. Families are an especially important source of information and insight.[51] As I have suggested, however, what counts as accurate evidence of core values and authentic decisions rests on uncertain empirical foundations.[52] It is natural for people to change their values and commitments over time, without sacrificing overall integrity, or to act on values and preferences that may be in transition. How consistent and stable must a person's values be over time? And what counts as evidence of instability?

A condition of reflective acceptance (or stability of values and preferences over time) is even more problematic as applied to advance directives than it is in the context of contemporaneous informed consent by the competent patient because questions about honoring advance directives ordinarily arise only at the time of implementation—after loss of decisional capacity.[53] From this retrospective vantage point, when the patient can no longer bear witness to the authenticity of his or her own choices, the effort to accurately determine whether a patient's treatment refusal is (was) consistent with reflectively accepted core values and commitments is extremely problematic. Thus, a condition of reflective acceptance invites suspect judgments by physicians who hold a contrary view of the patient's good. The problematic nature of accurately identifying the connection between treatment choices and the core self—of distinguishing authentic from inauthentic decisions—makes the integrity view of autonomy "notoriously uncertain and even dangerous."[54]

The intuitive appeal of the integrity (authenticity) view is that it raises a caution flag for families, proxies, and physicians, alerting us not to be too quick to honor treatment refusals that may be strongly influenced by depression, ambivalence, hidden family issues, or psychiatric problems.[55] Miller's narrow point that there is an obligation of further inquiry when such evidence exists is well taken. This point, however, requires no modification of the account of prospective decisional autonomy. To go further—to hold that the patient's intentional refusal of treatment should be ignored when there is reason to suspect it may not be grounded on authentic values—would be morally perilous.

The following case scenario helps to illustrate the relationship between these two ideas, and brings closure to the discussion of the two models of prospectively autonomous choice.

CASE SCENARIO: A RECENT CONVERSION

> Mr. G, a 55-year-old man, is admitted to the hospital with multiple injuries and internal bleeding after a car accident. His condition is stabilized for now, but he remains unresponsive to verbal communication. Surgery is required, and there is a strong likelihood that the surgery will save his life and put him on the path to complete recovery. The mobile intensive care unit team that brought Mr. G to the hospital has delivered a wallet-size living will along with other belongings found at the scene of the accident. Mrs. G has just arrived, and she anxiously awaits news of her husband. The physician explains to Mrs. G the need for surgery and the likelihood of recovery. The physician also explains that Mr. G has lost a lot of blood, and successful surgery is likely to require one or more blood transfusions. In the course of explaining Mr. G's condition, the physician hands Mrs. G the living will, which is titled "Declaration of Medical Preferences in the Witness Faith." The text expressly refuses blood transfusions, stating, "I understand that refusal of blood may mean that I will die. However, as a Witness I know that to willingly accept blood would be a sin against God and would deny me life everlasting. My life is in God's hands."
>
> Mrs. G is visibly distressed. She frantically begins to tell the story of how she and her husband had become Jehovah's Witnesses just two weeks earlier. "We weren't terribly religious for most of our lives. But we began to go to church with our friends Brian and Susan. We really liked the other

people in the congregation and felt like we were part of a community." With tears in her eyes, she asserts that her husband's commitment to their new-found religious faith is sincere. "I was there when he signed this card. I have one too."[56]

Here the likelihood that treatment can save the patient and return him to a normal healthy life makes the argument for overriding the directive on grounds of beneficence most compelling—for some commentators, dispositive.[57] Nonetheless, we have established that an autonomous directive takes precedence over others' views of the patient's best interests, even when the patient's choice may seem to be irrational, unreasonable, or even suicidal. There is no room to argue that Mr. G's instructions are ambiguous and fail to tell us the outcome he intends if his life depends on a blood transfusion. On the contrary, the terms of the directive are clear, and his wife confirms them. (The directive is an effective exercise of future-oriented autonomy under the standards developed at greater length in the following section.) Moreover, it is well-established that an adult Jehovah's Witness has the moral and legal right to refuse a blood transfusion.[58] Thus, resolution of the scenario depends on whether Mr. G's living will and its refusal of blood transfusion meets the conceptual criteria for a prospectively autonomous decision. It depends on whether we accept the document as an expression of Mr. G's intent or look beyond it to challenge his choice as inauthentic and nonautonomous.[59]

Without question, the exchange with Mrs. G gives us pause. The rational response is to want to know more. If we reasonably assume that prior to his conversion Mr. G would have chosen life, as would his wife on his behalf, it is natural to ask: Does the living will stand for the patient's settled values and commitments? Does Mr. G have a critical interest in whether these recently acquired religious beliefs are honored? Should we conclude that he has identified the interests and statements of the living will as *his* and has impressed his personal stamp of authorship on it? Mrs. G's presence at the bedside offers an easy resolution: Her judgment counts most, and she believes the living will should be followed. Yet it is also because of Mrs. G that we are able to learn more about the patient and pursue the difference between the intentionality and integrity views of prospective decisional autonomy.

On the intentionality view, it is reasonable to hold that the familiar teaching of the Witness faith has become a part of Mr. G's evaluational system (albeit one that has recently undergone substantial upheaval). Within this evaluational framework, Mr. G's reasoning can be described in the following way. "As a Jehovah's Witness I am prohibited from accepting blood or blood products. Doing so would be a sin against God and deprive me of everlasting life in God's kingdom. I know there is a risk that I may become seriously ill and suffer from a life-threatening disease at some time in the future or that I could be in a car accident tomorrow. The thing for me to do is to complete the living will prepared by my church. I can make sure that the religious beliefs I hold dear will be honored. And I know that my wife understands this, even though it will be very hard for her should this document ever be needed." Mr. G's living will is a statement of these values and commitments and manifests a clear decision.

Hypothetically, the search for explanation might indicate that Mr. G's living will is not autonomous. Perhaps he felt compelled (even coerced) by members of the congregation to sign the document as a testament to the sincerity of his faith. Perhaps he had recanted his conversion but was embarrassed to tell his wife and neglected to revoke it. No doubt other speculations could be added. That is not what Mrs. G is saying in our case, however. There is no evidence to vitiate the force of the living will.

Recall that the distinguishing feature of an integrity model of autonomous action is the condition of reflective acceptance. The issue is not whether Mr. G's living will expresses an intentional plan (although this factor is important) but whether his conversion should be understood as a genuine, authentic change of character and values that belong to *him*. In practical terms, the integrity view demands evidence of the patient's reflective acceptance of and identification with his or her decision as consistent with core values, commitments, and projects. In the absence of this identification at a higher-order level of the self, the patient's choice should be regarded as nonautonomous—and the health care team should proceed to save his life.

Attempting to make sense of Mr. G's case by pursuing this inquiry seems doomed to failure. Within the preceding two weeks, has Mr. G reflectively embraced the tenets of the Witness faith at a higher-order level of the self, concluding that he is and wants to be the kind of person who lives his life in fidelity to the tenets of his faith? Has he thereby repudiated at this deeper level prior contrary beliefs, setting his moral compass on a new course? Has he critically evaluated his new (changed) values and commitments and decided that he is and wants to be the kind of person for whom death with dignity means refusal of blood and staying the course to life everlasting, even at the cost of foreshortened worldly existence? Or was Mr. G's living will a deeply ambivalent act borne of a temporary triumph of newfound religious beliefs over the values, commitments, and interests acquired over 55 years of life?

There can be no persuasive answers to these questions. We will never know the full story of Mr. G's conversion; the attitudes, beliefs, and values that led him and his wife to this path; or the reasons and reasoning involved in his acceptance of these religious beliefs. Those who understand autonomy to require consistency and stability of preferences and values over time may well want to hold Mr. G's living will nonautonomous simply because his conversion occurred only two weeks before the accident. This is a quite slender reed, however, on which to invalidate Mr. G's living will and his wife's interpretation of his wishes. The fact that Mr. G's conversion occurred only two weeks earlier by itself is no reason to conclude that the document does not express an intentional plan. In fact, there is no necessary connection between the persistence of a person's values and beliefs and their sincerity. Even a person of lifelong devout religious faith may never have engaged in the process of reflective evaluation and identification demanded by the integrity view of autonomous actions. [60]

If Mr. G's case raises doubts—as it should—autonomy as integrity alerts us to important questions about the genuineness of choices expressed in a living will. Evidence that a patient's choice may be out of character raises a caution flag that prompts more thorough probing of the patient's wishes before honoring his or her advance directive.[61] The intentionality view of autonomy, however, does the necessary moral work of pointing the way to the appropriate treatment decision. We can seek assurance that Mr. G's conversion was voluntary and verify the intention of his living will without searching for the sort of higher-order reflection called for by autonomy as integrity. Attempting to justify disregard for the living will by appeal to integrity would indulge an empirically suspect (indeed imaginative) and morally perilous course to promote other peoples' views of Mr. G's best interests. For Mr. G, dying on the terms of his religious faith is a death with dignity. Performing the surgery and providing transfusions would work a horrible contradiction of Mr. G's life—no less than if he had lived 55 years as a Jehovah's Witness.

This analysis may appear to let paternalism sneak in through the back door because suspicion of an inauthentic choice is taken to justify questioning of the living will. There is a critical difference here between the integrity and intentionality models. The claim against the integrity model is that retrospective insistence on proof of reflective acceptance is notoriously uncertain, as Mr. G's case illustrates. Accepting this higher-order identification as a condition of autonomy clothes the physician's judgment of the patient's good in a different and suspect concept of autonomous action, allowing the physician wide berth to paternalistically insist that an otherwise autonomous treatment refusal in fact is nonautonomous (in effect, that the patient's considered intentional plan was the act of Frankfurt's wanton). On the intentionality model, by contrast, the approach to this case takes indicia of inauthenticity to justify a process of exploring the patient's intentions and plans in greater depth—but maintains that the intention of an advance directive should be respected. Evidence that the directive is not an intentional plan (for example, that it is nonvoluntary or that the patient was incompetent at the time of issuance) vitiates the force of the directive; evidence that the patient has not reflectively identified his or her decision as consistent with a core self does not. If more descriptive terms are needed to clarify the distinction, we may call the former, morally unacceptable act of overriding patient autonomy in the name of the patient's good "strong" paternalism and the latter, morally licit inquiry to seek greater assurance of the patient's intent "weak" or "limited" paternalism.[62]

The stark contrast in Mr. G's values pre- and postconversion in this scenario illustrates the difference between the two conceptions of prospective decisional autonomy. Proponents of an integrity-oriented model may respond, however, that it is not paradigmatic—that they are concerned primarily with more common situations involving patients who may be competent and whose interactions with others reveal reasons to believe the patient's expressed choice is not what he or she "really wants." A well-known study of critically ill patients in an intensive care unit conducted by David Jackson and Stuart Youngner is illustrative. Jackson and Youngner describe several cases in which the physician's resolve not to merely accept the patient's refusal of life support revealed to the physician and the patient hidden or unresolved motivations for refusing treatment—including ambivalence about treatment alternatives, depression caused by anticipated side effects of additional chemotherapy, fear of respiratory therapy, and depression brought on by perceived family abandonment—that the patient masked with a plea for death with dignity. In several instances, the patient subsequently consented to treatment. [63]

It is far from clear that these more familiar cases support an integrity model of autonomy. In a subsequent article, Jackson and Youngner correctly assert that it would be morally irresponsible to merely accept and honor the treatment refusals in these cases "while piously proclaiming respect for patient autonomy."[64] Nowhere, however, does the discussion articulate a conception of the necessary and sufficient conditions of autonomous choice, nor does it suggest that subsequent consent to treatment was grounded in higher-order reflection upon personal values and available options. Indicia that the patient's decision is out of character, inauthentic, or not "truly autonomous" raise a caution flag, counseling that implementation of a decision to forgo life support should be postponed to allow patients to confront ambivalence, depression, family conflict, or other factors that may be at work.[65] These cases show that seriously ill patients can change their minds, forming a different intention and plan. This is not going to be true of Mr. G—nor of many other incompetent, dying patients who are incapable of meaningful communication about their treatment choices.

WHAT MAKES AN ADVANCE DIRECTIVE EFFECTIVE?

The question that remains is what makes an intentional plan an effective plan; what makes an advance directive an effective exercise of prospective autonomy? In other words, what is the core pattern of a decisional process that translates the goal of death with dignity into effective action—into an effective advance directive? Closely connected to this question is another: What should we reasonably expect from instruction directives and proxy directives to consider them effective, autonomous, and worthy of respect? Our responses to these questions sharpen the inquiry into the moral weight of advance directives.

Initially, we must expand on the idea of an effective advance directive by introducing the concept of *materiality*. To make future-oriented decisions, the person should understand information that is *material* (important) to his or her decision, not all (possibly) relevant information. The author of a directive should have, of course, a correct understanding of important medical facts and the nature of the act of issuing an advance directive. Someone who refuses treatment "if I have cancer," holding the false belief that all cancers are untreatable and invariably cause death, has failed to appreciate a critical piece of information. A person who signs a durable power of attorney in the belief that the document grants a spouse authority to manage financial affairs cannot be said to have intended to authorize the spouse to serve as health care proxy, even if the document is later construed to include this authority. However, the author of a directive, not others, is the final arbiter of what is important for him or her to understand to make an informed decision. Materiality is at bottom a subjective standard. This rule holds for contemporaneous informed consent, and it should have equal force with regard to advance directives.[66] Moreover, the issue of what counts as material to the author of a directive should find its expression in the intentional plan(s) embodied in the written document.

Some of the problems with implementation of advance directives reflect a gap between what is material to the author of a directive at the time of writing and what is later considered material by those who are responsible for the patient's care. Writers who suggest that instruction directives must be very specific and meet standards of contemporaneous informed consent make the mistake of judging materiality retrospectively and from the physician's point of view rather than from the patient's prospective point of view.

Instructions for Future Care (The Living Will)

The intendment of instruction directives is best understood as outcome-oriented and condition-specific in nature. Effective instruction directives are best understood as outcome-oriented and condition-specific documents. These two connected premises are widely accepted, though they are rarely stated in this fashion. We can think of this conception as the *commonsense view*.[67] The only serious normative challenger to this position is the claim that advance directives must be treatment-specific and emulate a process of informed consent to be effective. As will become clear, we can think of this conception as the *reactionary view* because it has emerged as a response to the shortcomings of instruction directives revealed by past experience. I want to defend the commonsense view against this challenge.

To illuminate the distinction, consider more closely certain factual asymmetries between contemporaneous and prospective decision making. On the standard account of contemporaneous patient choice, the background conditions for the act of consent (or refusal) are specific to a diagnosed medical condition and the risks, burdens, and benefits of identified treatment options (including the option of no treatment). By contrast, in the exercise of prospective autonomy the background conditions for understanding what is being authorized typically are neither diagnosis-specific nor therapy-specific. Future-oriented decisions by definition are made in anticipation of a possible health care future, the central feature of which in the vast majority of cases is the irreversibility of illness and/or the inevitability of death.

The commonsense and reactionary views take these asymmetries seriously but in dramatically different ways. The former recognizes that these critical facts shape the information that is material to the author of a directive and what the author can reasonably expect a directive to accomplish. The latter responds to the difficulties of honoring condition-specific intentions encountered in clinical practice with the dual claims that advance directives should express treatment-specific choices and that the process of advance care planning should mirror that of contemporaneous informed consent. The strongest expression of this view co-opts the goals of informed consent into a condition of future-oriented autonomy, asserting that "[i]n other medical settings, we believe that a person's adequate understanding of the information relevant to treatment decisionmaking is a prerequisite to the exercise of true self-determination, . . . [w]e should take the same view of [the patient's] advance care planning."[68] Another advocate of this view states that "directives must meet standard criteria for real-time informed consent for medical decisionmaking."[69]

My position is that the commonsense view is an essentially correct (though not problem-free) way to understand what makes an advance directive an effective exercise of prospective autonomy and what we can reasonably and appropriately expect from instruction directives (and combined directives). Proponents of the alternative view are properly concerned with improving the nature and process of advance care planning, but they go too far when they graft an informed consent paradigm, translating laudable aspirations into necessary conditions for respecting advance directives.

An Outcome-Oriented Understanding (The Commonsense View)

The commonsense view has been expressed in various ways; it may be stated as follows. Issuance of an advance directive refusing life support involves a fundamental value judgment that there are some circumstances in which life support should be withheld or withdrawn and the natural dying process should be allowed to take its course. There are some states of affairs in which the quality of continued life is worse than death. What matters in the pursuit of death with dignity, what is material to the author of a directive, is whether the way in which one dies will bring serious mental impairment, severe disability and dependency, pain and suffering, loss of privacy, indignity, or other conditions that seriously diminish the quality of life. What matters is the goal of shaping the quality of the dying process (the process of both how and when we die) on one's own terms, in accordance with one's dignity and familial interests. In this sense, advance directives fundamentally are outcome-oriented documents.[70]

Most people would agree that it is unreasonable to attempt to specifically anticipate a wide range of specific potential medical conditions in which the nature and extent of progressive debilitation would be considered intolerable. This level of specificity is beyond the reach of normal anticipatory judgment. Hence, the usual approach to making these goals operational is to apply them to a range of possible *states of illness and disease*. In general form, the reasoning pattern that is characteristic of instruction directives may be phrased as a conditional statement: "If I am suffering from X and my condition is irreversible without reasonable hope of recovery, then I do not want life-sustaining treatment to artificially prolong my life." In the first clause X refers to a medical scenario—a possible future health state (illness or disease state)—rather than (typically) an actual diagnosis. The second clause expresses the author's intention and plan—the nexus between personal values and possible states or conditions. The familiar language of instruction directives attempts to capture what matters across this spectrum of medical circumstances through the use of descriptive categories (commonly, "terminal condition" and "permanent unconsciousness") to characterize conditions in which life support should be withheld or withdrawn. In this way, a condition-specific approach responds to the natural limitations of human foresight.

This understanding has shaped—and been shaped by—advance directive statutes nationally, which have uniformly used these descriptive categories (again, usually "terminal condition" and "permanent unconsciousness") to depict the parameters of the right to refuse treatment.[71] No statute nationally premises the right to refuse treatment on a diagnosis of cancer, heart disease, stroke, or other life-threatening illness or disease.

Of least significance to an intentional plan to refuse life-support is the rejection of specific treatment modalities. For most of us, death with dignity means "do not artificially prolong my life with medical interventions, but give me appropriate pain relief and keep me comfortable as I near the end of life." Mechanical breathing, surgery, chemotherapy, kidney dialysis, and so forth are life-sustaining treatments. Refusal of life-sustaining treatments as a class is the most direct means to achieve the desired outcome.

Again, the prevalence of this view is evident in past and present practice. Amidst the vast array of advance directive forms that have flooded the marketplace, relatively few call upon the author to make discrete choices to accept or refuse respiratory support, cardiopulmonary resuscitation, surgery, chemotherapy, antibiotics, or other medical modalities. Current state laws follow a similar pattern (again, there undoubtedly is a reciprocal relationship here), typically defining "life-sustaining treatment" broadly. The New Jersey statute is illustrative. It defines life-sustaining treatment to mean "the use of any mechanical device or procedure, artificially provided fluids and nutrition, drugs, surgery or therapy that uses mechanical or other artificial means to sustain, restore or supplant a vital bodily function, and thereby increase the expected life span of a patient."[72] Specific provision for refusing artificially provided fluids and nutrition is found in model forms in the handful of states that make specificity a legal requirement, but this approach typically has not been applied to refusal of other forms of life-sustaining treatment. (A place to specifically refuse feeding tubes sometimes is included in such forms, for the practical reason that this choice may alleviate the concerns of physicians who view artificial fluids and nutrition as basic and obligatory and need assurance of the patient's wishes to the contrary, even if such assurance is not required by law.)

Of course, a directive should specifically address matters of particular importance to the author. A person may wish to provide for organ donation; direct that care be given at a preferred hospital or nursing home or at home; affirm an underlying commitment to a religious faith; reject the determination of death on the basis of neurological criteria; direct that certain individuals be consulted to help interpret the document; or attempt to induce compliance by granting immunity to physicians or directing the proxy to take legal action to enforce the directive. Individuals who believe, for religious or other reasons, that artificially provided fluids and nutrition constitute basic sustenance that should always be provided should make this belief clear with an affirmative request or by excluding these medical interventions from the category of treatments that are considered to be life-sustaining. Together with the document's basic outcome orientation, these added particulars enhance the effectiveness of the directive in shaping the end of life to the patient's own conception of death with dignity (or avoidance of indignity).[73]

These more particular concerns essentially are fine-tuning, however. The center of gravity of an instruction directive's outcome-oriented plan lies in the connection between the author's dignity and familial interests and a condition-specific understanding of the sort described above. As Norman Cantor states (in one of the passages that begins this chapter), the crucial guidance in an instruction directive concerns what counts as an intolerable quality of life. Instructions should focus on desired outcomes with or without aggressive medical interventions, rather than the nature of the medical procedures themselves.[74] Under the standard of effectiveness, if the expression of this plan—of the outcome(s) desired by the patient—is sufficient to guide the people who are responsible for the patient's care, the instruction directive is effective and should be honored, trumping competing concerns for the patient's current experiential interests.

Over the years, advance directives have met with several pragmatic criticisms, which sometimes are referred to as the "practical problems" with advance directives. Most often, these critiques are aimed at instruction directives. The principal charge is that directives too often are vague and ambiguous and fail to provide instructions that effectively guide care. Among the reasons given are the inherent limitations of human foresight; the natural shortcomings of static written documents authored years earlier; the absence of meaningful communication among patient, family, and physician; and failures of draftsmanship. Critics also have observed that the patient's medical condition may be radically different than what he or she previously anticipated and that new medical advances may paint a very different clinical picture and hold the prospect of a very different outcome than the patient previously contemplated. These latter possibilities raise further questions about the effectiveness of instruction directives (and, to a lesser extent, proxy and combined directives), separate and apart from matters of ambiguity.[75]

The commonsense view acknowledges that instruction directives are imperfect instruments; that sound conceptual moorings cannot erase the genuine constraints of anticipatory judgments about a possible future; in sum, that there are limits to the effective exercise of prospective autonomy. Understanding advance directives as intentional, outcome-oriented plans is not a panacea. With this perspective in mind, these practical problems for the most part have been met with proposals for changes in practice, not theory. Among these proposals are recommendations for targeted education of the general public as well as health care professionals, integration of advance directive discussions into the physician-patient interaction, better patient-family communication, modification of institutional culture, use of a values history, use of narrative stories, and more careful draftsmanship.[76] The field is crowded with practice-reformers. In the main, these important efforts are and should remain grounded in the tone and tenor of this commonsense view. Placing advance care planning in the proper conceptual framework offers an essential grounding for making advance directives meaningful.

A small coterie of commentators have pressed further, suggesting that practice reforms be based on a fundamental conceptual shift in how we should understand effective advance directives. The *reactionary view* counters that advance directives should be aligned more closely with the model of contemporaneous informed consent and the making of discrete, specific choices. This construction has gained increasing currency, particularly among physicians. The following section presents this position and defends the outcome-oriented account against it.

Putting a Premium on Specificity (The Reactionary View)

Critics of the commonsense view make two related assertions. The first is that an effective instruction directive is treatment-specific. The second is that advance directives should meet standards of decision making that commonly are applied to contemporaneous informed consent. Implicit in each claim is the further premise that effective advance care planning must take place in consultation with a physician, as part of the physician-patient relationship. For the most part, these three claims must stand or fall together, though one could maintain the first and third premises but reject the proposition that effective directives are necessarily treatment-specific. (Logically one could hold that instruction directives should be treatment-specific but not insist that people consult with a physician. This combination seems implausible, however, because this arguably is where physicians' unique expertise and ability to explain the benefits and burdens of various treatment modalities would be most needed.) This position need not reject outright the posit of an outcome-oriented approach; its proponents hold, however, that the outcome-oriented approach is inadequate—that one or more of the three foregoing features also is a necessary condition of an effective instruction directive.

The most visible proponent of the reactionary view is Linda Emanuel. A 1989 article co-authored with her husband Ezekiel puts forward a treatment-specific document called the "Medical Directive" as the panacea for the familiar problems with living wills.[77] The document follows the path of the commonsense account to an extent, describing four medical scenarios in terms of mental disability and prognosis that are paradigmatic of the most common states in which patients have considered the quality of life worse than death. (The authors adapted these four illness scenarios from several leading court cases.) What distinguishes the Medical Directive is that it calls upon its author to choose from among 12 identified treatment modalities for each of the four scenarios. In effect, to use this document the person must complete a 48-choice grid matching each of the four scenarios to the refusal or acceptance of each of the 12 treatments.[78] Some other advance directive forms have used a different format to present a similar range of treatment-specific choices.

We have seen that treatment-specific decisions are not material to the core decisional process that is typical of advance care planning—but should they be? Treatment specificity may be counterproductive, in fact, because it obscures the importance of the patient's overall treatment goals in favor of attending to whether discrete interventions have been refused. As one physician-critic of specificity has noted, picking and choosing from among a menu of alternatives may lead to combinations of preselected interventions that in practice contradict the patient's goals. Moreover, a treatment-specific directive "runs the risk of promoting the selection or rejection of interventions because of their inherent characteristics, rather than as appropriate means to the ends that the patient would have wanted."[79] Compounding these difficulties, the treatment-specific directive gives the appearance of certainty where none may exist. In clinical practice, physicians interpreting such a directive may well infer from non-refusal of a particular intervention (e.g., antibiotics) that the intervention should be provided, failing to ask the most important question: Will the intervention serve the patient's goals? On the other hand, what now appear to be inconsistent choices may be taken to justify disregard for the document as ambiguous or unhelpful—again, cutting short the most significant inquiry into what outcome the patient would want.[80]

Through the lens of a medical ethos that cherishes technical proficiency, predictability, and certainty, the treatment-specific approach may appear to be a logical response to the historical uncertainties of living wills. It is not difficult to see that treatment-specific documents may be quite comforting to many clinicians who are reluctant to confront uncertainty about what the patient would want, nor why from this vantage point non-treatment-specific documents often are considered to be "unhelpful."[81] The quest for certainty is elusive and unrealistic, however. Insisting that only treatment-specific documents are effective pushes beyond reasonable boundaries of the reasonable exercise of anticipatory judgment under conditions of uncertainty. Furthermore, as a practical matter, documents such as the Medical Directive may well do more harm than good, giving false assurance of certainty and permission to treat (or not treat) and insulating those responsible for the patient's care from the duty to interpret the document with the patient's own goals and desired outcomes clearly before them. The result can be that the fundamental outcome orientation of the document is undermined, the patient's intentions subverted, and the patient's critical interests thwarted.[82]

The second claim of the reactionary view is that advance care planning with advance directives should meet familiar standards for the exercise of contemporaneous informed consent. Although some proponents of this view have implicitly and uncritically applied the informed consent paradigm to advance care planning, this position is made explicit by Linda Emanuel, who argues that "directives must meet criteria for real-time informed consent."[83] The unacknowledged assumption of this view is that advance directives are entitled to respect (or are "useful"—which amounts to the same thing) only if they come as close as is humanly possible to mirroring the contemporaneous consent or refusal of the competent patient.

There are good reasons to reject this position. One point of the prior discussion is that to expect prospective autonomy to mimic contemporaneous autonomy is simply unrealistic. Rigid insistence that advance directives satisfy this test suggests two untenable positions. Either we must embrace an almost irrational belief in the powers of human reason and foresight, or we must conclude that the exercise of prospective autonomy is beyond the reach of the average reasonable person and that very few advance directives are effective and entitled to respect.[84]

Furthermore, implicit in the informed consent model is the claim that effective use of advance directives requires consultation with a physician and presumably an ongoing physician-patient relationship. One group of Boston physicians advocates "comprehensive directives [by which they mean the Medical Directive], in which discussion between patient and physician can produce both documented treatment preferences based on the patient's response to specific scenarios and a durable power of attorney."[85] To be sure, there is widespread agreement that consultation with a physician is useful and advisable. The physician can explain important medical information, and this dialogue can engender mutual understanding—thereby giving the physician greater insight into the patient's wishes and fostering respect for what the patient would want. A frank dialogue also can identify value conflicts between physician and patient, in some cases suggesting that it may be advisable for the patient to seek a different physician.

Transforming this advice into a mandate is an altogether different matter, however. One objection to doing so is that it risks disenfranchising millions of Americans from the fundamental right to refuse treatment near the end of life. Most of the estimated 37 million Americans who are without health insurance at any given time (the number changes periodically but is consistently above 30 million) have no real physician-patient relationship; for many of us, contact with the health care system comes through the emergency room. For many others who have insurance, contact with a physician is intermittent and sporadic (especially for generally healthy people). Moreover, even assuming a physician-patient relationship, effective advance care planning presupposes a bond of trust that is the basis for meaningful communication about decisions near the end of life. Significant, practical barriers to effective communication have been well-documented.[86]

The reactionary view also mistakenly assumes that consultation with a physician is necessary because of the physician's unique knowledge and expertise. This position again ignores the wisdom of the commonsense approach. Again, what matters most to the author of an advance directive is an understanding of the relationship between personal values, critical interests, and possible future medical conditions that finds expression in an outcome-oriented directive. Most of us are able to reflect on and articulate certain principles that we hold dear, including what is in our dignity and familial interests. We are quite capable of having and expressing an understanding of a debilitated status that we would consider an intolerable quality of life. The many sources of information that shape this understanding are part of life's experience—among them personal experience with the death and illness of family and friends, as well as well-known court cases and news accounts that have become engrained in the public consciousness. The suggestion that physicians are needed to facilitate effective reasoning about these concerns is contrary to our common experience and improperly presumes that a professional and technological sophistication is essential to what in fact are very personal judgments. Certainly individuals *should* consult with family, friends, religious advisors, physicians, and others. Directives should be based on correct medical information that is material to the individual's intentions. Consultation serves the dual purposes of helping the individual to reach decisions and giving those who will be responsible for the person's care a better understanding of the directive's intendment. Again, however, there are good reasons not to cross the line from what *should* be to what *must* be.

To be clear: The informed consent model is an important yardstick for much-needed efforts to improve the use of advance directives and to make advance care planning a standard component of the physician-patient relationship. Documents developed in consultation with a physician (or other health care professional) may well be more informed than documents developed without such consultation. Recent work has begun to explore the use of *disease-specific* directives that allow patients to tailor instructions for future care to a diagnosed illness, disease, or condition. Advance care planning in these circumstances minimizes uncertainty and holds the promise of fostering more informed, less anticipatory decisions, particularly when such planning is conducted in consultation with a physician. This new direction in advance care planning may be most appropriate for a patient with a chronic, progressive illness with a relatively predictable clinical course in which the patient retains mental capacity for much of the period of illness.[87] Insisting, however, that all advance directives must satisfy informed consent standards to be effective, autonomous, and entitled to respect is mistaken and misleading. One consequence of this mistake has been the frequent but misguided insistence that directives should express highly specific treatment choices.

Thus, the reactionary view would render many otherwise autonomous instruction directives nonautonomous—first by insisting on treatment-specific instructions as a necessary vehicle for following the patient's intentions and satisfying the patient's goals and second by insisting that the process of advance care planning meet standards that mirror contemporaneous informed consent. This process can only unfold within the context of an established physician-patient relationship that is based on mutual trust—a feature that is absent from many people's experience with the health care system—and is most meaningful when it is tailored to a diagnosed illness or condition.

For all of these reasons, to the extent that the reactionary view posits further necessary conditions for the effective exercise of prospective autonomy, it runs the risk of thwarting rather than promoting prospective autonomy and the pursuit of death with dignity. Future efforts to improve advance care planning should continue to be grounded in the commonsense view of what makes an instruction directive an effective exercise of prospective autonomy. The goal of approximating contemporaneous informed consent should be understood as an ideal—but not a condition—for the exercise of prospective autonomy.

Appointing a Proxy

Appointment of a proxy is widely considered to be the preferred method of handling the uncertainties of future-oriented treatment choices. The use of a proxy avoids many of the problems that are endemic to committing anticipatory decisions to writing. Proxy directives do not rigidly bind others to the sometimes difficult task of faithful implementation when operative language is ambiguous or it is unclear whether anticipated circumstances have in fact materialized. Instead, a proxy entrusted with responsibility to "stand in the shoes" of the patient in the physician-patient encounter typically has authority to exercise judgment and discretion to make treatment decisions that are responsive to the patient's current medical condition. Close and caring family members and friends ordinarily are more familiar with the patient's wishes and values than anyone else and therefore are best able to decide as the patient would under the circumstances. As numerous courts and commentators have concluded, a close and caring family member or friend is best-positioned to know the patient's wishes and to faithfully implement those wishes in an informed and flexible manner that is responsive to the patient's developing medical circumstances. Another, more pragmatic, argument in favor of the proxy approach is that clear recognition of who has authority to decide simplifies the decision-making process and offers assurance to health care professionals.[88]

Several empirical studies have found that proxy and surrogate predictions of patient preferences are less reliable than is commonly believed; these findings offer a challenge to this familiar rationale.[89] In one study, proxy predictions were accurate only 50 percent of the time.[90] In another, 74 percent of surrogates accurately stated the patient's preferences for cardiopulmonary resuscitation (CPR), but only 50 percent correctly stated the patient's refusal of resuscitation more generally.[91] Some critics of the proxy approach have used these data to question the premise of the proxy's authority, claiming that "[w]hen families or other proxies cannot be relied on to choose as the patient would, they can no longer be said to be exercising the patient's right for the patient."[92] The Emanuels press this point a step further, suggesting that standards for end-of-life decisions that are based on community values ought to supplant the proxy, unless the proxy is expressly given authority to deviate from the patient's wishes.[93]

It is far from clear that these empirical findings support such a strong theoretical challenge to the foundations of the proxy's authority. A more plausible conclusion is that the data reinforce the need for better family communication about advance care planning, including the patient's wishes and expectations and the nature of the proxy's responsibilities.[94] Evidence of dissonance between patient wishes and family predictions also counsels more strongly that designated proxies should be provided with express instructions through the use of a combined directive. In fact, the combined directive has emerged as the best means to join express choices for treatment with flexibility and discretion, thereby offering greater assurance that autonomy will be recognized and respected. (A combined directive also may relieve some of the family stress that accompanies uncertainty about what the patient would choose when a proxy is without written direction and may be unguided by adequate prior conversations with the patient.)[95] Moreover, if the suggested choice is between family proxies or physician authority (with or without a proxy designation), the foregoing data give no warrant to the claim that physicians should fill this role. Studies also have shown that physicians' predictions of patients' wishes are less accurate than those of family members.[96] At least one study suggests that nurses and social workers are better able to predict patients' wishes than physicians, though they were less accurate in their predictions than family members.[97]

This critique also misses two important points about the proxy as an expression of prospective autonomy. First, as Hilde and James Lindemann Nelson observe, what is at stake in appointing a proxy is not just what will be decided but *who* will decide.[98] In designating a proxy, we *entrust* another person with important choices to be made in our behalf. The essence of the patient-proxy relationship is a fiduciary one. Grounded in personal and intimate relationships that span years, even lifetimes, selection of a proxy proclaims a trust and faith in the proxy's judgment. It is not the outcome alone that matters but also the autonomous agency of granting authority to a loved one.

A second and related point is that the critique crimps the substantive standard at work with the proxy directive. Although following the patient's previously expressed wishes and values is the proxy's primary charge, proxy authority ordinarily compasses as well discretion to apply a best interests standard on the patient's behalf—initially as a guide to interpreting the patient's wishes and, when this effort comes up short, as a basis for treatment decisions. Thus, the chief appeal of the proxy—its flexibility—springs from the fiduciary nature of the appointment. The point is forcefully made by one attorney whose practice has included assisting clients in planning for their health care futures:

> [Most] believe that the people who know them and love them understand their values enough to draw the cutoff lines, and they are willing to abide by the decision those people would make. They usually feel more strongly about the decisionmaker than the decision itself—they trust the decision their loved ones would make and do not trust a decision that would be made by others involved, including hospital personnel and (in the worst possible situation) courts. Thus, the most crucial aspect of the advance directive is the appointment of a health care representative.[99]

Our shared commitment to the place of this fiduciary bond finds expression in the vast majority of advance directive statutes and advance directive forms, which expressly presume a proxy's discretion not only to interpret the patient's wishes but also to act in the patient's best interests. (Law and practice also allow, of course, that a person may expressly limit the scope of the proxy's authority if a person chooses to do so.)[100]

At bottom, selection of a proxy demands a judgment about who the patient trusts with this responsibility and an intention to convey this trust and authority. An effective proxy directive chooses wisely; it gives authority to someone who knows the patient and is capable of faithfully and, if necessary, vigorously seeking to make the decision and achieve the outcome desired by the patient.[101] An effective proxy directive also defines with sufficient clarity the extent and boundaries of the proxy's authority to make treatment decisions. As Veatch notes, "Autonomy is preserved by the agent acting on the framework established by the person while competent."[102] Thus, the author of a directive should state whether the proxy is authorized to refuse life support; whether the proxy has (or does not have) authority to exercise judgment to interpret the patient's wishes (this authority ordinarily is assumed when the proxy is not given specific written instructions); and whether the proxy has (or does not have) authority to act in accordance with his or her judgment regarding what would serve the patient's best interests. It is especially important with the combined directive that the author make clear an intention to limit the proxy's authority to the written terms, as well as whether the proxy is permitted to override the literal terms of the directive on best interests grounds. The standard form language of proxy and combined directives commonly identifies and addresses these issues.

Some commentators suggest that the emotional and financial burdens of watching a loved one die present families with a conflict of interest, making them ill-suited candidates for proxy appointment.[103] It is precisely because of the especial bonds of family, however, that loved ones have long been recognized as the most appropriate surrogates for incompetent patients and that they are the unquestioned choice of the vast majority of people who issue proxy directives. Furthermore, entrusting a loved one to serve as proxy means assessing whether that person is likely to exercise sound judgment in fulfillment of this trust or be subject to distortions of judgment, succumb to self-interest, or act in bad faith—judgments that the patient (and perhaps the patient alone) is uniquely qualified to make. Such cases do occur; a person can choose a proxy unwisely. These rare situations offer no reason, however, to question wholesale our ability to understand and appreciate these concerns within our own families, nor to abandon the strong presumption of respect for proxy directives.[104]

Summary: Effective Advance Directives

We have now staked out an understanding of what makes advance directives effective. An effective, autonomous *instruction directive* is an outcome-oriented document that expresses an intentional plan whose center of gravity lies in the connection between the author's dignity and familial interests and a condition-specific understanding of possible future states of illness and disease. Specific intentions addressing matters that are material to the author should be set forth in the document, but treatment-specific instructions refusing particular medical modalities (implicitly accepting others) are not necessary to make clear the author's overall treatment objectives. The absence of treatment specificity provides no justification for disregarding the directive. An effective, autonomous *proxy directive* is an intentional plan that gives authority to a trusted family member or friend to make treatment decisions in the patient's behalf and expresses the author's intention to direct, limit, or extend that authority in ways that the author deems material. An effective, autonomous *combined directive* satisfies the criteria of effectiveness for an instruction directive and a proxy directive and should give sufficient guidance about whether the proxy is strictly bound by, or may deviate from, the terms of the instruction directive. The presence or absence of this authority ordinarily can be inferred even if not expressly stated.

When possible, advance care planning should approximate and aspire to a model of contemporaneous informed consent. Without question, consultation with others—family, religious advisors, or physicians—can facilitate more informed decision making and the writing of more effective directives. Holding all advance directives to a standard of contemporaneous informed consent or making consultation with a physician a necessary condition of an effective directive, however, is simply untenable.

The foregoing analysis also suggests that advance directives will not always qualify as effective and autonomous. Because of the natural limitations of human foresight, not all instruction directives will provide sufficient guidance to others to be effective. Effectiveness requires a *fit* between a previously articulated intentional plan and current circumstances, a fit that effectively bridges the temporal gap that is typical of advance directive practice.

Instruction directives can fail to have this fit—fail to be effective—in one of two ways. They can be too ambiguous (or vague, which amounts to the same thing) to provide sufficient guidance to those who are called upon to follow them, perhaps as a result of ill-conceived plans or poor draftsmanship. Another possibility is that divergence between previously anticipated and actual circumstances can be so radical that one cannot reasonably determine what the document's intention is. In rare cases, what medicine has to offer will have changed so dramatically that we cannot fairly say that the directive was meant to refuse life support and choose an earlier death. Although a proxy directive is almost always an effective exercise of prospective autonomy that rarely should be challenged, on occasion the proxy will find the burdens of decision simply overwhelming; will deviate so radically from the terms of an instruction directive as to fail in his or her fiduciary responsibilities; or will, in unusual cases, exhibit a palpable breach of trust. These failures of prospective autonomy play a central role in the discussion of the moral weight of advance directives that occupies chapter five, where they are recast as the (only) three grounds on which overriding a directive is justified.

CONCLUSION

Prospectively autonomous choice and advance directives are best understood as intentional plans that give concrete meaning to the pursuit of death with dignity. The intentionality view of prospective decisional autonomy resonates with our considered moral judgments and would qualify as autonomous a much broader and more acceptable range of health care decisions than the alternative integrity model. The latter view poses a serious threat to the authority of patient autonomy and advance directives as a shield against physician paternalism and as a sword wielding the right to control important decisions even when others may think such choices are wrong. Theoretical flaws and uncertain empirical foundations inherent in the integrity view of autonomous actions leave the gates open for people who disagree with a patient's treatment refusal to assert dubious judgments that reflective acceptance is absent and to override the patient's decision on the ground that it is nonautonomous. The fact that many physicians fail to take advance directives seriously suggests that this concern is far from hypothetical.

An autonomous and effective directive provides sufficient guidance to persons who are responsible for the patient's care to allow faithful implementation of the outcome intended by the directive's author. The competing conception—which holds that an effective directive mirrors contemporaneous informed consent, is developed in consultation with a physician, and sets forth specific and discrete elections of various treatment modalities— is unrealistic and would result in denying standing to many otherwise autonomous directives. This conception is out of keeping with the commonsense understanding of what matters most to the author of a directive. To take charge of how we die is to anticipate some range of future medical conditions in which the quality of life with aggressive interventions would be intolerable and to craft the outcome of the dying process in accord with our critical interests.

Two conclusions about the moral weight of advance directives emerge from the discussion in this chapter. First, an effective, autonomous directive should be honored and should trump competing views of what is best for the patient. Second, not all directives are autonomous. It may be justifiable to override an ineffective, nonautonomous directive in favor of the patient's current welfare interests. Hence, it is wrong to uniformly ascribe to advance directives the weight of precedent autonomy.

Each of these conclusions raises several important and controversial questions about the scope and limits of the duty to respect advance directives— the subject that occupies chapter five. Before traveling that path, however, I must address a different sort of conceptual challenge to the argument developed thus far. To develop the theory of prospective autonomy, I have set aside a very different line of philosophical inquiry. Drawing on personal identity theory, some critics of advance directives claim that some incompetent patients—in particular, those who are severely demented or permanently unconscious—are no longer the same person who authored the prior directive and that the document therefore has no moral authority to dictate current treatment decisions. In chapter four, I present this philosophical challenge and go on to argue that this position is mistaken and morally perilous.

NOTES

1. Norman L. Cantor, *Advance Directives and the Pursuit of Death with Dignity* (Bloomington: Indiana University Press, 1993), 60.
2. Joan M. Teno, Hilde Lindemann Nelson, and Joanne Lynn, "Advance Care Planning: Priorities for Ethical and Empirical Research," *Hastings Center Report* 24, no. 6 (November-December 1994): S32.

3. For discussion of this distinction, see Tom L. Beauchamp and James F. Childress, *Principles of Biomedical Ethics*, 4th ed. (New York: Oxford University Press, 1994), 121–25; Ruth R. Faden and Tom L. Beauchamp, *A History and Theory of Informed Consent* (New York: Oxford University Press, 1986), 235–37.

4. An analogous distinction exists between competence and autonomy. In the broadest sense, competence refers to the ability to perform a task—such as balancing a budget, writing a book, or deciding to undergo surgery. Beauchamp and Childress, *Biomedical Ethics*, 134 (quoting Charles M. Culver and Bernard Gert, *Philosophy in Medicine* (New York: Oxford University Press, 1982). Possessing the requisite capacities (being a competent person), however, does not necessarily mean that the patient will exercise those capacities and make an autonomous (competent) treatment decision.

   The consensus generally has failed to attend to another important aspect of the distinction between competence and autonomy. The concept of competence also serves a gatekeeping function whereby persons with authority to make their own decisions (competent patients) are distinguished from those who do not have this authority (incompetent patients). The presumption of competence involves a normative judgment that qualifies the patient to make certain decisions. Beauchamp and Childress, *Biomedical Ethics*, 132–33. A determination of incompetence (overcoming this presumption) shifts the locus of decisional authority from the patient to an advance directive; a surrogate decision maker (if no proxy has been designated); or, in some cases, a court-appointed guardian—generally in this order of priority. Here the consensus has fallen into a conceptual error, similar to the failure to attend to the distinction between autonomous persons and their actions. The dominant focus of the consensus, particularly in law, has been to establish a parallelism and equivalence between the rights of competent patients and those of incompetent patients. In the same way that the presumption of competence fixes decisional authority with the patient, the presumption that the author of a directive was competent at the time of writing has qualified the decisional authority of advance directives. There is no reason to question this well-established rule of presumption. Failure to appreciate this point has contributed, however, to the misguided assumption that if an individual was competent when the directive was written, no further inquiry about autonomy is required.

   The concept of competence (or decision-making capacity) is treated at length in several sources, including Allen E. Buchanan and Dan W. Brock, *Deciding for Others: The Ethics of Surrogate Decision Making* (Cambridge: Cambridge University Press, 1989), chapter one; Beauchamp and Childress, *Biomedical Ethics*, 132–41; President's Commission for the Study of Ethical Problems in Medicine and Biomedical and Behavioral Research, *Making Health Care Decisions: The Ethical and Legal Implications of Informed Consent in the Patient-Practitioner Relationship* (Washington, D.C.: GPO, 1982), chapter three.

5. Faden and Beauchamp, *Informed Consent*, especially chapter seven.

6. Beauchamp and Childress, *Biomedical Ethics*, especially chapter three.

7. I discuss only the first two of these three conditions. The condition of understanding is construed as secondary to the question of effectiveness of advance directives. I assume but do not argue that to be autonomous, an advance directive must be issued without controlling influences that determine the person's actions. In general, this means that a person's choices may be affected by a range of influences—among them, the wishes and emotional appeals of loved

ones, physicians' attempts to persuade, even threats of abandonment from family or health care professionals if the person chooses in one way rather than another. Most often, these influences are properly characterized as attempts at persuasion; on rare occasion they may be regarded as efforts at manipulation. These factors generally are compatible with autonomy; rarely are they coercive and controlling. The discussion of advance care planning assumes that the condition of noncontrol is satisfied. The question of whether a person has voluntarily written and signed an advance directive or, conversely, has had his or her choices determined by the controlling influences of others, rarely is at issue. (We might imagine, by analogy to testamentary wills, the greedy family member coercing the choice of an earlier death in the hope of an earlier inheritance.) Some writers interpret the concept of voluntariness to raise questions about freedom from psychological and emotional influences such as depression, fear of pain, compulsions, disorders, and the like. I consider questions of psychological influences in a different way in chapter five, in connection with intentional treatment decisions that nonetheless may appear to be inauthentic. For extensive discussion of the condition of noncontrol, see Faden and Beauchamp, *Informed Consent,* chapter ten; Beauchamp and Childress, *Biomedical Ethics,* 163–70. Both sources discuss the condition of noncontrol (voluntariness) as consisting of a continuum of degrees of influence that is analyzable in terms of coercion, manipulation, and persuasion.

8. It bears emphasis that my inquiry is limited and normative. A full theory of prospective decisional autonomy would have to address a series of related questions, such as how individuals should acquire necessary understanding; with whom a person should consult; how the physician-patient-family dialogue should be structured to facilitate more effective use of advance directives; or, more generally, the practical barriers to effective advance directive use. These issues figure prominently in what has become a virtual cottage industry of theoretical and empirical research about advance directives. See, e.g., the collected essays in "Dying Well in the Hospital: The Lessons of SUPPORT," *Hastings Center Report* 25, no. 6, supplement (November-December 1995); "Advance Care Planning: Priorities for Ethical and Empirical Research," Special Supplement, *Hastings Center Report* 24, no. 6 (November-December 1994). I touch on these questions at various points, but they do not receive separate extended attention here.

9. See generally Jon Elster, ed., *Rational Choice* (New York: New York University Press, 1986).

10. My point here should be understood to define the scope of the analysis to follow, not as a normative claim about autonomy. Some people believe by definition that a recent directive is more effective than one written longer ago. To be sure, there is practical wisdom in revisiting and updating the document to ensure that it accurately reflects one's current wishes. In truth, however, there is no direct correlation between the date of a directive and its effectiveness, which may be one reason advance directive laws do not require updating as a condition of validity or legislate expiration dates for directives.

11. Gerald Dworkin, "Autonomy and Behavior Control," *Hastings Center Report* 6, no. 1 (February 1976): 23.

12. Faden and Beauchamp, *Informed Consent,* 237–41.

13. See Faden and Beauchamp, *Informed Consent,* chapter seven, arguing that autonomous informed consent of the competent patient demands substantial—but not full—autonomy.

14. This approach borrows from Faden and Beauchamp's analysis of understanding as a condition of autonomous informed consent. Faden and Beauchamp describe *understanding* in terms of a continuum on which full and complete understanding and full ignorance are at either end. Substantial understanding marks a portion of the upper half of the range, short of full and correct apprehension, and characterizes the extent of understanding necessary to call an action substantially autonomous and therefore to be respected as autonomous. See Faden and Beauchamp, *Informed Consent*, 251–52. In this sense, substantial understanding is "merely a rough benchmark." Ibid., 302. As used here, sufficiency, or effectiveness, also is intended as a rough benchmark.

15. There are at least two senses in which a directive might be regarded as effective but not necessarily autonomous. One would be that the document is legally effective—in other words, binding—regardless of whether it meets criteria for autonomous choice. That is not the meaning of effectiveness I use here. There also is the theoretical possibility that a directive could be effective—that is, provide on its terms sufficient guidance to others—but be based on insufficient, even incorrect, understanding. Arguably, such a directive would be effective but nonautonomous. The latter sort of scenario, if it were supported by enough evidence, could provide grounds to override a directive, but such cases would be extremely rare.

16. Advocates of advance directives will rightly point to the danger that in a climate in which advance directives are not taken seriously, paternalistic physicians and critics of advance directives will seize on the suggestion that some directives are nonautonomous. I share this concern, especially in the aftermath of the much-publicized study of the SUPPORT investigators, which found (confirming several earlier smaller studies elsewhere) that a majority of physicians at five major medical centers ignored patients' wishes for end-of-life care, even after a targeted intervention that was designed to enhance physicians' awareness of patients' wishes. See SUPPORT Principal Investigators, "A Controlled Trial to Improve Care for Seriously Ill Hospitalized Patients: The Study to Understand Prognoses and Preferences for Outcomes and Risks of Treatments (SUPPORT)," *Journal of the American Medical Association* 274, no. 20 (November 22/29, 1995): 1591–98. The pro-directive camp has a strong argument that policy should insist that all advance directives carry the weight of precedent autonomy because any diminution in their authority opens the door to unjustified paternalism. As will become clear, the vast majority of directives do, or can, satisfy the conditions for prospectively autonomous decision making I discuss here. To advance the current debate and respond to the truly troubling cases in which directives fail to provide sufficient guidance, a coherent theory of decision making with advance directives that straightforwardly acknowledges the limits of effective advance care planning and the implications for the moral weight of advance directives is required.

17. Faden and Beauchamp, *Informed Consent*, 243 (emphasis in original). The meaning of formulating and performing an intentional plan (acting intentionally, or with intention) should be distinguished from the ideas of "having an intention," "intending," or other uses of the concept of intention that refer to "mental acts" or states of mind that have not (yet) been translated into performative acts.

18. Wayne A. Davis, "A Causal Theory of Intending," *American Philosophical Quarterly* 21, no. 1 (January 1984): 43–52.

19. Donald Davidson, "Intending," in *Essays on Actions and Events* (New York: Oxford University Press, 1980).
20. Faden and Beauchamp, *Informed Consent*, 242.
21. The clause "whether the act [outcome] is wanted or not" clarifies that the operative concept of intentionality is based on a model of willing rather than wanting. For some philosophers, actions that are not wanted are not intended. Whatever validity this view may have in the moral life generally, insisting on such a close connection between intending and wanting is especially ill-suited to the context of health care decisions. Patients who intentionally consent to treatment cannot be said to want or desire the discomfort and pain of surgery, dialysis, and so forth. A person who refuses treatment in an advance directive does not *want* to burden loved ones with decisional authority or the anguish of a prolonged bedside vigil. Nonetheless, the patient's refusal of treatment is an intentional decision and should be described as an intentional treatment refusal accompanied by unwanted (or tolerated) and foreseeable consequences. For more extensive analysis of this point, see Faden and Beauchamp, *Informed Consent*, 244–47.
22. I assume but do not argue that an action is either intentional or not. In other words, the concept of intentionality is not variable and admitting of degrees; one action is not more intentional than another. For discussion of this point, see Faden and Beauchamp, *Informed Consent*, 247–48.
23. Ibid., 242.
24. This line of thought is suggested by Gary Watson's essay "Free Agency," in *Moral Responsibility*, edited by John Martin Fischer (Ithaca, N.Y.: Cornell University Press, 1986), 81–96. Watson distinguishes a person's *valuational* system from his or her *motivational* system. The former term refers to "that set of considerations which, when combined with his factual beliefs (and probability estimates), yields judgments of the form: The thing for me to do in these circumstances, all things considered, is *a*." The latter term refers to "that set of considerations which move [the agent] to action." Ibid., 91. I collapse these distinctions under the rubric of a person's evaluational system.
25. I use the term "judgment" here and elsewhere to express the general idea of a process of reasoning; I do not intend it to have any special analytical significance.
26. This view parallels that of Faden and Beauchamp, *Informed Consent*, 242–48, who analyze informed consents and informed refusals of the competent patient as particular types of intentional actions. See also James F. Childress, *Who Should Decide? Paternalism in Health Care* (New York: Oxford University Press, 1982), 78, stating that "consent is an intentional act."
27. J. L. Austin, "Three Ways of Spilling Ink," *Philosophical Review* (October 1966): 438–39.
28. Ibid. Austin writes, "So with human activities; we can assess them in terms of intentions, purposes, ultimate objectives, and the like, but there is much that is arbitrary about this unless we take the way the agent himself did actually structure it in his mind before the event."
29. Ronald Dworkin, *Life's Dominion: An Argument About Abortion, Euthanasia, and Individual Freedom* (New York: Alfred A. Knopf, 1993), 224: "The integrity view of autonomy does not assume that competent people have consistent values

or always make consistent choices, or that they always lead structured, reflective lives."

30. Teno, Nelson, and Lynn, "Advance Care Planning," S34.
31. Terrie Wetle, "Individual Preferences and Advance Directives," *Hastings Center Report* 24, no. 6 (November-December 1994): S6. See also Linda L. Emanuel et al., "Advance Directives: Stability of Patients' Treatment Choices," *Archives of Internal Medicine* 154 (January 24, 1994): 209–17 (emphasizing the importance of stability of choices and alluding to Frankfurt's hierarchical model).
32. Harry G. Frankfurt, "Freedom of the Will and the Concept of a Person," *Journal of Philosophy* 68 (1971): 5–20; Harry G. Frankfurt, "Identification and Externality," in *The Identities of Persons*, edited by Amelie O. Rorty (Berkeley: University of California Press, 1976), 239–51; Gerald Dworkin, "Autonomy and Behavior Control"; Gerald Dworkin, "Autonomy and Informed Consent," in President's Commission for the Study of Ethical Problems in Medicine and Biomedical and Behavioral Research, *Making Health Care Decisions*, vol. III, 63–81. Frankfurt and Dworkin are concerned largely with developing a conception of autonomous persons, but their ideas can be applied readily to autonomous actions. Although neither uses the term *integrity*, their analysis is similarly grounded in the idea of reflective acceptance as a condition of autonomy.
33. Frankfurt, "Freedom of the Will," 8–10. The term *desire* is not intended to introduce a conceptual distinction among desires, values, preferences, and commitments. Authenticity theorists often use these terms synonymously.
34. Ibid., 11.
35. Ibid., 13, note 6.
36. Gabriele Taylor, *Pride, Shame and Guilt: Emotions of Self-Assessment* (New York: Oxford University Press, 1985), 113–14.
37. Gerald Dworkin, "Autonomy and Informed Consent," 71.
38. Ibid., 25. See also Taylor, *Pride, Shame and Guilt*, 114 (arguing that consistency of identifications that marks integrity includes seeing one's actions under a general description that expresses a pattern of what the person values, such as "helping others" or "being a good neighbor").
39. Taylor, *Pride, Shame and Guilt*, 114 (claiming more strongly that the persistently shallowly sincere person lacks any identity as an evaluating agent). Taylor makes the additional claim that someone who repeatedly acts contrary to his or her evaluations—who repeatedly acts out of character—is not a person of integrity because he or she does not manifest a consistency of identifications that evidences valuing something. Ibid., 117–19. Although this claim is intuitively plausible, it may go too far. Arguably, a person's core self-identification could be of the form, "I am the kind of person who thrives on new experiences and surprising others; acting 'out of character' is my true character." Or, as Robert Jay Lifton suggests in *The Protean Self: Human Resilience in an Age of Fragmentation* (New York: Basic Books, 1993), many of us may be proteans—shapeshifters whose essential self is regularly in a state of variation, adjustment, and transformation. Identifying a core protean self that remains stable over time may be difficult, yet the capacity for transformation, resiliency, and integrated change are consistent features of such a self. Related questions about integrity that are more directly relevant to decisions near the end of life arise with individuals who have recently undergone a significant upheaval and restructuring of core

commitments—for example, a recent conversion to a religious faith such as I discuss at the end of this chapter.
40. Ronald Dworkin apparently believes that decisions near the end of life occasion the kind of reflection about critical interests and death with dignity that are the hallmarks of integrity. Dworkin's focus, however, is on autonomous persons, and he offers no real analysis of what it means to act autonomously in particular instances.
41. Frankfurt, "Freedom of the Will," 16.
42. Ibid. Frankfurt states: "When a person identifies himself *decisively* with one of his first-order desires, this commitment 'resounds' throughout the potentially endless array of higher orders. . . . The decisiveness of the commitment he has made means that he has decided that no further question about his second-order volition, at any higher order, remains to be asked" (emphasis in original).
43. John Martin Fischer, "Responsibility and Freedom," in *Moral Responsibility*, edited by John Martin Fischer, 48. Fischer observes that conflicts between second-order desires logically must be resolved at a higher order. To simply stop the analysis at the second level is arbitrary; the problem of infinite regress cannot be avoided.
44. Adrian M. S. Piper, "Two Conceptions of the Self," *Philosophical Studies* 48 (1985): 176–77; Watson, "Free Agency," 94–95.
45. Note that the difficulty here lies in the conceptual framework of a hierarchical motivational structure. This issue is separate from the issue of whether decisions should be held to a standard of *full* considered reflective acceptance and *full* integrity to be worthy of respect.
46. Faden and Beauchamp, *Informed Consent*, 265.
47. Beauchamp and Childress, *Biomedical Ethics*, 123. For the most part, beyond generalized duties not to interfere with the liberty of others, the exercise of autonomy and correlative obligations to respect autonomy acquire real meaning only in the context of specific actions and choices. Although I believe that an intentionality view of prospective autonomy is important in other areas of the moral life, I do not expressly argue for this position. My concern is with advance care planning for end-of-life decisions.
48. This illustration is given by Faden and Beauchamp, *Informed Consent*, 265, in support of the same general thesis.
49. Bruce L. Miller, "Autonomy and the Refusal of Lifesaving Treatment," *Hastings Center Report* 11, no. 4 (August 1981): 27.
50. Emanuel, et al., "Advance Directives," 214. See also Wetle, "Individual Preferences and Advance Directives."
51. For discussion of this point, see Mark Siegler, "Critical Illness: The Limits of Autonomy," *Hastings Center Report* 7, no. 5 (October 1977): 13.
52. Miller, "Autonomy and the Refusal of Lifesaving Treatment," 24, also recognizes this concern: "It will not always be possible to label an action authentic or inauthentic, even where much is known about a person's attitudes, values, and life plans." This point is underscored by empirical studies (noted below) showing that proxies do not always reliably predict what patients would want—a task that is *less* problematic than confidently assessing a person's settled values and authentic choices.

53. Stability of preferences over time and reflective acceptance are not necessarily identical measures of integrity and authenticity. It is difficult to see the practical difference here, however, because indicia of instability invite the query, "Is this what the patient really wants?" and a search for evidence of identification with and reflective acceptance of the treatment decision at a deeper level of the self. Emanuel et al., "Advance Directives," 215 (claiming that patients' preferences should be stable over time and suggesting that Frankfurt's hierarchical model offers a way to understand whether a person has changed his or her mind). Modifying the integrity standard to require that treatment decisions be consistent with settled values and commitments over time does little to obviate the above difficulties. In short, this condition, like reflective acceptance, would render nonautonomous many advance directives, rests on uncertain empirical grounds, and invites suspect scrutiny of advance directives by paternalistic physicians at a time when the person who is uniquely qualified to make this judgment—the patient—cannot reliably do so. Faden and Beauchamp, *Informed Consent,* 266 (noting and rejecting this possible reformulation of an authenticity condition, and arguing that this revision would nonetheless "render nonautonomous many choices that are worthy of respect as autonomous").

54. Childress, *Who Should Decide?* 85 (discussing authenticity as a condition of contemporaneous autonomy).

55. Cases such as these are discussed in David L. Jackson and Stuart J. Youngner, "Patient Autonomy and 'Death with Dignity:' Some Clinical Caveats," *New England Journal of Medicine* 301 (August 1979): 404–408. See also Stuart J. Youngner and David L. Jackson, "Family Wishes and Patient Autonomy," *Hastings Center Report* 10, no. 5 (October 1980): 21–22.

56. The premise for this case was suggested by Robert Veatch. The facts, though hypothetical, are based in several respects on *In re Osborne*, 294 A.2d 372 (D.C. App. 1972), which was one of the early cases recognizing a Jehovah's Witness patient's right to refuse a life-saving blood transfusion. *Osborne* and other similar cases almost always have involved refusals of blood transfusions by competent patients.

57. Baruch Brody, *Life and Death Decision Making* (New York: Oxford University Press, 1988), 128–32. Brody presents a similar case in which the patient converted to the Jehovah's Witness faith less than one year previously and had verbally expressed her intent to refuse blood during a prior hospital admission. Brody's conclusion is that an appeal to consequences—primarily the benefit of saving life—should prevail in favor of the procedure and transfusion in question in this case.

58. For a summary of leading cases, see Norman L. Cantor, *Legal Frontiers of Death and Dying* (Bloomington: Indiana University Press, 1987), 22–24; see also Ruth Macklin, "The Inner Workings of an Ethics Committee: Latest Battle over Jehovah's Witnesses," *Hastings Center Report* 18, no. 1 (February/March 1988): 15–20 (describing development of institutional policy that includes recognition of the right of a Jehovah's Witness to refuse blood by means of an advance directive).

59. Of course, there is the option of seeking a court-ordered transfusion. For conscious patients who are ambivalent about the choice between faith and life, this approach has allowed the conflict of conscience to be reconciled on the ground that the transfusion was coerced and not chosen. The claim is that the transfusion was given "against my will" and that its receipt was not a sin. See

Macklin, "The Inner Workings of an Ethics Committee." This practical approach is not available here without violating Mr. G's autonomy and his moral and legal right to refuse treatment.
60. Note that if Mr. G also had written his testamentary will post-conversion, the law's response to a probate challenge would be similar. The court would not rest a judgment to overturn Mr. G's estate distributions on the authenticity of his expressed wishes, nothwithstanding the timing of his conversion. Judges do overturn testamentary wills, however, if the evidence shows that issuance of the document was coerced or otherwise nonvoluntary.
61. Childress, *Who Should Decide?* 64.
62. Tom L. Beauchamp, "Paternalism," in *Encyclopedia of Bioethics*, edited by Warren Reich (New York: Free Press, 1978), 1194–95; Childress, *Who Should Decide?* 102–03.
63. Jackson and Youngner, "Patient Autonomy and 'Death with Dignity.'"
64. Youngner and Jackson, "Family Wishes and Patient Autonomy," 21–22.
65. Youngner and Jackson reach a similar conclusion: "By postponing an irreversible decision until important issues can be clarified, physicians may not be violating the true autonomy of their patients." Ibid., 22.
66. This formulation slightly overstates the majority legal rule. The law of informed consent and the scholarly literature have been more interested in the physician's duty to disclose information about the risks, benefits, and burdens of treatment options than in what the patient actually understands—an emphasis that is attributable largely to the law's historical origins in lawsuits in battery or negligence that allege wrongdoing by the physician. Most courts have framed the physician's duty of disclosure in terms of what information would be material to the *average reasonable patient* under the circumstances—a patient-centered but not purely subjective standard. The leading case is *Canterbury v. Spence*, 464 F.2d 772 (D.C. Cir. 1972). Yet the issue of what information is material for a patient to understand (as opposed to what the physician must disclose) is a purely subjective question. Faden and Beauchamp, *Informed Consent*, 300–304, also use a subjective criterion of materiality in their analysis of the condition of understanding in the context of contemporaneous informed consent. On their view, to give informed consent (or refusal) the competent patient should substantially understand *that* he or she is authorizing that others provide (or not provide) treatment; and material information about his or her medical condition and the risks, benefits, and burdens of available treatment options sufficient to understand *what* is being authorized.
67. Note that the consensus around the commonsense view is not necessarily the same consensus about the moral weight of advance directives as I describe in chapter one. Recall that my analysis is grounded in an intentionality view of prospective autonomy that has received very little attention.
68. Rebecca Dresser, "Dworkin on Dementia: Elegant Theory, Questionable Policy," *Hastings Center Report* 25, no. 6 (November-December 1995): 34. Dresser goes on to briefly sketch a conception of understanding that is quite similar to the standard approach to informed consent.
69. Linda L. Emanuel, "What Makes a Directive Valid?" *Hastings Center Report* 24, no. 6 (November-December 1994): S27.
70. Cantor, *Advance Directives*, 25 (taking a similar position and describing advance directives as outcome-oriented).

71. The point here is descriptive; it is not intended as a statement of patients' substantive rights to refuse treatment, which have constitutional and common law bases that are independent of statutory recognition. As I note in chapter one, the law of many states is restrictive in its statutory limitation of the right to refuse treatment to conditions of terminal illness and permanent unconsciousness. Exceptions include Florida, New Jersey, and Oregon. Advance directive forms, especially those developed by organizations within the state, often mirror the statute on this point. Forms published and widely distributed by the New Jersey Bioethics Commission are among the few to encourage individuals to state what *terminal condition* means to them (suggested choices range from "I will die within a few days" to "I have a life expectancy of approximately one year"). They also give individuals the opportunity to identify conditions of incurable and irreversible but nonterminal illness and disease, such as Alzheimer's dementia or other progressive debilitating conditions, in which they would consider the burdens of continued life to outweigh its benefits. New Jersey Commission on Legal and Ethical Problems in the Delivery of Health Care, *Advance Directives for Health Care: Planning Ahead for Important Health Care Decisions* (Princeton: New Jersey Commission, 1991) (brochure).
72. N.J. Stat. Ann. 26:2H-55 (West 1996).
73. Further discussion of various options a person may wish to consider can be found in Robert M. Veatch, *Death, Dying and the Biological Revolution: Our Last Quest for Responsibility* (New Haven, Conn.: Yale University Press, 1989), 151–55, and Cantor, *Advance Directives*, 61–71. Some organizations have made available advance directive forms that are designed to facilitate decisions in accordance with a religious faith. Examples of so-called religious directives include The Rabbinical Assembly, Committee on Jewish Law and Standards, *Jewish Medical Directives for Health Care* (1994) (brochure containing a combined directive in the Conservative Jewish tradition); Agudath Israel of America, "Halachic Living Will" (form, 1990); and Center for Health Care Ethics, St. Louis University Medical Center, "Advance Directive for Future Health Care Decisions: A Christian Perspective" (brochure with forms in the Christian tradition, 1991).
74. Cantor, *Advance Directives*, 60. Cantor believes that specific instructions are important if they are material to the directive's author.
75. The literature on these and other practical aspects of advance directives is legion. A selection of valuable sources is Cantor, *Advance Directives*; Nancy M. P. King, *Making Sense of Advance Directives*, rev. ed. (Washington, D.C.: Georgetown University Press, 1996); Robert F. Weir, "Advance Directives as Instruments of Moral Persuasion," in *Medicine Unbound: The Human Body and the Limits of Medical Intervention*, edited by Robert H. Blank and Andrea L. Bonnicksen (New York: Columbia University Press, 1994), 171–87; Ezekiel Emanuel and Linda Emanuel, "Living Wills: Past, Present, and Future," *Journal of Clinical Ethics* 1 (spring 1990): 9–20; Joanne Lynn, "Why I Don't Have a Living Will," *Law, Medicine & Health Care* 19, no. 1–2 (Spring-Summer 1991): 101–04.

On the topic of physician-patient communication, see Dale G. Larson and Daniel R. Tobin, "End-of-Life Conversations: Evolving Practice and Theory," *Journal of the American Medical Association* 284, no. 12 (September 27, 2000): 1573–78 (summarizing the literature); Lawrence Markson et al., "The Doctor's Role in Discussing Advance Preferences for End-of-Life Care: Perceptions of Physicians Practicing in the VA," *Journal of the American Geriatrics Society* 45 (1997): 399–406; Jaya Virmani, Lawrence J. Schneiderman, and Robert M. Kaplan, "Relationship of Advance Directives to Physician-Patient Communication," *Archives of Internal Medicine* 154 (April 25, 1994): 909–913; Kent Davidson, Chris Hackler, Delba Caradine, and Ronald S. McCord, "Physicians' Attitudes on Advance Directives," *Journal of the American Medical Association* 262, no. 17 (November 3, 1989): 2415–19.

76. See generally "Dying Well in the Hospital: The Lessons of SUPPORT," *Hastings Center Report* 25, no. 6, supplement (November-December 1995): S1–S36. For a seminal discussion of the Values History, see Pam Lambert, Joan M. Gibson, and Paul Nathanson, "The Values History: An Innovation in Surrogate Decision-Making," *Law, Medicine & Health Care* 18 (Fall 1990): 202–12. The idea of using narrative stories as an aid to completing an advance directive is discussed in Rita Kielstein and Hans-Martin Sass, "Using Stories to Assess Values and Establish Medical Directives," *Kennedy Institute of Ethics Journal* 3, no. 3 (September 1993): 303–25. Extensive analysis of the problems associated with drafting advance directives and a proposal for making advance directives more effective instruments through careful draftsmanship is offered by Norman L. Cantor, "Making Advance Directives Meaningful," *Psychology, Public Policy, and Law* 4, no. 3 (1998): 629–52.

77. Linda L. Emanuel and Ezekiel J. Emanuel, "The Medical Directive: A New Comprehensive Advance Care Document," *Journal of the American Medical Association* 261, no. 22 (June 9, 1989): 3288–93. This article boldly proclaims that "the problems of existing living wills . . . can all be substantially relieved by the use of the Medical Directive" (3289).

78. In fact, the grid has two additional line items: one to indicate being undecided, the other to state, "I want a trial: If no clear improvement, stop treatment." These items raise more questions about the effectiveness of a directive than they answer, but we can set these added concerns aside.

79. Allan S. Brett, "Limitations of Listing Specific Medical Interventions in Advance Directives," *Journal of the American Medical Association* 266, no. 6 (August 14, 1991): 826.

80. I made these points in an earlier presentation of an outcome-oriented approach and critique of treatment-specificity in Robert S. Olick, "Approximating Informed Consent and Fostering Communication: The Anatomy of an Advance Directive," *Journal of Clinical Ethics* 2, no. 3 (Fall 1991): 181–95. One study has found that treatment-specific documents create precisely these sorts of dilemmas. The authors advise caution in refusing specific treatment modalities. Marion Danis et al., "A Prospective Study of Advance Directives for Life-Sustaining Care," *New England Journal of Medicine* 324, no. 13 (March 28, 1991): 882–88.

81. Many physicians with whom I have spoken feel strongly that advance directives should be clear and minimize uncertainty as much as possible. They also say that the Medical Directive is not the solution and that they would not offer this document to their patients. Their chief complaint is the document's dominant treatment-specific orientation—a complaint that can be generalized to other documents of different form that share this same orientation.

82. Some proponents of this feature of the reactionary view also appear to be motivated by the belief that to be legally effective, an advance directive must provide clear and convincing evidence of the patient's wishes. See Linda Emanuel, "Advance Directives: What Have We Learned So Far?" *Journal of Clinical Ethics* 4, no. 1 (Spring 1993): 9. As I argue in chapter one, this position simply misstates the law in the vast majority of states. Of course, we should aspire to

making advance directives as clear, convincing, and effective as possible. As Brett, "Limitations of Listing Specific Medical Interventions in Advance Directives," 827, notes, however, the further danger of promoting documents such as the Medical Directive as the "gold standard" is that "patients without advance directives or those who completed less complex documents may find themselves even more vulnerable to the imposition of unwanted life-sustaining measures."

83. Emanuel, "What Makes a Directive Valid?" S27. Dresser holds a similar position. See also King, *Making Sense of Advance Directives*, 58–60, noting and rejecting the claim that advance directives should mirror informed consent.

84. As Elster has noted, in the Kantian tradition "the first task of reason is to recognize its own limitations and draw the boundaries within which it can operate." He refers to "the irrational belief in the omnipotence of reason" as "hyperrationality." Jon Elster, *Solomonic Judgments: Studies in the Limitations of Rationality* (Cambridge: Cambridge University Press, 1989), 17.

85. Emanuel et al., "Advance Directives for Medical Care," 889.

86. See Larson and Tobin, "End-of-Life Conversations" (discussing barriers to end-of-life conversations and summarizing the literature). Markson and colleagues' survey of physicians' roles in advance care planning in the Veterans' Administration system found that systemic factors that make effective advance care planning discussions less likely include clinic scheduling policies (21 percent), productivity pressures (23 percent), and discontinuity of care (34 percent). James A. Tulsky et al., "Opening the Black Box: How Do Physicians Communicate About Advance Directives?" *Annals of Internal Medicine* 129 (1998): 441–49, found that conversations about advance directives averaged 5.6 minutes and rarely explored patients' values. Some physicians have suggested that they be reimbursed for the time they spend discussing advance directives with their patients, just as attorneys are paid for the same consultation with their clients. Linda Emanuel, "Structured Advance Care Planning: Is It Finally Time for Physician Action and Reimbursement?" *Journal of the American Medical Association* 274, no. 6 (August 9, 1995): 501–03. This recommendation is worthy of further study. Perhaps managed care plans should be required to adopt such a policy and to cover such consultations. Coupled with the assertion that effective directives are issued in consultation with a physician, however, the reactionary view would have us attach a fee to the exercise of the right to refuse treatment.

87. See generally *Jahrbuch fur Recht und Ethik/Annual Review of Law and Ethics* 4 (1996): 329–557, collecting papers from the Volkswagen Project on Advance Directives and Durable Powers of Attorney. For an example of a disease-specific document for patients with amyotrophic lateral sclerosis, see Robert S. Olick, "A Disease-Specific Advance Directive for Amyotrophic Lateral Sclerosis Patients," in that issue, 553–57. Documents expressly designed for patients on dialysis, with chronic obstructive pulmonary disease, and with HIV appear in Peter A. Singer, "Disease-Specific Advance Directives," *Lancet* 344 (August 27, 1994): 594–96.

88. This standard rationale for favoring the health care proxy appears in numerous sources, some of which I have cited in connection with the discussion of instruction directives. An especially good and extensive discussion is Robert Swidler, "The Health Care Agent: Protecting the Choices and Interests of Patients Who Lack Capacity," *New York Law School Journal of Human Rights* 6

(Fall 1988): 1–61 (focusing on New York's proxy law). It is worth noting that the law generally imposes few restrictions on a person's choice of proxy. One exception is that many states prohibit the patient's physician from simultaneously serving as the patient's proxy. The primary rationale for this limitation—the potential conflict of interest if the patient's wishes are contrary to the physician's best interests judgment—is straightforward. In practical terms, the patient must choose whether his or her physician will be physician or proxy. The validity of this limitation is challenged in Arti Rai, Mark Siegler, and John Lantos, "The Physician as a Health Care Proxy," *Hastings Center Report* 29, no. 5 (September-October 1999): 14–19.

89. Ezekiel J. Emanuel and Linda L. Emanuel, "Proxy Decision Making for Incompetent Patients: An Ethical and Empirical Analysis," *Journal of the American Medical Association* 267, no. 15 (April 15, 1992): 2067–71.

90. Much of this data concerns elderly patients and their families. See, e.g., R. F. Uhlmann, Robert A. Pearlman, and K. C. Cain, "Physicians' and Spouses' Predictions of Elderly Patients' Resuscitation Preferences," *Journal of Gerontology* 43, supp. (1988): M115–M121; Allison B. Seckler et al., "Substituted Judgment: How Accurate Are Proxy Predictions?" *Annals of Internal Medicine* 115 (1991): 92–98.

91. Peter M. Layde, Craig A. Beam, Steven K. Broste, et al., "Surrogates' Predictions of Seriously Ill Patients' Resuscitation Preferences," *Archives of Family Medicine* 4 (June 1995): 518–23.

92. Emanuel and Emanuel, "Proxy Decision Making," 2069.

93. Ibid., 2069–70.

94. Joanne Lynn, "Procedures for Making Medical Decisions for Incompetent Adults," *Journal of the American Medical Association* 267, no. 15 (April 15, 1992): 2082–84.

95. An opinion to the contrary is that it is better *not to* put specific treatment wishes in writing because the absence of a writing shields the proxy's decision from physician scrutiny on the ground that it does not represent what the patient would want. George J. Annas, "The Health Care Proxy and the Living Will," *New England Journal of Medicine* 324 (April 25, 1991): 1210–13.

96. Joel Tsevat et al., "Health Values of the Seriously Ill," *Annals of Internal Medicine* 122, no. 7 (1994): 514–20; Uhlmann, Pearlman, and Cain, "Physicians' and Spouses' Predictions of Elderly Patients' Resuscitation Preferences"; Seckler et al., "Substituted Judgment."

97. Joseph G. Ouslander, Alexander J. Tymchuk, and Bita Rahbar, "Health Care Decisions Among Elderly Long-Term Care Residents and Their Potential Proxies," *Archives of Internal Medicine* 149 (June 1989): 1367–72.

98. Hilde Lindemann Nelson and James Lindemann Nelson, *The Patient in the Family: An Ethics of Medicine and Families* (New York: Routledge, 1995), 90–95.

99. Letter from Ellen Friedland, attorney and consultant to the New Jersey Bioethics Commission, to Norman L. Cantor (December 1991), quoted in Cantor, *Advance Directives*, 56.

100. Often overlooked is that some persons with strong religious convictions may prefer to designate a rabbi or minister as their proxy to assure that decisions are made in accordance with their religious faith. A good example is the "Halachic Living Will" published by Agudath Israel of America, which allows

a person to designate his or her rabbi as proxy, with authority to decide in accordance with Orthodox Jewish law.

101. Ideally, the document also will designate one or more alternates in anticipation of the possibility that the primary designee will become unable or unwilling to serve in this capacity or for some reason will be unavailable. Anticipating the possibility of family disagreement or tension, some people consider giving proxy authority to two or more family members jointly. My own recommendation is that choosing one person to exercise this authority and directing that other loved ones be consulted is a better approach. These questions of strategy, however, do not speak to the core pattern of what makes for an effective proxy directive.

102. Robert M. Veatch, *A Theory of Medical Ethics* (New York: Basic Books, 1981), 210.

103. See Emanuel and Emanuel, "Proxy Decision Making," 2068 (summarizing objections to proxy decision making). More cynical voices contend that families have an inherent conflict of interest and that the presumption of trust should be reversed—or, more strongly, that families are morally disqualified from service as health care proxy.

104. John Hardwig offers a different critique of this view of health care proxies. Hardwig contends that the duty to follow the patient's wishes ought to be constrained by concerns for justice and fairness within families and that the proxy has a duty to those affected by end-of-life choices that should override the patient's wishes in cases of serious conflict. He also asserts that patient autonomy entails patient responsibility and that patients can abuse their autonomy by neglecting the interests of loved ones. John Hardwig, "The Problem of Proxies with Interests of Their Own: Toward a Better Theory of Proxy Decisions," *Journal of Clinical Ethics* 4, no. 1 (Spring 1993): 20–27. Hardwig's interesting proposal deserves greater attention. Under the theory of prospective autonomy presented here, the proxy's obligations are patient-centered and do not run to loved ones except as considered morally relevant by the patient. The theory would allow end-of-life choices that selfishly, but autonomously, disregard the interests of family members—a result Hardwig seeks to prevent.

Chapter Four

THE PROBLEM OF PERSONAL IDENTITY

Nancy Beth Cruzan

Most Loved

Daughter—Sister—Aunt

Born July 20, 1957

Departed Jan. 11, 1983

At Peace Dec. 26, 1990

From the headstone of Nancy Beth Cruzan [1]

> I can only wait for the final amnesia, the one that can erase an entire life, as it did my mother's.... You have to begin to lose your memory, if only in bits and pieces, to realize that memory is what makes our lives. Life without memory is no life at all.... Our memory is our coherence, our reason, our feeling, even our action. Without it, we are nothing.
>
> Luis Buñuel, Spanish filmmaker[2]

INTRODUCTION

For Nancy Cruzan's family and friends, the Nancy they once knew was lost after the motor vehicle accident that took her consciousness, leaving her in a PVS. Similar feelings of profound loss are experienced daily by families of people who have fallen prey to the ravages of Alzheimer's disease or the many other disorders that cause progressive, severe dementia. The loss of self, which sometimes is personally experienced by the patient, is most profoundly felt by family and loved ones whose anguish is captured only partially by the perception that Mom or Dad is no longer the person she or he once was.[3]

Pressing a philosophical turn to the personal and social insights of these two passages, a small group of commentators have suggested a deeper challenge to the theory of prospective autonomy. The moral authority of an advance directive, they argue, presupposes that the now-incompetent patient is the same person who previously authored that directive. For some patients, however, we cannot make this claim because incompetence brings a loss of psychological continuity and connectedness with the prior competent self, thereby destroying the conditions necessary for personal identity. We should conclude, the argument goes, that a prior directive has no moral weight in these instances because its author no longer exists, and the document has no moral (nor should it have legal) authority to govern treatment decisions for the *new person* or the *nonperson* that the incompetent patient has become.

Law professor Rebecca Dresser asserts that an incompetent patient "who is now a different person" should not "be burdened by a treatment decision consistent with the former person's preferences." She holds that the earlier person is "no longer in existence."[4] This radical and sweeping position, apparently also entertained by law professor John Robertson, links the question of personal identity with the claim that the competent person's interests do not survive loss of competence (discussed at length in chapter two) and purports to undermine the moral authority of a prior directive for the vast majority of incompetent patients (perhaps all).[5]

Philosophers Allen Buchanan and Dan Brock, who generally support advance directives, suggest that loss of psychological continuity with a former self diminishes the moral authority of advance directives for some— but by no means all—incompetent patients. Although Buchanan and Brock acknowledge that some cognitively impaired patients might be regarded as new persons, they appear to hold that loss of personal identity should be taken to diminish but not invalidate the moral authority of a prior directive for individuals who, in their view, have become nonpersons. The clear example is patients who, like permanently unconscious patients, have irreversibly lost all cognitive function and interactive capacity and thus have suffered such profound and permanent dementia as to no longer possess one or more characteristics necessary to the ascription of personhood.[6] Significantly, in contrast to the Dresser/Robertson view, Buchanan and Brock simultaneously hold that the personal identity objection is valid *and* that the self who authored the directive has interests in how he or she is treated that survive loss of personal identity. As we shall see, these dual commitments lead to a tortured argument that the author of a directive has surviving interests in what happens to the "nonperson successor" who inhabits his or her (former) body. These interests are considered to be akin to property rights but less weighty than the autonomy-based interests that are at stake when personal identity remains intact.[7]

My purpose in this chapter is to show why we should reject the *personal identity challenge* to the place of advance directives in deciding for incompetent patients, in all of its forms. Fortunately, we need not travel the thorny path of attempting to establish a definitive theory of personal identity. The critical analysis in this chapter is essentially moral, not ontological. As proponents of the personal identity argument themselves have done, I accept *arguendo* the psychological continuity view of personal identity over time; I then critique this position on its own terms. I accept, as have others, that arguments about public policy and our approach to decisions near the end of life are inherently moral arguments that can be judged on moral grounds.

Proponents of the psychological continuity thesis deny much of what is important in the account of autonomy as integrity and the importance we attach to taking charge of how we die. One ready response is to revisit the compelling moral case for honoring prospective autonomy and advance directives in the care and treatment of incompetent patients. In short, there is no good reason to reject the autonomy paradigm in favor of the personal identity alternative. Other commentators have made this case persuasively.[8] The discussion here goes a step further. I suggest several ways in which the theory of prospective autonomy implicitly acknowledges and might be grounded in a morally acceptable view of personal identity over time, though I do not attempt to justify these theories on ontological grounds.[9]

The central focus of my critical response lies elsewhere, however. As will become clear, the pivotal posit of the argument from personal identity is that in cases of psychological discontinuity with the past, the person who authored the directive no longer exists. The logical implication of this discontinuity, which supporters largely have ignored, is that death behavior is now appropriate. Yet the body of the severely demented patient still lives; indeed, according to defenders of the discontinuity thesis, it is now inhabited by a new and different self. Thus, the psychological continuity view is committed to a radical distinction between the death of the person and the death of the body—in stark contravention of our Judeo-Christian heritage in which declaration of a person's death triggers funeral and burial rites as integral components of the mourning process. As we shall see, this core premise is conceptually flawed. Its adoption as policy would necessitate morally unacceptable revisions of social institutions and practices.

Given the line of argument I follow here, we also need not establish the definitive conditions that are necessary and sufficient for the ascription of personhood (a debate with a long and contentious history in philosophy). This is not to say, however, that the distinction between new persons and nonpersons is irrelevant. Calling the patient a new person rather than a nonperson suggests that the former has a more significant moral status. For our purposes, however, this distinction is construed most usefully as a question about the strength of the patient's interests in continued life—including the capacity to experience pain and pleasure and to interact with others—that are the basis for that moral status, not as a metaphysical question about which patients satisfy the conditions for personhood. For this reason, I use the term *nonperson* narrowly to refer to permanently unconscious patients who are uncontroversially not persons. I take the term *new person* to refer to (severely) demented patients who retain some capacity for interaction with the world around them and hence have more significant interests in continued life, albeit truncated interests. The discussion touches on but does not engage the more contentious question of whether some severely demented patients have suffered such serious cognitive impairment that they have become nonpersons. To proceed with the analysis, we need not agree on where to place the line separating new persons and nonpersons—only that we agree *arguendo* that there is such a line.[10]

THE ARGUMENT FROM PERSONAL IDENTITY

Statement of the Argument

Modifying Buchanan and Brock's syllogistic formulation (in language but not in substance), we can state the *argument from personal identity* in the following way:

1. One person's advance directive has no moral authority to determine treatment decisions for another person.

2. Some patients suffer such severe and permanent neurological damage that psychological continuity is so disrupted that the person who issued the advance directive no longer exists.

3. The patient who has suffered such neurological damage is a different and new person (or a nonperson).

4. Therefore, the advance directive issued by the former, no longer existing, person has no moral authority to determine treatment decisions for the neurologically damaged patient who has become a new person (or a nonperson).[11]

The first premise is uncontroversial on its face. *Simpliciter*, one person has no authority to decide for another, absent role-relationships that confer that authority (physician-patient, proxy-patient, parent-child). The heart of the debate lies in premises 2 and 3, which we may call jointly the *discontinuity thesis*. We must first understand the underlying claim of these conjoint premises—namely, that psychological continuity is a necessary condition of personal identity.

Psychological Continuity and Personal Identity

Without undertaking the task of constructing the "correct theory" of personal identity—which would include a full account of necessary and sufficient conditions for personal identity over time—Buchanan and Brock accept for the sake of argument that "psychological continuity is (at least) a necessary condition for personal identity"; they note that the psychological continuity view is "widely held and well-supported in the philosophical literature."[12] They assert that psychological continuity is an essential feature of the *unity relation* that allows us to say that the stages of a person's life are stages of the *same* person's life. Applied to decisions near the end of life, to state that the life of the now-incompetent patient is a stage (part) of the life of the competent person who wrote an advance directive, that they are stages in the life of the same person, a condition of psychological continuity between the two "person life-stages" must obtain.[13] On this view, the fact that a seriously ill patient, Wilson$_2$, has the same body and brain as Wilson$_1$ of years ago (albeit a very much changed body) is not sufficient ground to hold that they are the same person. Physical (bodily) continuity over time may be a necessary condition of personal identity, but it is not a sufficient condition for personal identity.[14]

An obvious next question is, How much psychological continuity is enough for the preservation of personal identity? Before exploring that question and looking at the meaning of the personal identity thesis for decisions near the end of life, we need to give more content to the concept of psychological continuity and the thesis that psychological continuity is the defining feature of the unity relation between person life-stages. To do so, we can look to the work of Derek Parfit, who is widely regarded as the leading contemporary proponent of a psychological continuity thesis.[15]

To begin, we may see persons as agents in the world (essentially active) and as subjects of experience (essentially passive); both are true of our nature.[16] The theory of prospective autonomy emphasizes the former aspect of what we are. Thinkers who, like Parfit, take psychological continuity to be a necessary condition of personal identity over time tend to emphasize the latter and proceed from the presupposition that a person is a subject of experiences. What makes me the same person today as I was on March 24, 1996, is some important connection between experiences at these two points in time that justifies saying that I have had both experiences—that justifies calling both experiences *mine*. This connection should be located within the psychological states of the self who has these experiences, not externally from the point of view of others. For Parfit, personal identity over time necessarily involves or consists of two general relations: Psychological connectedness and psychological continuity. He states that *"psychological connectedness* is the holding of particular direct psychological connections." Psychological continuity over time is defined in terms of these connections: "Psychological continuity is the holding of overlapping chains of *strong* connectedness." Hence, psychological connectedness is "more important both in theory and in practice" because the presence of this connectedness is constitutive of psychological continuity.[17]

To explain what *psychological connectedness* means, it is useful to briefly contrast—as Parfit himself does—psychological continuity with an experience-memory theory of personal identity. What chiefly distinguishes Parfit's view of the meaning of psychological continuity from a straightforward experience-memory theory of personal identity such as that in the seminal writings of John Locke is the concept of "overlapping chains of memories" or of other psychological states such as intentions, beliefs, or desires. Under Locke's classic memory theory, there must be "direct memory connections" if we are to justifiably say that $Wilson_2$ today and $Wilson_1$ 20 years ago are the same person.[18] It follows from a strict application of this view that if $Wilson_2$ does not have memories of particular experiences of $Wilson_1$ 20 years ago, they are not one and the same person—a conclusion widely considered to be a major flaw in Locke's theory.[19] Parfit takes a different tack, which he sees as a response to this objection and a revision of Locke's theory. Psychological connectedness consists in overlapping chains of memories that are causally related in an appropriate way to a person's experiences and that persist over time:

> [E]ven if there are *no* such direct memory connections, there may be *continuity of memory* between X now and Y twenty years ago. This would be so if between X now and Y at that time there has been an overlapping chain of direct memories. In the case of most adults, there would be such a chain. In each day within the last twenty years, most of these people remembered some of their experiences on the previous day. On the revised version of Locke's view, some present person X is the same as some past person Y if there is between them continuity of memory.[20]

The concept of an overlapping chain of direct memories is meant to express a logically transitive relation between present and past experiences. In other words, if X is connected to Y and Y is connected to Z, then X is connected to Z. There need not be a direct connection between X and Z for psychological continuity to obtain. To illustrate the distinction, on a Lockean theory a patient suffering from amnesia or senile dementia who cannot remember particular past events, such as signing an advance directive, is not connected to this past self and has become a new person. On Parfit's view, a series of overlapping memories might supply the requisite connectedness of person life-stages. Connectedness and continuity also might be located in chains of beliefs that are held over time, even if Wilson$_2$ today does not hold the same beliefs as Wilson$_1$ 20 years ago and may not even remember having formerly held certain beliefs. Parfit's inclusion of other psychological states besides memory, such as intentions and beliefs, is an added revision of Locke's theory.

Note that the criteria of connectedness are not the same as criteria that commonly are applied to determine incompetence—a point of special relevance to treatment decisions. It is perfectly plausible that cognitive impairment resulting from serious illness might rob the person of the ability to properly perform the task of reasoning about medical information and choosing from among treatment options but leave intact enough chains of connected memories, beliefs, and so forth to preserve psychological continuity. Decisional incapacity and psychological continuity are concerned with different types of cognitive functions that are not necessarily co-extensive. This distinction is a serious problem for anyone who would broadly equate a break in psychological continuity with incapacity to make health care decisions.[21]

In sum, the unity relation (which Parfit calls Relation-R) that is constitutive of personal identity over time is the holding of these sorts of overlapping chains of connectedness of psychological states over time. Clearly, however, not all memories, beliefs, and intentions are held with equal strength. For example, it is common for a person to have many and vivid memories of important events from five years ago but fewer and weaker memories of less significant but more recent experiences. Connectedness is a matter of degree.[22] On the psychological continuity thesis, the unity of past and present stages in a person's life consists of possession of *enough* psychological connectedness over time; this connectedness is what matters in personal identity.

The next step is to determine how much connectedness over time is sufficient to establish continuity. In the context of end-of-life decisions, how strong must connectedness be to conclude that the incompetent patient and the author of a prior directive are the same person—or, conversely, that psychological continuity has been so disrupted as to warrant the conclusion that the incompetent patient is a new person (or nonperson)?[23]

How Strong Must Psychological Connectedness/Continuity Be?

Answering this query requires that we undertake two inquiries. The first is an evidentiary issue that raises concerns about whether we can make such judgments reliably. The second involves a moral judgment about where to place the threshold of continuity that sorts patients into two categories: those who are the same person they once were and those who have become new persons (or nonpersons).

With regard to the first point, there is good reason to doubt whether such determinations can be made accurately and consistently from patient to patient, at least in cases in which the patient retains some level of cognitive function. Parfit claims that psychological continuity requires overlapping chains of *strong* connectedness, but he does not explore how we are to distinguish strong connections from weak ones. In fact, he believes that "[s]ince connectedness is a matter of degree, we cannot plausibly define precisely what counts as enough."[24] Dresser, who relies heavily on Parfit's theory, notes that "[o]bservers will usually be unable to ascertain with accuracy the strength of connection between a patient's past and present selves when the patient has become unconscious or otherwise incapacitated."[25]

Buchanan and Brock are more optimistic. Although they note that psychological continuity is "inherently vague," they believe that appropriate lines can be drawn. One clear example is a permanently unconscious patient who has lost all capacity to have psychological states (but is not, under extant law, dead).[26] Whether the same is true of those with severe dementia, however, clearly is controversial. Although some thinkers believe that severe dementia destroys psychological continuity,[27] others note that even severely demented patients who are unable to communicate effectively may appear to maintain some continuity with their former selves.[28]

If end-stage dementia is taken to mark a loss of personal identity with the past, when has a patient deteriorated to this final stage? When the patient appears to live his or her life entirely in the present, with virtually no connection to the past? Sooner than this? The problem here is not simply conceptual, it is practical and empirical. No reliable criteria for measuring psychological continuity/connectedness in these gray areas exist.[29]

Setting these practical concerns aside, the personal identity argument demands that we choose a threshold level of continuity that is sufficient for personal identity. Doing so requires on one hand a judgment about the continuing moral status of formerly competent persons and their autonomy-based rights and interests. On the other hand, it calls for a judgment about the moral status of now-incompetent patients and their rights and interests. What is fundamentally at stake is a decision about whether to look to a patient's advance directive or to his or her current experiential interests in making treatment decisions.

If the threshold for preservation of psychological continuity (personal identity) is set high, there will be very few cases in which the conclusion that the incompetent patient and the author of the directive are the same person in the moral sense will be justified. Thus, there will be very few cases in which advance directives will be honored. Conversely, a low threshold will more often warrant the conclusion that the life of the formerly competent author of a directive and the life of the now-incompetent patient are stages in the life of the same person. Thus, many more advance directives will be honored. If we take seriously the psychological continuity view as a plausible metaphysical account of what matters in personal identity, further justification is still required to show why this view should inform revisions of existing policy and practice and a different approach to end-of-life decisions for at least some incompetent patients.[30]

Using degree of psychological impairment as an indicator, three logically distinct points on the continuum of psychological continuity might be candidates for such a threshold. The first and most *conservative* choice would be to set the threshold extremely low—at the point at which only permanently unconscious patients who have suffered the most severe neurological damage such that we can most confidently view them as (living) nonpersons, would be regarded as having lost personal identity.[31] A second stopping place on the continuum would be to extend the conservative criterion to bring within its reach demented patients who have suffered severe cognitive impairment but retain some limited mental functions, including capacities to experience pleasure and pain. These patients have more significant interests in what happens to them than those who are permanently unconscious. We can call this position the *extended conservative threshold*. This sort of middle threshold sets the line a bit higher; a prior directive would have no moral authority for a wider scope of patients than on the most conservative criterion, and this broader group of patients would include some (severely) demented patients. A third option would be to set the line even higher (the *high threshold* position), so that virtually all incompetent patients would no longer be considered the same person as their former selves.[32]

The fact that attempts to distinguish incompetent patients who have lost psychological continuity/connectedness with the past from those who retain it rest on highly uncertain empirical grounds is sufficient reason to reject this approach. Even strong advocates of the psychological continuity view are skeptical of attempts to define how much connectedness/continuity is enough for personal identity. Descriptively and metaphorically, a severely demented patient clearly is not the person he or she once was; he or she is a different (new) person. Until reliable and widely accepted criteria and methods for assessing psychological continuity/connectedness emerge (if ever), however, there is good reason to reject this position in all but the most clear-cut cases.

A related concern is that for all other patients, the discontinuity thesis extends to physicians (and others), who are reluctant to follow a patient's documented treatment refusal, an invitation to challenge a directive by observing that "he is not the person he once was." Any attempt to define as new persons a segment of the population suffering from a form of dementia in a way that attaches moral significance to these terms sanctions arbitrary judgments that invalidate advance directives and violate prospective autonomy. Only the most conservative continuity threshold survives these objections without controversy because PVS and irreversible coma can be diagnosed with a high degree of accuracy and certainty.[33]

In the remainder of this chapter I turn to a series of moral objections to the personal identity argument and show why we should reject this position in its entirety and in all its forms, including its most conservative application to permanently unconscious patients only. I emphasize that the continuity threshold marks the beginning of the new person (or the nonperson) and the end of the former person. The argument is not merely that the incompetent, new person and the formerly competent author of a directive are not the same person; the personal identity argument holds that the formerly competent person has ceased to exist. Recall the second premise of the syllogism: Psychological continuity is so disrupted that the person who issued the advance directive no longer exists.[34] If that is so, then social policy, practice, and behavior must respond appropriately to the moral status of new and former persons.

At the center of the argument that follows is the fact that, carried to the limits of its logic, the discontinuity thesis leads to the radical conclusion that the death of the person is a separate and distinct event from the death of the body. Acceptance of this view would require morally unacceptable revision of important social institutions and practices, including our understanding of family life and the family unit. In addition, centuries-old religious and cultural practices of funeral rites, burial, and mourning would be disrupted and, for many people, denied altogether. Furthermore, on the discontinuity thesis there is no meaningful place for respect for persons in the treatment of incompetent new persons whose person-lives begin as severely demented dying patients with no history of values, interests, or choices, nor for permanently unconscious patients who are simply nonpersons. The thesis readily lends itself to the treatment of these patients as if they were objects and wards of the state.

MORAL OBJECTIONS TO THE DISCONTINUITY THESIS

A Paradigm Scenario

A case scenario is helpful as a concrete point of reference for the discussion. Proponents as well as critics of the personal identity argument often appeal to cases of advanced dementia in which the patient previously has refused treatment but appears to have meaningful interests in continued life, albeit a severely diminished life.[35] Consider the following scenario:

Mr. S suffers from progressive Alzheimer's dementia, which was diagnosed 18 months ago—a few days after he celebrated his 55th birthday and 30th wedding anniversary (which are one week apart). Mr. S is an independent small businessman with a wife and two children; with years of hard work and dedication, he built a successful advertising agency and was able to send his children to the colleges of their choice. Mr. S is finding it increasingly difficult to greet members of his family by name and to remember that his family visited the day before, though he seems to enjoy their visits while they last. He is unable to engage in conversation about his business but has almost vivid memories of trips to Yankee Stadium and idolizing Mickey Mantle. He still seems to derive pleasure from watching baseball games on television, but he cannot tell a visitor who won last night's contest. As his illness progresses, Mr. S will soon reach the point at which his capacities for memory, intention, and other psychological states have been virtually destroyed by neurological damage, yet he will retain at least a basic perceptual awareness of the world around him. He is not in serious pain and does not appear to be suffering.

Assume a prior, effective advance directive that appoints Mrs. S as health care proxy and refuses life support "if I should be suffering from an advanced stage of Alzheimer's dementia." Assume further that the directive is based on conversations among Mr. S, Mrs. S, their children, and his personal physician and that Mr. S has expressed on numerous occasions the desire not to have his life artificially maintained should he suffer serious and irreversible mental and physical incapacity. His wishes are understood, and there is no discord within the family. If Mr. S becomes unable (perhaps unwilling) to eat and a feeding tube becomes necessary to sustain his life, should it be placed? If it has been started, should it be stopped?

Without question, these cases are among the most difficult in which decisions about life support must be made. Such cases pose genuine dilemmas and pull at our heart strings. Yet they also require a response, however uncomfortable. The foregoing case is constructed purposely with an effective advance directive in place to eliminate the question of whether prospective autonomy has been effectively exercised. (Indeed, the directive's language is exceptionally clear.) The question is whether the discontinuity thesis offers a morally preferable and conceptually coherent resolution of cases such as these.

I already have presented the moral case for Mr. S's advance directive. When Mr. S wrote his directive, he looked ahead and saw his life including a possible future of Alzheimer's dementia. He regarded this illness as a critical stage in a single unified life that is his to live and as an event in his life that will have a profound impact on others, most centrally his family. We see his life in the same way. On the theory of prospective autonomy, illness, incapacity, and death are all stages of a single unitary life. Mr. S is a person who has become demented, not simply a demented person. We should respond to him as a person with a past, a present, and a future that are connected in important ways and are uniquely his own—as a person with a history whose life is understood as involving goals, projects, and commitments, many of which are embedded in relationships with others.

Honoring Mr. S's advance directive honors his right and earned prerogative to exercise dominion over his life as a whole and recognizes the unity of his life and his right to shape the stages of *his* life.[36] First, this means recognizing his wife's authority to decide as his designated proxy. Second, it means honoring his refusal of life support in these circumstances. If Mrs. S should be ambivalent, it may well be because she honestly struggles to balance dual obligations to decide as her husband would and to do what is best for him while coming to terms with his final days.

When ambivalence turns to resolve and a decision to forgo a feeding tube is made, the family's "death watch" will begin. When Mr. S dies, his funeral and burial (or cremation) will be in accordance with his own preferences, and he will be remembered with love by family, friends, and colleagues for the full life he has had. The way he is remembered will be shaped in part by how he dies. Respect for Mr. S's advance directive honors his deeply felt desire for a dignified dying process that is controlled by and consistent with the values, beliefs, and character that have shaped his entire life.

For the discontinuity theorist, Mr. S's advance directive is irrelevant. We should resolve this case first by finding that Mr. S is a new person (presumably on the basis of one or more psychiatric consultations). From this finding flow the conclusions that his former self—the person who authored the directive—no longer exists and that the directive therefore has no moral authority and should be ignored. A decision about whether to place the feeding tube therefore will depend on how we evaluate Mr. S's current experiential interests in continued life. It also follows that the S family should be informed that Mr. S has died, even though his body is now inhabited by a new person, S_2.

Before turning to the fatal flaw of the discontinuity argument—the claim that Mr. S has died but that his body is now inhabited by a new person—it is worthwhile to probe more fully the question of the unity of a life over time. Indirectly, what proponents of the personal identity position allege is that the consensus view assumes rather than justifies the position that the self who authors the directive and the self who is now demented are selves at different stages of a single unitary life. The suggestion is that our commitment to prospective autonomy is conceptually flawed.

Although the bioethics literature has devoted scant attention to articulating a theory of personal identity *per se* in support of the moral authority of advance directives, it is wrong to suggest that such a theory cannot be developed and defended. In the following section, I briefly sketch several ways in which a theory of the unity of a life might be constructed in support of the prospective autonomy consensus. I do not attempt to offer a rigorous defense of any of these alternatives on ontological grounds; such an enterprise would require much more extensive analysis. Instead, the discussion is intended to show that the consensus is not conceptually flawed in the way its critics suggest—because one or more plausible theories of personal identity, each with more morally acceptable implications for policy and practice, can be supplied—and to make out a stronger case for the moral authority of advance directives. I then go on to directly critique the discontinuity thesis.

On the Unity of a Life

Parting company with the psychological continuity theorist, we might hold that bodily continuity is what matters in personal identity over time (or, at least, that bodily continuity is sufficient for identity). Bodily continuity is essential to being a living human being. As long as the same body is living, the same person is alive. When the body is determined to be dead, on the basis of either of the two legally recognized standards for declaring death (irreversible loss of cardiorespiratory functions or irreversible loss of all functions of the entire brain, including the brainstem), the person and his or her body are dead.

Bodily continuity is fundamental in the Judeo-Christian tradition that informs much of our religious and cultural understanding of death and death behavior. As William May has written, in this tradition "a man not only *has* a body, he *is* his body."[37] Death rituals presuppose that the person dies when the person's body is declared dead, not before, and that therefore it is fitting to bury (or cremate) the corpse. A modification of this view that gives greater voice to the place of cognitive capacities in what makes us distinctively human is suggested by thinkers who consider possession of the embodied capacity for social interaction to be essential to being a living human being. On this understanding—most clearly and forcefully articulated by Robert Veatch—the capacity for embodied consciousness over time provides the unity of a person's life. When that capacity is irreversibly lost, as it is for permanently unconscious patients, the person has died. Death should be declared, and the body should be released to the family.[38]

On either account, the death of the person and the death of the body are a unitary event. Thus, both positions are compatible not only with the consensus approach to termination of treatment but with traditional beliefs about death, mourning, and burial rites.[39] It may be that in philosophical circles a bodily continuity theory of identity (or variations thereof) no longer can be considered the "majority" position. As will become more clear, however, there are good moral, social, and practical grounds for maintaining commitment to this understanding for the purposes of legal and moral judgments about when death has occurred.[40]

Implicit in the theory of prospective autonomy is another sort of conception of the unity of a life. Recall our dual nature as subjects of experience and as moral agents. Rather than focus on the former, we can focus on the latter aspect of our natures. From this standpoint, we can construct an alternative description of what it means to identify having desires, intentions, beliefs, plans, relationships and so on as mine, as parts of a single, perduring self. Through this lens, choosing one action over another is intelligible only on the presupposition that not only what I do is chosen by my self at a given moment but that it will have consequences for this same self immediately and in the future.

I drive to work each morning because I have a job and a family and am invested in my professional projects. The trip to work is intelligible for these reasons. Why should I rise each morning and labor through the day if I will be a different person at the end of the day; if my weekly paycheck goes to the bank account of a future person who is not me; or if my pension, savings, and investments will benefit a future person who is not me? In short, investing in a possible future presupposes that I will continue to be the same person in that future. Creating a syllabus for a semester course, writing this book, and planning a family vacation upon its completion make sense because I project a unity of self between present and future. The point becomes more compelling when we consider pursuit of our critical interests and projects that ordinarily demand substantial investment over many years. As Korsgaard argues, "In choosing our careers, and pursuing our friendships and family lives, we both presuppose and construct a continuity of identity and of agency."[41]

In one sense, this argument is about the intrinsic nature of human persons. It also is a practical argument, however. A rational presupposition of life's activities—in particular, the exercise of prospective autonomy—is that what I do today has implications for a future self that will be me. Without this presupposition of unity, many of the things we do in pursuit of a good life (or simply a life) would not be intelligible. As Bernard Williams writes, "That a man should have some interest now in what he will do or undergo later, requires that he have some desires or projects or concerns now which relate to those doings or happenings later."[42] That a future person will be me and not someone else inhabiting my body is good reason to care about the future. More strongly, from the standpoint of practical reason, this presupposition is necessary to make sense of having and pursuing life plans. Moreover, to the extent that many present actions anticipate a possible future, connectedness to a future self may be a necessary condition for the unity of a single self in the present.[43] When I plan for a future knowing that I will undergo changes such as serious illness and incapacity, the present project of issuing advance care instructions makes sense only if I understand those changes as belonging to *my* life.[44]

Similar themes resonate in Alasdair MacIntyre's conception of the unity of a life as "the unity of a narrative embodied in a single life."[45] Rather than see ourselves as subjects of experience, we can see ourselves as subjects of a history (past, present, and future) in which choices, actions, and relationships play a central part. What binds the various stages of a person's life is a narrative that makes that life intelligible. That narrative must include the aspect of our natures that involves moral agency. On one hand, the intelligibility of an individual's life story presupposes that its chapters are part of the life of the same person and thus presupposes personal identity over time. On the other hand, however, we cannot make sense of the stages of a person's life without a story. Hence, narrative, intelligibility, and personal identity are said to exist in relationships of mutual presupposition. We cannot speak exclusively of one without the others. To understand personal identity over time independently of a narrative that provides intelligibility, as proponents of the psychological continuity view would have us do, is to leave out something important.[46]

This account also is consonant with two other important features of the way we ordinarily see the unity of a person's life. Most of us live our lives embedded in various social relationships. Indeed, in significant ways family life involves not just a collection of individuals pursuing their respective life projects but a conception of a possible shared future.[47] The story of a person's life that binds an individual's person-stages into a narrative of a single life can be told from the point of view of others, especially families. It does not depend on the conscious ability to tell one's own story—through memory, experience, and so forth—reflectively or to others. If I suffer serious illness, the fact that this illness is an event in my life is seen and related through the eyes of others even if I am unable to consciously articulate the same connection. Moreover, because my life is connected in important ways to the lives of others, my narrative is a part of their narrative. My terminal illness is not just an event in my life; it is an event in the lives of family and friends as well. And how I die is a part of the story of my life and theirs.[48]

To summarize, there is an initial choice to be made concerning which aspect of our nature—that of being moral agents or being subjects of experience—will ground how analysis of the unity of a life unfolds. There is no decisive normative reason to consider one aspect of our nature more fundamental than the other.[49] Proponents of the personal identity challenge to advance directives posit that what matters in the unity of a life starts from the premise that we are subjects of experience. A strong—indeed compelling—argument can be made, however, that it is a rational presupposition of the moral life that my actions have meaning for a future person who will still be me and that our lives as moral agents would not be intelligible without this presupposition. An account of personal identity over time that is grounded in moral agency of the sort depicted (but by no means fully developed) here resonates with centrally important themes of the moral life. It also explains and justifies time-honored and considered judgments about the lives of persons, about the value of prospective autonomy, and about our obligations to respect persons' surviving interests and their quest for death with dignity that are pillars of the consensus. Like an embodiment view, this account is entirely compatible with the understanding that the death of the person and legal determination of death of the body are the same event.[50]

In the following sections, I directly critique the personal identity challenge, offering additional reasons why it fails to provide a plausible and persuasive alternative. As Buchanan and Brock themselves acknowledge, the discontinuity theorist bears a heavy burden of persuasion if we are to change the consensus approach to decisions near the end of life on the basis of the psychological continuity account.[51] The argument that proponents of this position fail to carry this burden centers primarily on three points. First, the central premise of the discontinuity thesis—that the author of the directive no longer exists—entails the morally unacceptable conclusion that the death of the person occurs before (perhaps well before) the death of the body. Acceptance of this premise would require radical revision of a range of existing social institutions and practices. Second, the discontinuity thesis cannot offer a satisfactory explanation of the place of surviving interests and surviving obligations in making decisions for incompetent patients who have, proponents argue, become new persons. Third, the further consequence of the argument—unintended by its proponents—is that new persons and nonpersons should be regarded as wards of the state divorced from a personal history, family, and relationships with others—who may therefore be treated, in effect, as property.

The Newly Dead

Assume that we were to embrace the extended conservative threshold view of personal identity in policy and practice and that prior to the time when a feeding tube becomes necessary, Mr. S is determined to have lost connectedness and continuity with his former self. Any concern for his advance directive—for Mr. S's own values, interests, and beliefs about how or when he would die—has been extinguished. If Mr. S had insisted instead on continued treatment, perhaps out of deeply held convictions about the sanctity of life, these values also would be undermined. The attending physician's responsibility is to declare Mr. S dead and inform Mrs. S and her children that he has died.[52] Ordinarily, bereavement and death behavior would begin. Yet there can be no funeral. The body of Mr. S cannot be buried because it is still living and breathing, even engaging in rudimentary forms of communication. (Again, we can refer to the new S as S_2.) What sort of grieving process are family and friends to have at this point?

Defining Mr. S as newly dead redefines the death of the person as a separate event from the death of the body. This definition may have some intuitive appeal in a metaphorical sense. The S family has most likely come to regard Mr. S as a different person than he once was. Yet they see him as a loved one who has become demented and who continues to occupy the same body he has always had, the ravages of illness notwithstanding. There is a powerful reason for this state of affairs. In the Judeo-Christian tradition, the individual and the body are integrally and inseparably connected. Traditional death rituals rest in large measure on the understanding that the death of the individual and the death of the body are a unitary phenomenon: "[T]he funeral service (which includes fitting disposition of the corpse) presupposes and reinforces a certain continuity between the person [and] his mortal remains."[53] It further presupposes and reinforces a continuity with the family unit. Social recognition of this unity grounds the family's right to provide for fitting disposition of the corpse. Moreover, recognition of the family's rightful place in shaping the funeral and burial and in otherwise determining how the corpse will be treated (ordinarily in a fashion that honors the deceased's own wishes) holds a central place in the family's process of social and psychological detachment, mourning, transition, healing, and return to the larger community.[54]

The discontinuity thesis flies in the face of these time-honored religious and cultural norms. In fact, it is not clear that Mr. S's family will ever be able to physically bury his body. Presumably, what the law calls Mrs. S's "quasi-property right" that entitles her to release and custody of her husband's body has been extinguished with his loss of personal identity. After all, S_2 is a new person. Not only is he still living, he is not married to Mrs. S. She became a widow when Mr. S, the former self, died. If Mrs. S wants to go to the bedside to see the body of her former husband, her request might be granted as a courtesy, but it is no longer her right (she is not Mrs. S_2). The same is true for family and friends.

To amplify: Suppose Mr. S is Jewish, and suppose further that he and his family take seriously the mandate of Jewish law that the body must be buried within 24 hours of death (unless that would fall on the Sabbath or a holiday). His family knows him as a Jew and knows that these beliefs are important to who he has been and how he will be remembered. Are we simply to say to the S family and all other families whose beliefs and practices command a funeral, burial, and other death rituals that the body must remain in the hospital because it is now S_2 and not S at all? [55]

Ex hypothesi, the new system would dishonor Mr. S's religious beliefs but honor the beliefs of those for whom death of the person and death of the body correspond—such as victims of sudden heart attack or a fatal accident—and those whose death from illness and disease comes before loss of psychological continuity. Thus, not only does the proposed redefinition of death stand in bald contradiction of traditional religiously and culturally based beliefs and practices defining appropriate death behavior, it also would commit us to unequal respect under the law for those cherished beliefs and practices. There is no good reason to wreak havoc with religious and cultural freedoms that are so deeply embedded in our social fabric.[56]

Other interrelated legal institutions and rules that concern time of death also would be affected, some more substantially than others. Perhaps Mr. S's testamentary will could be read and his property and assets distributed to his next of kin. Family law could be modified to make clear that S's family is not the family of S_2. Life insurance contracts could be revised to conform to this new definition of death. No doubt changes in estate tax laws would quickly follow suit. Some mechanism also could be developed to continue to pay S_2's health care costs because S's health coverage expires with his death. (Perhaps, as I discuss further below, new persons who have no other legal relations would now be the responsibility of government under the Medicare/Medicaid programs.)

If transition to this new system has the appearance of relative ease, it is only because talk of enacting new legal rules oversimplifies what is at stake. All of these rules and practices presuppose a legal definition of death. All depend in important ways on the closure that comes with a funeral, burial, grieving, and other behavior that follows the declaration of death. It is difficult to imagine redefining death to trigger all of these legal mechanisms while denying loved ones a crucial means of closure. The cost of doing so would be a substantial sacrifice of human compassion and decency. [57]

As the President's Commission for the Study of Ethical Problems in Medicine and Biomedical and Behavioral Research noted in its report *Defining Death*, society has a strong interest in a uniform, reliable legal standard of death. Any change in that legal standard has substantial societal implications.[58] Proponents of the discontinuity thesis suggest a radical redefinition of death that is neither uniform nor reliable. Moreover, the discontinuity thesis ignores deeply held values and beliefs about when and how we should die and when appropriate death behavior should begin. Adoption of this thesis would necessitate substantial restructuring of important social, cultural, and religious institutions, practices, and values—all premised on a stark distinction between the death of the person and the death of the body.

To illustrate the magnitude of the potential impact, researchers have estimated that more than 2.4 million patients in the United States suffer from severe dementia—a number that is projected to increase to 7.4 million by the year 2040.[59] This statistic says nothing of the thousands, perhaps millions, of other patients who are afflicted with less severe forms of dementia but arguably have become new persons. Moreover, these numbers only suggest the potential implications for the much wider circle of families, friends, and colleagues of patients with severe dementia. There are no compelling reasons to follow this road, and many good reasons not to.

Proponents of the discontinuity thesis might respond to this critique by adducing other prudential reasons to continue to give individuals and families special say in our response to the dead and the disposition of dead bodies—that is, to grant families a privileged place at the bedside of the new person-patient. As I have suggested, perhaps other institutions and practices—such as various forms of insurance, reading of the deceased's will, and so forth—could be modified accordingly. I do not attempt to construct this line of supplementary argument here, but I note that it would bear a heavy burden of justification. More important to the present discussion, the challenge for proponents of the discontinuity thesis is to show why we should give *any* moral weight to the claims of former persons and/or their families, while maintaining that former persons (and by implication their families) have no special claim to this authority—the central posit of the discontinuity thesis. Buchanan and Brock suggest a way out of this puzzle by drawing our attention to the claims of a (former) person's interests that survive loss of personal identity. In the following section, I argue that this attempt at reconciliation is flawed. Although the discussion is concerned with the place of surviving interests in treatment decisions for *living* new persons, the conceptual analysis is equally applicable to the question of our response to the newly dead.

Treatment of New Persons: Surviving Interests and Obligations

Proponents of the discontinuity thesis must respond to the argument that Mr. S's directive embodies interests and imposes obligations that survive loss of psychological continuity. It would be logically consistent to assert that if the author of a directive no longer exists, the interests of that former person as embodied in the directive also have been extinguished. Mr. S has no surviving interests when neurological damage destroys the person he once was. This position—advocated by Dresser and Robertson—is untenable, however. In chapter two I argue that our critical interests in what happens to us in dying and in death survive the ravages of severe cognitive impairment and death itself. I also argue that obligations to the formerly competent person survive in the same way. I have bolstered that account by briefly articulating several alternative understandings of what is important in personal identity over time, which easily accommodate the concepts of surviving interests and obligations.

The claim that S_2 is a new person does nothing to support the erroneous insistence that critical interests and obligations do not survive and do not matter. The real issue is how the relative weight due critical surviving interests and experiential interests shape our obligations to the now-incompetent patient. Once the question is construed as one of balancing interests, the concept of personal identity and the discontinuity thesis do nothing to advance the analysis and only confuse it. Talking about critical interests and experiential interests as interests of the same person and talking of corresponding obligations as obligations to the same person simply makes more sense. The discontinuity thesis serves only as a misguided makeweight effort to deny the fact and importance of surviving interests and obligations.

Buchanan and Brock see the problem differently. They attempt to reconcile the position that some interests survive death with the claim that personal identity matters in such cases. Their argument proceeds roughly in the following way. Surviving interests cannot be construed as rights of *self*-determination because this self no longer exists. We should hold, they argue, that the former self has a "right of disposal" over "what is to happen to one's living, nonperson successor"—a right we can conceive "as something like a property right in an external object." This right of disposal asserts interests in treatment decisions for the new person (nonperson) as well as interests in disposition of the dead body.[60]

Buchanan and Brock's main point is to distinguish the *self*-determination interest of a self in what happens to that same self (person) from the interest a self has in what happens to "a thing that is not only not that self, but not a person at all." The former interests have greater moral weight than the latter.[61] This distinction is intended to show that not all instances of self-determination have equal weight and to argue that although a best interests analysis must take surviving interests into account, "not all surviving interests are of equal weight."[62] A further concern is to lay some of the groundwork required to assert that the just claims and interests of others justifiably might take precedence over these surviving interests—for example, to prolong life (presumably contrary to the terms of a prior directive) for the purpose of organ retrieval for the benefit of others.

Speaking of a right of disposal may make sense in some contexts, such as disposition of a dead body for burial (recall Mrs. S's quasi-property right in her husband's body), but use of this concept here amounts to philosophical gerrymandering. The core premise of the discontinuity thesis is that destruction of psychological connectedness/continuity means the ending of one person's life and the beginning of another's. One person, proponents of the thesis argue, has no moral authority to decide the medical fate of another different person (or nonperson). If this thesis is so, as the author of a directive I should not have *any* right to control treatment choices for a self that now inhabits my body but is *not me*. By whatever name, a so-called right of disposal must admit some morally relevant connection between the person who holds this right and the individual whose life is affected by its exercise. Proponents of the personal identity thesis cannot plausibly allow this connection without violating the core premise that severs it.[63]

The same conclusion follows from the discussion of a person's relationships with others. It is hard to see why this right of disposal should be held by a proxy or by family members. These relationships were established with the former self who has died, not with the new person whose person-life began with the destruction of identity with a former self. We sometimes regard family members as custodians of seriously ill and dying loved ones, and law and society have long recognized the family's rights to control disposition of the body of a deceased loved one. The basis for this custodial relationship and this right, however, is the family relationship, and this family relationship presupposes that a person is the same person—morally and legally—until burial.[64]

Furthermore, if the concern is to allow that an advance directive might be justifiably overridden to avoid undue harm or secure an important benefit, it is far from clear why such a tortured analysis is required.[65] It is far more plausible to recognize the duty to take seriously the autonomy-based *and* experiential interests of a person with a past, present, and future (albeit brief and dim) and to hold that these interests must be balanced in appropriate cases with the just claims of others who might suffer harm if a directive is followed or benefit if it is overridden. That there is a balance to be struck presupposes that surviving critical interests and current experiential interests are interests of the same person (or interests of selves that are stages in the life of the same person). Depending on the weight assigned to competing interests, respect for patient autonomy might yield to more weighty claims of others, such as potential organ recipients. Holding that the claims of others should be balanced against the rights of disposal that belong to a self (or his family) that no longer exists but whose body is now occupied by a new person merely confuses the issue.[66]

Treating New Persons as Persons

I argue in chapter two that once the incompetent patient is stripped of his or her past values, interests, and expressed wishes, we cannot maintain that basing treatment decisions on the patient's current experiential interests treats the patient as a person. To regard S's advance directive and the interests it embodies as irrelevant is to deny the profound significance of moral agency and authorship of a complete life, divorcing S from his historicity and reducing him to a subject of experiences. The current interests approach dehumanizes and objectifies the life of incompetent patients.

This objectification is even more stark on the discontinuity thesis. The successor new person S_2 has no personal history. His person-life begins as a severely demented dying patient whose life will be extremely short. He has no family, no friends, no one who has been a part of his life and is able to act on his behalf in a way that takes a personal history into account. Respect for autonomy and respect for the person that he was and is has been reduced to the question of what obligations are owed to a dying patient with truncated interests in continued life who has no past (other than that of being a dying individual), no relationships, no future. According S_2 the status of new person identifies him as the bearer of some rights (which presumably can be exercised on his behalf by a court-appointed guardian, if needed). It also connotes that we owe S_2 certain obligations, among them obligations to alleviate pain and suffering and to preserve function and opportunity for experiences that appear to have meaning and enjoyment for him.

We might hold (as Dresser and Robertson do) that we should sustain life as long as the patient retains some relational capacity and doing so would not impose significant pain or discomfort on the patient. Certainly there would be the hypothetical obligation to provide any new treatments or procedures that hold the promise of significant reversal, even cure, of dementia. Calling S_2 a new person, however, and embracing a best interests approach hardly rescues the discontinuity thesis from the charge that S_2 and all others like him have become merely subjects of experience, totally separated from a past life that ordinarily gives meaning and intelligibility to the patient as a person and allows us some insight into who he is. Without any narrative of the prior stages of S_2's life, it is difficult to see how respect for persons even enters the equation.

This concern is magnified when we pause to consider that new persons will be wards of the state. After all, their person-lives have just begun, and they have no family. It follows that health care coverage is now fully state-funded under Medicare or Medicaid (if that is not already the case). Without intending to be coarse, the discontinuity thesis opens the door to a radically different conception of severely demented patients than its proponents appear to intend. Pressed to the limits of its logic, it might hold that severely demented, irreversibly dying wards of the state are (quasi?) property of the state. After all, autonomy no longer functions as a constraint on what others may do to the patient, including under the guise of state authority.

Consider, for a moment, that the new definition of death would throw into turmoil our entire approach to organ donation, retrieval, and transplantation. On the discontinuity thesis, Mr. S cannot be an organ donor because he has no right to control disposition of the body now inhabited by his successor. Nor can consent be obtained from the family whose rights have similarly expired. By the time S_2 is near death and becomes a viable candidate for organ retrieval (assuming this is a medical option in his case), it will be up to the state (or, perhaps, the hospital, presumably based on recognized legal authority) to decide in the exercise of the right of eminent domain whether organs will be harvested. It also will be up to the state or its agents—again, presumably acting through promulgated laws—to dispose of the dead body. (Again, proponents of the discontinuity thesis might offer other arguments for privileging family control over the dead body, including for purposes of organ donation. They cannot rely, however, on the claim that S has surviving interests in what happens to S_2 without falling into inconsistency.)

In sum, one cannot plausibly maintain that in reducing severely demented patients to mere subjects of experience the discontinuity thesis respects severely demented new persons as persons. By contrast, precisely because the consensus approach sees the patient as a person who has become demented—as a person for whom a past competent self and a present incompetent self are stages in the life of a single person— it can honor the principle of respect for persons.

Permanently Unconscious Nonpersons

One must grant that patients who have suffered permanent and irreversible loss of cognitive functions and are no longer able to interact with their environment have ceased to be psychologically connected to their former selves. Furthermore, PVS and irreversible coma can be diagnosed reliably, with a highly accurate prognosis.[67] Thus, practical objections to the psychological continuity view are not applicable here.[68] Nonetheless, there are good reasons to reject the most conservative threshold of continuity.

On the psychological continuity view, a permanently unconscious patient is a living human being but not a person. Again, there is a choice between regarding the patient as a person who has become irreversibly comatose or simply as someone who is irreversibly comatose. If we regard him as someone whose life as an irreversibly comatose patient has just begun, many of the foregoing objections hold here as well. By separating the death of the person from the death of the body, this policy and practice would do serious violence to longstanding religious and cultural traditions. The S family is expected to engage in appropriate death behavior but has no body to bury. In fact, PVS patients can live for many years, even decades, with appropriate life support. When does the bereavement process end?

Proponents hold that once diagnosis and prognosis have been reliably confirmed, treatment should be discontinued, and the patient should be allowed to die.[69] They argue that a permanently unconscious patient has no relational capacities and no interests in continued life; nor do we have obligations to sustain the biological life of a patient who can derive no benefit from that life. Some proponents have supported this position by asserting that this result does not offend a person's prior values and advance directive because the vast majority of people would refuse life support if they were permanently unconscious.[70]

It is not entirely clear why a discontinuity theorist would want to make this claim; the posit of the argument is that prior values are irrelevant. This claim also is factually inaccurate, however. Termination of treatment would still offend the values of people who hold dear a commitment to the sanctity of life and believe that life has value and should be sustained at all costs. This reaction also is not the only potential response to the permanently unconscious patient. Again, given that the patient is now a nonperson ward of the state with no history, no family, and no interests in what happens to him or her, we might instead hold that before we terminate life support we should salvage any viable organs for transplantation or harvest tissue (perhaps DNA samples) for medical research. As with severely demented patients, autonomy has no place as a constraint. Respect for persons does not apply because the permanently unconscious patient is a nonperson who has never been a person. Moreover, because permanently unconscious patients have no capacity to experience pain or suffering, prohibitions against doing harm also seem to offer no moral constraints on how we should treat the vegetative body. Thus, the discontinuity thesis opens wide the door to treating these wards of the state not as mortal remains but as organ banks for the benefit of others. On the other hand, it takes little imagination to see that if we understand the patient as a person who has become permanently unconscious, continuation of life support for the benefit of others when the person finds a vegetative existence to be intolerable would be a horrible offense to that person's life.

The contention is not that shifting the current presumption in favor of life that governs treatment of a permanently unconscious patient, absent patient or family refusal, is necessarily bad policy. Such an assertion would require much more extensive argumentation. Some proponents have argued on grounds of justice that law, policy, and practice should reverse the presumption in favor of treatment, claiming that health care resources ought to be used to serve the interests of others in need.[71] Others take the position that there simply is no obligation to provide futile care in such cases.[72]

Any movement in this direction, however, should continue to recognize—as most people do—that the permanently unconscious patient is still the same person as in the past. By doing so, we continue to recognize that family members have a proper place at the bedside during care and treatment and that when death is declared, the body is to be released to them for burial. Holding firm on this point makes sense of proposals to carve out an exception to a new rule that reverses the presumption—one that honors prior autonomy and moral and religious values by allowing patients who cling dearly even to vegetative life or do not want to donate their organs (perhaps believing that the body should be buried as a whole) to "opt out."[73] Maintaining our current understanding of the unity of a person's life undergirds the fundamental premise that my body is my property (and my family's), not the property of the state and community. These options are not open to the discontinuity theorist, who must remain committed to a temporal disjunction between the death of the person and the death of the body—and the morally unacceptable conclusions that follow.[74]

CONCLUSION

Proponents of the argument from personal identity deny much of what is important in the moral life and much of what is important in the living of a full and unitary life. They cannot adequately account for the value we attach to surviving interests and obligations that is manifest in the exercise of prospective autonomy and the pursuit of death with dignity. Expanded to the limits of its logic, the discontinuity thesis posits a stark separation of the death of the person from death of the body and calls for radical revision—indeed, a rejection—of time-honored, deeply held religious and cultural values and practices concerning death and appropriate death behavior. Furthermore, by treating incompetent "new persons" as mere subjects of experience, divorced from any personal history, this view not only fails to respect the patient as a person, it suggests precisely the opposite—that severely demented patients should be seen as property of the state. The most conservative continuity threshold, under which only permanently unconscious patients would be considered to have lost continuity with their former selves, does not escape these criticisms. For all of these reasons, even if agreement could be reached on clear and reliable criteria for determining when a patient has ceased to be connected to the former self who authored a directive (itself a dubious proposition), the argument from personal identity should be rejected in its entirety.

NOTES

1. A picture of Nancy Beth Cruzan's headstone with this inscription appears on the cover of the *Bioethics Forum* 11, no. 3 (Fall 1995).
2. Luis Buñuel, *My Last Sigh*, trans. Abigail Israel (New York: Alfred A. Knopf, 1984), 4–5.
3. David H. Smith, "Seeing and Knowing Dementia," in *Dementia and Aging: Ethics, Values, and Policy Choices*, ed. Robert H. Binstock, Stephen G. Post, and Peter J. Whitehouse (Baltimore: Johns Hopkins University Press, 1992), 46.

4. Rebecca Dresser, "Life, Death and Incompetent Patients: Conceptual Infirmities and Hidden Values in the Law," *Arizona Law Review* 28 (1986): 379–81. See also Rebecca Dresser, "Relitigating Life and Death," *Ohio State Law Journal* 51 (1990): 432 (defending the claim that a living will may express the wishes of a different person from the now-incompetent patient).
5. This position is suggested in Rebecca S. Dresser and John A. Robertson, "Quality of Life and Non-Treatment Decisions for Incompetent Patients: A Critique of the Orthodox Approach," *Law, Medicine & Health Care* 17, no. 3 (Fall 1989): 236–37. This more radical view of who has lost personal identity and become a new person emerges because of the way these authors link with personal identity theory their reliance on a strong distinction between the current experiential interests of the incompetent patient and the autonomy-based but no longer surviving interests of the formerly competent person. It is unclear whether they would press the point this far solely on the basis of loss of psychological continuity. This radical position is more strongly identifiable in Dresser's writings. More recently she has appeared to confine this argument to dementia patients, though without analysis of the concept of personal identity. See Rebecca Dresser, "Dworkin on Dementia: Elegant Theory, Questionable Policy," *Hastings Center Report* 25, no. 6 (July-August 1996): 32–38. For Robertson, the idea of present and former selves at times seems to be more a way of talking about interests than an argument about a theory of personal identity. See John A. Robertson, "*Cruzan* and the Constitutional Status of Nontreatment Decisions for Incompetent Patients," *Georgia Law Review* 25, no. 5 (Summer 1991): 1166 (rejecting the importance commonly assigned to the incompetent patient's long prior history, including authorship of a directive, and embracing the view that "respect for the incompetent patient requires that she be regarded as she now is and not as she previously was").
6. Allen E. Buchanan and Dan W. Brock, *Deciding for Others: The Ethics of Surrogate Decision Making* (Cambridge: Cambridge University Press, 1989), 185. For the authors' conclusions, see pp. 184–89. This chapter of *Deciding for Others* is a significantly modified version of Buchanan's earlier article, "Advance Directives and the Personal Identity Problem," *Philosophy and Public Affairs* 17, no. 4 (Fall 1988): 277–302. Buchanan and Brock suggest that severely demented patients might be considered new persons, or nonpersons, depending on the extent of neurological damage and cognitive impairment.
7. Buchanan and Brock, *Deciding for Others,* 166.
8. Norman L. Cantor, *Advance Directives and the Pursuit of Death with Dignity* (Bloomington: Indiana University Press, 1993), 109–12; Ronald Dworkin, *Life's Dominion: An Argument About Abortion, Euthanasia, and Individual Freedom* (New York: Alfred A. Knopf, 1993), 222–29.
9. Some proponents of the personal identity argument have suggested that the moral authority of advance directives rests on a presupposition of the identity of persons over time that has been assumed rather than justified. A portion of my analysis is intended to show that several plausible accounts of identity over time that are compatible with the consensus approach to decisions near the end of life might be constructed. My purpose here is not to fully argue that any particular alternative theory of personal identity is necessarily more philosophically sound, although I suggest that each of these alternatives offers a more plausible and morally acceptable grounding for our approach to decisions near the end of life.

10. These are not the only ways to describe the person status of PVS patients. One might think of PVS patients prior to confirmation of the diagnosis as "pilgrim persons," meaning that as long as recovery of the necessary properties for ascription of personhood is considered possible they may again possess the status of person. We also might think of PVS and other permanently unconscious patients as "previous persons," meaning that they once possessed the properties of personhood but have irretrievably lost these properties (based on the medical evidence). These variations on the person/personhood theme are suggested by Robert F. Weir, *Abating Treatment with Critically Ill Patients: Ethical and Legal Limits to the Medical Prolongation of Life* (New York: Oxford University Press, 1989), 406.
11. Buchanan and Brock, *Deciding for Others*, 157–58.
12. Ibid., 155–56. Dresser makes the same assumption; see, e.g., Rebecca Dresser, "Advance Directives, Self-Determination, and Personal Identity," in *Advance Directives in Medicine*, ed. Chris Hackler, Ray Moseley, and Dorothy Vawter (New York: Praeger Publishers, 1989).
13. Buchanan and Brock, *Deciding for Others*, 155. The authors state that "[t]he unity relation for persons [means that] two or more 'person life stages' are stages of the *same* person's life if and only if these conditions obtain." The terms *unity relation* and *person life-stages* are borrowed from John Perry, "The Problem of Personal Identity," in *Personal Identity*, edited by John Perry (Berkeley: University of California Press, 1975), 3–30.
14. For further discussion of this point, see Dan W. Brock, "Justice and the Severely Demented Elderly," *Journal of Medicine and Philosophy* 13 (1988): 85–86. Other than this brief discussion, proponents of the discontinuity thesis offer no analysis of the bodily continuity theory of identity. Although it is unclear whether they consider bodily continuity a necessary condition of personal identity, they must hold that it is not a sufficient condition. There is no suggestion that radical physical changes caused by serious illness destroy bodily continuity *and* identity. Given the way the argument has been framed, however, bodily continuity apparently is at least assumed to be present. I discuss this point further below.
15. Proponents of the personal identity argument in bioethics have relied heavily on Parfit's theory as authoritative, although they have not offered any sustained analysis of Parfit's position. See e.g., Dresser, "Advance Directives, Self-Determination, and Personal Identity," 157–59; Buchanan and Brock, *Deciding for Others*, 156, note 2 (citing Derek Parfit, *Reasons and Persons* [Oxford: Oxford University Press, 1984] as an influential discussion of a psychological continuity theory).
16. This analytical distinction is suggested by the discussion and critique of Parfit's theory in Christine M. Korsgaard, "Personal Identity and the Unity of Agency: A Kantian Response to Parfit," *Philosophy & Public Affairs* 18, no. 2 (Spring 1989): 101–32. The importance of this distinction will surface again later.
17. Parfit, *Reasons and Persons*, 206 (emphasis in original).
18. Locke's classic formulation of the memory theory of personal identity, originally published in 1690 as chapter 27 of his *Essay Concerning Human Understanding*, is reprinted as chapter 2 of the collected essays in Perry, *Personal Identity*, 33–52.
19. See, e.g., Perry, "The Problem of Personal Identity."

20. Parfit, *Reasons and Persons*, 205 (emphasis in original).
21. In support of my point here, see Brock, "Justice and the Severely Demented Elderly," 92 (describing moderately demented patients as "still having memory function and/or other psychological continuity sufficient for maintaining personal identity . . . though as often suffering from cognitive disabilities sufficient to leave them incompetent to make at least some decisions about their health care"); Norman L. Cantor, "Prospective Autonomy: On the Limits of Shaping One's Postcompetence Medical Fate," *Journal of Contemporary Health Law and Policy* 8 (1992): 31 (noting that incompetent patients often retain a significant measure of long-term memory).
22. Parfit, *Reasons and Persons*, 206; Buchanan and Brock, *Deciding for Others*, 156.
23. Parfit, *Reasons and Persons*, 262, adds that psychological connectedness/continuity should have "the right kind of cause." For our purposes, we can assume that having memories, intentions, and other psychological states involves the continued existence of a living brain—or what is sometimes called the "normal cause" of psychological continuity. Ibid., 208. The personal identity challenge to advance directives seems to make this same assumption. The normal cause is entirely compatible with the way the argument has been presented because it frames the factual context for the debate. Therefore we need not press the point further and challenge this assumption by posing questions such as, "If my brain patterns were replicated and transferred to another brain and body, would that still be me?" Parfit develops a hypothetical scenario along these lines in an effort to establish that psychological continuity, not personal identity, really matters. The essence of this argument is that the replicated person would not be *me* because he would be living in an entirely different body—but that this fact would not matter in asking the question whether "I" have survived the replication procedure. To pursue this inquiry, Parfit allows that psychological continuity can have *any* cause and uses the concept "in its widest sense." Ibid., 208.

    There is another sense in which causation is important, which concerns whether someone's memories, beliefs, and so forth are *genuine*. On one hand, if a person comes to have a set of memories and beliefs and to believe that he or she has had a set of experiences because he or she has been "brainwashed," we would not say that these experiences are genuine—nor that he or she is the same person who in fact had these prior experiences (assuming anyone, in fact, has). On the other hand, a person who is consistently delusional may not in fact have had a set of experiences that he or she believes he or she has had, yet this person may at least be the same person over time who holds a connected series of delusional beliefs and memories. The present inquiry can safely set these questions aside.
24. Parfit, *Reasons and Persons*, 206. Parfit goes on in the next sentence to make the curious claim that "there is enough connectedness if the number of direct connections, over any day, is *at least half* the number that hold, over every day, in the lives of nearly every actual person." Enough direct connections make for strong connectedness. Parfit does not develop this point, and it is hard to see its utility for constructing an approach to assessing the personal identity of incompetent patients. At most, Parfit's position—though it is not developed with incompetency in mind—would appear to be that strong connectedness (whatever that means) is an appropriate threshold.

25. Dresser, "Advance Directives, Self-Determination, and Personal Identity," 162. Dresser apparently believes that this sweeping practical objection to the use of a psychological continuity criterion in clinical practice supports her attack on advance directives because she believes the standard presumption in favor of prospective autonomy should be reversed. In other words, if we cannot be sure that the incompetent patient and the former competent person are the same person, we should adopt a current best interests approach as the standard of decision. If we retain—as we should—a strong presumption in favor of the authority of advance directives, however, this line of reasoning seems to be a devastating critique of her own position.
26. Buchanan and Brock, *Deciding for Others*, 156. The authors state that "the fact that there is a twilight does not show that we cannot distinguish between noon and midnight."
27. Ibid., 185.
28. Stephen G. Post, "Alzheimer Disease and the 'Then' Self," *Kennedy Institute of Ethics Journal* 5, no. 4 (December 1995): 307.
29. Nancy M. P. King, *Making Sense of Advance Directives*, rev. ed. (Washington, D.C.: Georgetown University Press, 1996), 85 ("Our current scientific ignorance alone should be enough to make sufficient agreement [about how much psychological continuity is enough] impossible"); Cantor, "Prospective Autonomy," 31 (making the related point that none of the current literature defines the degree of loss of psychological continuity that would make an incompetent patient a new person).
30. Buchanan and Brock, *Deciding for Others*, 160–61, also take the issue to be fundamentally moral, noting that the moral and metaphysical concepts of persons cannot be neatly separated.
31. Ibid., 159.
32. A fourth option, which follows from rigorous application of Parfit's position, would be to acknowledge that psychological continuity is strictly a matter of degree and to accord weight to advance directives in proportion to the degree of psychological continuity present. This policy would be utterly unworkable. Among other problems, without any markers on the continuity continuum, people could have no reasonable expectations about when their advance directives would be followed or even when they would cease to be the same person with the same spouse, children, job, and so forth. On this last point, see my critique of the personal identity thesis. The fourth option and a possible compromise are discussed in Buchanan and Brock, *Deciding for Others*, 178–84.
33. Arguably, judgments that psychological continuity has been destroyed in severely demented patients can be made with some reliability, but we should be highly skeptical of our ability to identify a bright line that tells us when a patient has crossed the continuity threshold (assuming that we were to agree on where this line exists). Policy and practice would have to be extremely vigilant in safeguarding against the risk of abuse by those who would too quickly attach the label of "new person" or "nonperson" to a certain stage of dementia; perhaps motivated by a document that directs forgoing of life support for a patient who appears to have present interests in continued life.
34. Parfit's conclusions in *Reasons and Persons*, especially 202 and 323, are the same.

35. See Buchanan and Brock, *Deciding for Others*, 157 (a patient with advanced Alzheimer's disease); Dworkin, *Life's Dominion*, 220–21 (the case of Margo, a woman with Alzheimer's dementia); Dresser, "Dworkin on Dementia" (offering a different analysis of Margo's case); Cantor, *Advance Directives*, 102 (a sociology professor who suffers a debilitating stroke); Sanford H. Kadish, "Letting Patients Die: Legal and Moral Reflections," *California Law Review* 80 (1992): 871–72 (the case of Composer Then and Composer Now—a woman with senile dementia).
36. Cantor, *Advance Directives*, 111; Nancy K. Rhoden, "The Limits of Legal Objectivity," *North Carolina Law Review* 68 (1990): 860.
37. William F. May, "Attitudes Toward the Newly Dead," *Hastings Center Studies* 1, no. 1 (1973): 3.
38. Robert M. Veatch, *Death, Dying and the Biological Revolution* (New Haven, Conn.: Yale University Press, 1989), 28–30. See also Robert M. Veatch, "The Whole-Brain-Oriented Concept of Death: An Outmoded Philosophical Formulation," *Journal of Thanatology* 3 (1975): 13–30. Veatch would recognize a right of conscientious objection to declaring death on this basis; see, e.g., Robert M. Veatch, "The Impending Collapse of the Whole-Brain Definition of Death," *Hastings Center Report* 23, no. 4 (July-August 1993): 21–22. I briefly discuss below the question of redefining death to include permanently unconscious patients who have lost the capacity for embodied consciousness. Whether such a redefinition of death should be adopted as public policy is beyond the scope of this book.
39. Veatch's writings suggest another sort of analysis that also is compatible with the consensus and with traditional mores about death behavior. We might distinguish the death of a human person from that of a human individual. We might go on to hold that the life of an individual is the same life up to and including death as determined in accordance with the accepted definition of death. Thus, the death of the individual and the death of the body are a unitary event. On this understanding, we also might accept that loss of personal identity marks the death of the person while we maintain that the life of the individual survives death of the person the individual once was. One consequence of this understanding would be to acknowledge that psychological continuity matters in personal identity but that loss of personal identity does not matter in our moral and legal response to death and death behavior (personal communication with Robert Veatch). For the purposes of the present argument, I need not develop this line of reasoning further.
40. Critiques of the bodily continuity theory often use a "puzzle case" involving the transfer of one person's memory, personality, and other psychological states into the body of another person. Perhaps the most famous scenario is Locke's posit of a prince who awakens one morning in the body of a cobbler but still believes himself to be the prince of the land. The point of such cases is to show that there are strong intuitive reasons to believe that the person now inhabiting the cobbler's body is in fact the prince, not the cobbler. We can reach this conclusion only if we hold that psychological continuity—the possession of psychological states over time—matters, not the sameness of the body over time. Just as the choice of a continuity threshold involves a moral judgment, not a purely metaphysical one, however, so too does the choice of what matters in the unity of a life involve a moral judgment, especially when being alive or dead depends on that judgment. Until brain transplants become a reality, there seems to be no good reason to revise our current understanding.

41. Korsgaard, "Personal Identity and the Unity of Agency," 113.
42. Bernard Williams, *Moral Luck* (Cambridge: Cambridge University Press, 1981), 8.
43. Korsgaard, "Personal Identity and the Unity of Agency," 113–14. Korsgaard stresses that grounding personal identity in the unity of agency rests on the necessity of practical reason to render intelligible our natures as moral agents. She also claims that this theory "requires no metaphysical support." I need not develop this position further here. Again, I mean to suggest that approaching personal identity from the standpoint of moral agency offers a more persuasive alternative account of what matters in the moral life. Korsgaard's point is similar.
44. Williams, *Moral Luck,* 10. Summarizing the necessary connection between the present and the future from the standpoint of moral agency, Williams states: "[O]ne's pattern of interests, desires and projects not only provide the reason for an interest in what happens within the horizon of one's future, but also constitute the conditions of there being such a future at all." Ibid., 11.
45. Alasdair MacIntyre, *After Virtue* (South Bend, Ind.: University of Notre Dame Press, 1984), 218.
46. Ibid., 216–18.
47. Ibid., 215.
48. For a discussion of a narrative view of unity that emphasizes a communitarian understanding of the self, see Mark G. Kuczewski, "Whose Life Is It Anyway? A Discussion of Advance Directives, Personal Identity, and Consensus in Medical Ethics," *Bioethics* 8, no. 1 (1994): 27–48.
49. Korsgaard, "Personal Identity and the Unity of Agency"; Kuczewski, "Whose Life Is It Anyway?" 42 (arguing that a narrative view of unity over time reveals that the psychological continuity view is not definitive). There is a further dichotomy of approach between the two views. The Parfitian view puts the question of identity over time under a retrospective lens. By contrast, the standpoint of the unity of agency is largely prospective. There is no intrinsically better choice between these two vantage points.
50. David DeGrazia, "Advance Directives, Dementia, and 'The Someone Else Problem,'" *Bioethics* 13, no. 5 (October 1999): 373–91, argues that proponents of the psychological continuity view make a different sort of fundamental error. He contends that they incorrectly assume that we are fundamentally persons. To the contrary, we are fundamentally human animals and as such continue to be the same human animal over time despite severe cognitive impairment.
51. Buchanan and Brock, Deciding for Others, 174: "We would have to have extraordinarily weighty reasons for giving up the view of personal identity upon which [existing institutions and practices] are founded."
52. Ibid., 175. See also Michael B. Green and Daniel Wikler, "Brain Death and Personal Identity," *Philosophy and Public Affairs* 9, no. 2 (Winter 1980): 105–33 (arguing that total destruction of psychological continuity in the persistent vegetative state patient justifies redefining death to include the permanently unconscious). I discuss the Green/Wikler position further below.
53. May, "Attitudes Toward the Newly Dead," 7.
54. Ibid., 9.
55. For a similar point, see Cantor, *Advance Directives*, 111. Cantor argues that the incompetent persona is regarded as an extension of the former self and hence continues to be regarded as a Jew, a Catholic, and so on.

56. May, "Attitudes Toward the Newly Dead," 9. In discussing various proposals concerning organ transplantation policy—including those to shift to a system of routine salvaging of organs—May argues that "[t]he social and psychological price exacted by this partial or total elimination of mourning rites may be high." He notes that such a policy would alter our understanding of the individual's and the family's relationship to the corpse and cloud the issue of when it was appropriate to express grief and begin the bereavement process. The price would be extremely high on the discontinuity thesis for the many families who would be deprived of any formal occasion and ritual to mark the loss of a loved one and the beginning of the mourning process.
57. This new definition of death also would have important implications for criminal law (when has a murder occurred?) and tort law (has there been a wrongful death?), though not in Mr. S's case.
58. President's Commission for the Study of Ethical Problems in Medicine and Biomedical and Behavioral Research, *Defining Death* (Washington, D.C.: G.P.O., 1981). I have argued elsewhere that this interest in uniformity is not absolute and that it can and should yield to accommodate religious and moral objections to a determination of death on the basis of neurological criteria held by a very small number. Robert S. Olick, "Brain Death, Religious Freedom, and Public Policy: New Jersey's Landmark Legislative Initiative," *Kennedy Institute of Ethics Journal* 1, no. 4 (1991): 275–92. The discontinuity theorist proposes a radical redefinition of the basic legal standard of death, not a limited exception to the general rule.
59. Congress of the United States, Office of Technology Assessment, *Losing a Million Minds: Confronting the Tragedy of Alzheimer's Disease and Other Dementias*, OTA-BA-323 (Washington, D.C.: G.P.O., 1987), 3, 16.
60. Buchanan and Brock, *Deciding for Others*, 166. This argument is meant to apply to the severely demented patient as well as the permanently unconscious patient, both of whom the authors consider to be nonpersons.
61. Ibid.
62. Ibid., 167–68.
63. Helga Kuhse, "Some Reflections on the Problem of Advance Directives, Personhood, and Personal Identity," *Kennedy Institute of Ethics Journal* 9, no. 4 (December 1999): 347–64, makes a similar point in her critique of the Buchanan/Brock analysis. Apparently in agreement with the philosophical tenets of the psychological continuity view, the main point of her argument is that personhood, not personal identity, should count in treatment decision making for the severely demented. Forgoing of life support is justified because nonpersons—which for Kuhse includes severely demented patients—have no interests in continued existence.
64. One possible road out of this dilemma, as I have suggested, would be to embrace a distinction between individuals and persons. Doing so would allow that as the individual who is the author of a directive, I (and my family) have continuing interests in decisions near the end of life for an individual who is still *me*, and those interests survive loss of psychological continuity—even loss of personhood. On this view, however, proponents of the personal identity argument would have to give up, or substantially modify, the moral significance for advance directives that they attach to loss of psychological continuity/connectedness. In short, this approach is incompatible with the discontinuity thesis as it has been formulated.

65. Buchanan and Brock, *Deciding for Others*, 166, also express an opposite concern—that refusals of treatment will not be honored precisely because a right of disposal carries less moral weight than a right of self-determination. One result might be continued treatment that imposes great financial and emotional distress on family members. To avoid this outcome, they assert that this quasi-property right would have the same force as ordinary property rights, requiring good reasons to override it. Again, it is hard to see why the concept of quasi-property rights is needed at all. We can address these same concerns in a more coherent fashion by continuing to call the right to refuse treatment a right of prospective autonomy and self-determination, while treating the moral weight of that right and the duty to respect it as a separate question.

66. It does not help the argument to hold, as Buchanan and Brock do, that severely demented patients who have lost continuity with their former selves are nonpersons. The main posit remains that there is a right of disposal over treatment decisions for a patient who is not the same person as the author of a prior directive. The issue here is not the significance of the patient's interests but the question of why, on the discontinuity thesis, the wishes of a former self that has ceased to exist should count at all.

67. See the two-part set of articles by the Multi-Society Task Force on PVS: "Medical Aspects of the Persistent Vegetative State," *New England Journal of Medicine* 330, no. 21 (May 26, 1994): 1499–1508; "Medical Aspects of the Persistent Vegetative State," *New England Journal of Medicine* 330, no. 22 (June 2, 1994): 1572–79.

68. There still is reason to be concerned with the highly unusual case of misdiagnosis or recovery. What of patients who have lost psychological continuity but later recover cognitive function—of a radically altered nature—and subsequently return to society to lead a normal life? Is there a new person inhabiting the same body? Should that person return to his or her family? See Veatch, *Death, Dying and the Biological Revolution*, 28 (giving the example of severe amnesia); President's Commission, *Defining Death*, 40. It would seem that a waiting period to rule out the possibility of such occurrences is appropriate before the death of the former person should be declared. The hypothetical situation also suggests the question of how to respond to an arguably new person (such as in the amnesia case) who emerges from a serious illness or injury with intact cognitive function and now repudiates a prior directive (perhaps has no memory of writing the document and of its being his or hers). On the new person view, we are compelled to say that indeed the prior directive is not the patient's and was written by a different person. There is a more plausible way to handle such a scenario, however. We could simply hold that the now-competent patient has changed his or her mind and has the right to revoke his or her prior directive, regardless of whether he or she still possesses the same beliefs, values, and memories as before. I discuss the question of an incompetent patient's change of mind in repudiating a prior treatment refusal in chapter five, without the baggage of the personal identity problem.

69. Reliable confirmation of PVS usually occurs within months, not days, of the initial diagnosis. Thus, the former person will have ceased to exist long before a decision to terminate treatment is made. See the articles by the Multi-Society Task Force on PVS cited in note 67.

70. Brock, "Justice and the Severely Demented Elderly," 80 ("nearly all persons who reflect on this question conclude that . . . continuing to sustain the life of

the patient's body is of no benefit whatever to the patient"). See, e.g., "Bioethics Debate," *National Law Journal* (May 13, 1991), 1. This *National Law Journal*/Lexis poll found that 80 percent of respondents would want their life support discontinued almost immediately (58 percent) or after a few months (22 percent) if they were in irreversible coma. There is no indication that popular sentiment rests on any appreciation of personal identity theory.

71. Brock, "Justice and the Severely Demented Elderly," 79–81. An especially cogent analysis of this question is provided in John D. Arras, "Beyond *Cruzan*: Individual Rights, Family Autonomy and the Persistent Vegetative State," *Journal of the American Geriatrics Society* 39, no. 10 (October 1991): 1018–24.

72. Steven H. Miles, "Informed Demand for 'Non-Beneficial' Medical Treatment," *New England Journal of Medicine* 325 (1991): 512–15.

73. Arras favors a policy that reverses the current presumption but also recognizes the right of a "vitalist" to insist on continued treatment.

74. Some writers have relied on a psychological continuity theory to argue that the permanently unconscious patient should be considered dead. Green and Wikler, "Brain Death and Personal Identity," 127, argue that "a given person ceases to exist with the destruction of whatever processes there are which normally underlie that person's psychological continuity and connectedness." They argue that "irreversible cessation of upper-brain functioning constitutes the death of that person." Although this position has little to do with the challenge to the moral authority of advance directives, it is worth noting that if public policy is to move in the direction of considering permanently unconscious patients morally and legally dead, there are several reasons not to ground this ongoing debate on the concept of psychological continuity. Even on the prudential judgment that diagnosis of permanent unconsciousness must be certain before death is declared (and there is some disagreement about whether this diagnosis can be made with the requisite certainty), the discontinuity thesis still cannot account for the right of the family to bury the body without admitting some alternative view of identity (such as bodily continuity) as the basis for their relationship. Nor can it account for why the deceased's or the family's wishes for the funeral, burial, or other death behavior should control or for religious or moral objections to a determination of death on the basis of loss of psychological continuity. The only coherent way to obviate this difficulty and to honor deeply held religious and cultural convictions is to identify the time of death for legal and moral purposes with death of the body and to regard death as a single event in a unitary life of the person. There also is a more conceptually coherent way to make the case. We might hold that "death is most appropriately thought of as the irreversible loss of the embodied capacity for social interaction" and that one's social nature and embodiment are truly essential to being a living human being. Veatch, *Death, Dying and the Biological Revolution*, 28–30. On this understanding, a permanently unconscious patient who has suffered irreversible loss of higher-brain functions (sometimes called "neocortical death") would be dead—the same result sought by the discontinuity theorist. The emphasis on embodiment makes clear, however, that this position is entirely compatible with the unitary existence of an individual's life and traditional death behaviors. For additional, comprehensive analysis of the redefinition of death debate and the various arguments in favor of a higher-brain-death formulation, see Karen Grandstand Gervais, *Redefining Death* (New Haven, Conn.: Yale University Press, 1986).

Chapter Five

RESPECTING ADVANCE DIRECTIVES: PUTTING THEORY INTO PRACTICE

> Advance directives placed in the medical records of seriously ill patients often did not guide medical decision-making beyond naming a healthcare proxy or documenting general preferences in a standard living will format. Even when specific instructions were present, care was potentially inconsistent in half of the cases.
>
> Joan Teno et al., for the SUPPORT Investigators, 1997[1]

> I found that I was dealing with a bewildering array of medical specialists trained to prolong lives, not to let patients die. . . . [S]he had given me durable power of attorney for health care. . . . I was told that my mother had had a stroke and that she would not recover from her hemiparalysis. The physicians hoped to fit her with a tracheostomy tube and send her to a nursing home. . . . I knew that she did not want such a life. Yet my mother's wishes, as they were understood by her family physician and her daughter, were now subject to the approval of strangers: the cadre of cardiologists, neurologists, and pulmonologists who attended her.
>
> "A Letter from a Patient's Daughter," 1996[2]

INTRODUCTION

What would taking prospective autonomy and advance directives seriously in daily clinical practice mean? My goal in this chapter is to put theory into practice and thereby to develop a further, more concrete understanding of the duty to honor advance directives. I prescribe several policy and practice emendations to the consensus, each designed to ensure that advance directives are given the full measure of respect to which they are entitled in the care of dying patients.

Beneath the surface of debate about advance directives is a shared disquiet with the ambiguity and uncertainty involved in end-of-life decisions. Although such uncertainty is understandable, improvement in care of the dying demands that we confront and resolve uncertainty, not hide from it. There are strong moral and policy reasons to look to proxies and families to shoulder this responsibility. Earnest respect means recognizing the full scope of proxy and family authority to exercise judgment and discretion on the patient's behalf. Building on the argument of chapter three, in the first part of this chapter I argue that we should forthrightly recognize an *ethic of judgment*, and I describe its basic parameters.

Taking prospective autonomy seriously also means giving true voice to the presumptive weight of advance directives. I take up an oft-overlooked question: What rules should govern decisions *not* to honor advance directives? My response builds on a critical posit of the theory of prospective decisional autonomy—namely, that there are *three substantive grounds* on which an advance directive may justifiably be overridden. In the second part of the chapter, I contend that these three grounds should be translated into policy standards to govern bedside decisions *not* to follow advance directives. The three tests are Hopeless Ambiguity, Radical Change of Circumstances, and the Rebel Proxy.

More precise definition here of what I mean by *overriding* a directive will facilitate understanding of what follows. Consistent with what seems to be the popular understanding, I take overriding a directive to mean that the document is held not to possess decisional authority or, more simply, that the document is set aside and is not followed. When an instruction directive is overridden on one of the first two grounds, what justifies this choice is the fact that the directive is nonautonomous; hence, there is no violation of autonomy. Setting aside an instruction directive for other reasons, including to promote the patient's best interests, violates prior autonomy and therefore is unjustified. When a proxy appointment is overridden, what justifies this choice is the proxy's own actions in disregard of his or her entrusted authority. Although the patient may not have chosen wisely in such instances, a proxy directive nonetheless expresses an autonomous decision (at least in the vast majority of cases), and overriding the directive on this ground also counts as a violation, albeit justified, of prior autonomy.

Central to the inquiry are two procedural questions: Who should bear the burden of responsibility for challenging an advance directive (in legal terms, the burden of proof and the burden of going forward), and what process should be followed when such a decision is contemplated? In the latter part of the chapter, I contend that making respect for advance directives truly meaningful requires that *the burden of meeting one of these standards rest squarely with those who would override the directive*. To achieve this objective, the choice to override a directive should be *subject to mandatory prospective review* by an institutional ethics committee or a court, with judicial review as a final arbiter if necessary. Each of these procedural rules should be embraced, legitimated, and enforced by the law.

After presenting the argument for each of these prescriptions, I conclude the chapter with several case analyses. The first scenario explores the problems of interpreting an ambiguous advance directive—the most common concern of health care professionals—and illustrates the role of an ethic of judgment. The second scenario draws attention to a series of issues; it devotes special attention to the often-ignored and particularly challenging question of the moral weight due an incompetent patient's contemporaneous expressions in favor of life. The final scenario illustrates the problem of the rebel proxy. Any analysis of cases, of course, is selective. All of the scenarios I discuss in this chapter are based on real-life stories (two were courtroom dramas). Collectively, the scenarios serve two important purposes: They press the limits of the developed theory, and they further demonstrate its practical application.

TOWARD AN ETHIC OF JUDGMENT

When the terms of a directive provide clear and unambiguous guidance, the task of ascertaining the patient's intention and plan is essentially administrative. Implementing the patient's wishes should be unproblematic. What should be done, however, if the terms of a directive are less clear and the meaning of the directive is open to some interpretation? What if the document seems vague or ambiguous on its face? How should we respond to treatment refusals that appear to be inconsistent with statements made at an earlier time in the patient's life? On the surface, these questions are very familiar; they are readily identified with the practical problems with advance directives I note in the discussion of what makes a directive effective. At a deeper level, each of these queries raises a more fundamental question that too often has been sidestepped: What obligations do proxy, family, and physician have when applying an advance directive means confronting uncertainty?

The moral and policy argument for proxy and family discretion makes clear that persons who are responsible for the patient's care have the duty and responsibility to make their best efforts to determine and give effect to the patient's intention(s) and plan. If the patient's intention cannot be determined, a best interests approach should be followed, taking into account what is known of the patient's wishes and values. Numerous advance directive laws explicitly charge proxies with these responsibilities.[3] A pragmatic look at these obligations reveals the basic parameters of an *ethic of judgment* that should be at work in end-of-life decisions.

A common concern is whether the person acting on the patient's behalf should look beyond the "four corners" of the document. The Florida case *In re Guardianship of Browning v. Herbert* is illustrative.[4] Mrs. Browning was an elderly PVS patient who was being sustained by a nasogastric tube. She had issued a living will instructing that life support be forgone "if at any time I should have a terminal condition and if my attending physician has determined that there can be no recovery from such condition and that my death is imminent." A second cousin and close friend, Mrs. Herbert, who had lived with Mrs. Browning for several years and who was appointed as her guardian, petitioned the court for removal of life support on the basis of the living will.

First and foremost, Mrs. Herbert's duty as guardian was to look to the terms of the directive. To stop there, however, and interpret the directive strictly and literally—reading the document to be refusing treatment only in the event of terminal illness and imminent death—would lead to the morally offensive result that Mrs. Browning should be maintained in a vegetative state, perhaps indefinitely. May Mrs. Herbert, in her capacity as guardian, look beyond the text of the document to determine whether Mrs. Browning intended to refuse treatment and be allowed to die if she were in a PVS? Should Mrs. Herbert consider Mrs. Browning's past statements made after visiting seriously ill friends ("I would never want to be like that") or personal knowledge of Mrs. Browning's values, commitments, and attitudes that inform her directive?

The answer to these queries must be yes. Here, continued struggle against inexorable decline and progressive debilitation was considered an intolerable existence. To hold that Mrs. Browning would find permanently unconscious life acceptable or that life support must be continued absent clear written refusal contemplating precisely these medical circumstances would be an affront to her autonomy and dignity. There is no reasonable basis for thinking this was the outcome Mrs. Browning intended. The *Browning* court reached the same conclusion. After receiving testimony from Mrs. Herbert and others, as well as evidence that Mrs. Browning had reaffirmed and updated an earlier identical living will, the court ruled that the language of the living will should be applied to the current circumstance of PVS and authorized withdrawal of life support.

Significantly, the court also resolved the living will's apparent ambiguity by finding that Mrs. Browning's condition in fact was terminal.[5] This assessment typically is not the case with PVS patients, who may survive for several years (even decades) on life support. This aspect of the case points to another important and often-neglected way in which the language of a directive can be imprecise and require the exercise of judgment to give effect to its meaning. Advance directives commonly use the critical term *terminal illness* without defining it.[6] How imminent must death be from the patient's point of view before treatment is withheld or withdrawn? Is the patient's intent to relinquish only the last few weeks of life, or is the prospect of six months of progressive debilitation and incapacity an intolerable quality of life? Clearly, Mrs. Herbert's understanding of what her close friend meant by this phrase should control.[7]

Consider one further example. Operative language in a "next generation" advance directive jointly published in 1995 by the American Bar Association Commission on Legal Problems of the Elderly, the American Medical Association, and the American Association of Retired Persons provides the following language as one of the options for refusal of treatment:

> I do not want my life prolonged . . . if the treatment will leave me with no more than some ability to think or communicate with others, and the likely risks and burdens of treatment outweigh the expected benefits. Risks, burdens and benefits include consideration of length of life, quality of life, financial costs, and my personal dignity and privacy.[8]

When called on to implement this provision, how are persons who are responsible for the patient's care to decide when no more than *some* ability to think or communicate remains? How are they to determine when this combination of factors—length and quality of life, costs of continued care, and invasions of personal dignity and privacy—are so burdensome that they outweigh the benefits of continued treatment?

One point of the integrity view of autonomy is that in the task of implementing advance directives, we should regard the patient as a person who has lived a whole life. Doing so requires us to take into account the values and commitments that are manifest in the course of a person's life history; the type of person he or she has been; and, in particular, prior statements made before and after issuance of a directive. It also requires us to take into account the patient's current experience as a dying person—including pain, suffering, pleasure, contentment, indignity, and other factors that are relevant to weighing the burdens and benefits of treatment and quality of life. Certainly the purpose of this language is to direct the proxy (or family member) to do precisely this—to exercise sound judgment within the bounds of his or her authority. (This process sometimes is referred to as following the intent and spirit of the directive.)

Suppose, however, that the patient has no close and caring person— no "bonded surrogate"—acting on his or her behalf, and the express terms of the living will do not provide clear guidance. In some instances, the physician-patient relationship is a real partnership in which the physician can and should fill the role of bonded surrogate. A physician who is caring for a chronically ill patient over an extended period may come to know the patient as a person who has become ill and be qualified to faithfully interpret and implement the patient's intention within the larger context of the patient's life as a whole. The image of the old-school family physician is still real for many people. On the other hand, a relationship of moral distance (the stranger in a white coat) is a far more prevalent norm for physician and patient in today's health care system. Here, the scope of the physician's discretion to interpret the patient's intention should be more limited.[9] As a practical matter, the way to protect patients against abuse of this discretion in favor of treatment that a physician deems to be in the patient's best interests ("the living will is ambiguous, and life support benefits the patient") is to ensure that the choice to disregard the directive is justified to others through a mandated review process.

One may counter that these illustrations show the ambiguity of advance directives. There is obvious merit in this observation. To acquiesce to *prima facie* ambiguity, however, despairing the lack of precision in future-oriented autonomy, is to miss the forest for the trees. The morally licit response is to recognize that honoring the judgment entrusted to the proxy and/or family member honors the patient's prospectively autonomous decision. At the same time, physicians and other health care professionals have important responsibilities not only to advise the proxy but to safeguard the patient's interests by being alert to the boundaries of the proxy's authority. The latter responsibility includes the possibility that the proxy may overreach in good-faith efforts to make sense of hopelessly ambiguous instructions.

It is far from clear that this view is as widely shared as one might think. Ardent advocates, fearful of opening the door to challenges, insist that directives are absolutely binding and deny that they require interpretation and judgment to be effective. Where discretion is admitted, it is reposed absolutely in proxy and family, excepting only clear instances of ill will and blatant self-concern. For people who believe that the written document *ipso facto* stands for clear and convincing evidence, there is no need to look further than the document itself; the need to do so is considered to diminish the directive's probative value. By contrast, those who are invested in the quest to make advance directives increasingly precise instruments betray an underlying disquiet with the need for judgment in the face of uncertainty. The law has been of little help in shaping the appropriate understanding here. Although case law applying a substituted judgment standard has uniformly allowed a broad range of evidence to be considered (substituted judgment would have no meaning otherwise), statutory law governing advance directives is largely silent and neither expressly permits nor prohibits resort to other evidence to interpret a directive.[10]

Explicit and uniform recognition of an ethic of judgment, in law and practice, would be an important step in the direction of resolving apparent conflicts and assuring greater respect for advance directives. This stride alone is unlikely to secure substantial progress in respect for patients' wishes, however. New rules are needed to make plain the presumptive moral and legal authority of directives and to require that decisions to override be clearly articulated and justified. In the following section, I sketch the basic parameters of the approach that ought to govern when the authority of an advance directive is challenged.

CHALLENGING AN ADVANCE DIRECTIVE: PROCESS AND PROCEDURE

Changing Incentives, Changing Behavior

Given the presumptive weight of advance directives, the burden of showing why prospective autonomy should *not* be honored properly rests with those who would override the directive. Although a substantial portion of the medical profession acknowledges the gravamen of patients' end-of-life decisions, there is considerable evidence that the opposite norm—which accords this presumption limited practical import—is more characteristic of the prevailing medical culture. That culture freely allows physicians and hospitals who are unwilling to honor a treatment refusal to shift to the proxy and family the burden of challenging the provider's judgment. Legal rules and ethical principles notwithstanding, many health care providers feel safe, even comfortable, when they just say no. This reality was laid bare by the SUPPORT study, which found that a controlled intervention that was designed to foster respect for patients' treatment refusals made no difference in the alarming frequency with which dying patients' wishes were ignored,[11] even when patients had written advance directives.[12] In the words of one commentator, a sizable body of empirical work shows that patient choice at the end of life is an "illusion."[13]

If law and ethics have failed to effect corresponding behavior patterns, what should be done? The flurry of commentary in the aftermath of publication of the SUPPORT study's early findings offers an extensive menu of recipes for change: We should produce better advance directive forms; encourage better physician-patient communication about end-of-life care; enhance efforts to educate health care professionals; strive through education to change the culture of medicine; place greater emphasis on hospice and home care; develop more effective practice guidelines to trigger consideration of limiting care for the dying; and pursue more aggressively a societal dialogue about the place of death in human life and the proper goals of medicine.[14]

Certainly all of these strategies hold some promise of improving care of the dying and are worthy of investment. Some objectives clearly are more ambitious than others. At the turn of the 21st century, efforts to change practice, if not culture—through education, outreach, and engagement at the community level—have taken center stage. (These efforts have been helped immensely by the Robert Wood Johnson Foundation's initiatives Last Acts and the foundation's funding of Community-State Partnerships to Improve End-of-Life Care, as well as the PBS program hosted by Bill Moyers, *On Our Own Terms*.) For the most part, however, each of these prescriptions relies on the subtle persuasive forces of education and culture as the agents of change. None would give a stronger voice to the role of law in shaping professional behavior. (Not surprisingly, much of this literature comes from physician-commentators with a shared disdain for legal intervention.)

Noticeably absent from the list is any serious attention to the consequences of not honoring an advance directive or the role of law and policy in enforcing patients' rights.[15] Few commentators have proposed a direct response to the simple question: What happens if a physician refuses to honor a patient's advance directive? One law professor, George Annas, eschews the soft sell. Annas suggests deploying the engine of the law to impose penalties for noncompliance in the hope that fear of litigation will bring about more direct and meaningful change in physicians' behavior. What is needed, he contends, is an army of law firms committed to suing doctors for monetary damages (not just a declaration of patients' rights) when they fail to honor refusals of treatment near the end of life.[16]

Annas is correct in his focus on the consequences of noncompliance and in his call for bench and bar to play more effective roles in enforcing patients' rights. The old maxim that for every violation of a right there ought to be a remedy cannot be gainsaid. The idea that the specter of civil litigation is the answer to the problem is largely untested, however, and it should be received with more than a modicum of caution.

To date there have been few lawsuits seeking to recover monetary damages for violation of a patient's right to refuse treatment, and these cases have sent mixed messages. Patients' rights advocates frequently cite an early appellate case from Ohio, *Estate of Leach v. Shapiro*,[17] for its recognition of a civil cause of action for wrongful continuation of life support, although the case ended with an unreported settlement. A more recent decision from Ohio's highest court leaves the significance of *Leach* in considerable doubt, however. In *Anderson*[18] (also known as *Winter* because Anderson sued as administrator of patient Edward Winter's estate), the court strongly rejected a "wrongful living" cause of action, holding that "continued living" is not a compensable injury.[19] The Ohio Supreme Court embraced the proposition (as did the court in *Leach*) that continuing (or starting) treatment after it has been refused may constitute a battery (that is, an unauthorized intrusion upon the body) but seriously limited recovery of damages to actual harm (broken bones, tissue burns) caused by the life-sustaining intervention, stating that "[w]here the battery was physically harmless . . . the plaintiff is entitled to nominal damages only."[20] In effect, as long as resuscitation or other measures are performed competently, health care professionals in the Buckeye state seem to have little to fear when they override a treatment refusal.[21]

A 1996 Michigan jury verdict awarding $16 million in damages for wrongful continuation of aggressive treatment might have sent shock waves through the halls of critical care units if it had been officially reported and received more publicity at the time. The basis for the verdict was that continuing life support contrary to the repeated requests of the patient's mother, who was legally appointed as proxy (the Michigan term is "patient advocate"), constituted a battery. The impact of *Osgood*[22] was significantly diminished on appeal, however; the circuit court reduced the award to approximately $1 million (still a substantial sum but more than likely within the policy limits of applicable insurance). More important, following *Anderson* the Michigan court rejected a cause of action for wrongful life and limited recovery to "nominal damages."[23] On a related issue, *Osgood* allowed recovery for the costs of care after wrongful resuscitation. On the other hand, courts in New York and North Carolina have been unreceptive to efforts to force health care facilities to pay for the costs of continued treatment that was refused by the patient.[24]

Future developments in end-of-life damage actions cannot be reliably predicted on the basis of these scant precedents. Moreover, the legal issues are far more complicated than the foregoing summary suggests, as evidenced by the prominence of this topic in the law reviews over time.[25] One critical and untested set of complexities concerns how advance directive statutes themselves parse liability. As I note in chapter one, some statutes grant legal immunity to physicians and other health care professionals who act in good faith to honor a patient's directive—suggesting that liability would have to be premised on bad-faith behavior, if not blatant noncompliance. On the other hand, several states grant legal immunity for continuing life support even if the patient's directive refuses it. These laws create no legal incentive to honor a written treatment refusal and, absent unusual circumstances, would bar completely an award of monetary damages for violation of the patient's rights. In sum, extant law hardly is cause for enthusiasm among patients' rights advocates who are hoping for a litigation explosion.[26]

Even granting Annas's premise that a litigation assault ultimately would carry the day for patients' rights, we would do better to chart an alternative course that looks to the combined efforts of legislatures and courts but does not blaze a path to the courthouse.[27] Creating more effective (and less threatening) legal incentives to honor patients' wishes requires explicit policy guidance to set forth rules for overriding an advance directive. By the same token, rules for overriding would define more clearly when not honoring a directive is a violation of a patient's rights.

The law should expressly recognize the position I suggest in chapter three—namely, that there are three, and only three, substantive grounds for overriding an advance directive. I call these grounds the Hopeless Ambiguity Standard, the Radical Change in Circumstances Standard, and the Rebel Proxy Standard. Clear policy is required to govern the process to be followed when a decision to override a directive is contemplated. The way to ensure that the burden of meeting one of these standards clearly rests with those who would set aside a directive (most often physicians and hospitals but possibly proxy or family) is to subject this decision to mandatory review by an institutional ethics committee or a court of law. (This argument is not to suggest, of course, that physicians and hospitals should not be held legally responsible for failure to comply with a dying patient's expressed treatment refusal.) The discussion that follows expands on these prescriptions.

It bears emphasis that these prescriptions are a call to move from ethical norms to legal and policy norms in order to shape clinical norms and behavior. Implicitly, the case for specific and limited standards for overriding directives (like the theory of prospective autonomy presented in chapters two and three) also is an argument for removing restrictions on patient and proxy authority contained in many advance directive statutes, such as those that authorize forgoing of life support only when the patient is terminally ill or permanently unconscious or that impose added requirements for removal of feeding tubes. I suggest in chapter one that restrictions such as these are not only ethically suspect, they are vulnerable to legal challenge. Nonetheless, I acknowledge here that if a directive's treatment refusal is out of keeping with a particular state's current law, this discrepancy may present a fourth ground for overriding it, arguably justified on legal (perhaps risk management), not ethical, grounds. I do not undertake here the sort of detailed analysis of various state laws required to address this question.

Substantive Grounds for Overriding an Advance Directive

Hopeless Ambiguity

When advance directives are properly understood as condition-oriented and outcome-oriented intentional plans, and the interpretive authority and responsibility of proxies and family members are straightforwardly recognized, only the occasional directive will prove *hopelessly* ambiguous and fail the test of sufficient guidance. Critics who fail to appreciate these points and wrongly assert that the written terms of the document must be highly specific, fit the current medical circumstances with great accuracy, mimic informed consent, and leave little (if any) room for uncertainty and interpretive judgment are prone to exaggerate the scope of the problem of ambiguity. The case for an ethic of judgment makes plain that proxy and/or family should and can resolve apparent ambiguities. It also makes patent the absurd consequence of rigid adherence to one or more of these alternative conceptions of what we should reasonably expect from advance care planning.[28]

Nevertheless, that a directive may prove hopelessly ambiguous is by no means a mere theoretical possibility. There are and will be instances where one simply cannot determine what the patient would want. Ambiguity is of particular concern when health care providers are called on to interpret a living will for a patient with no proxy and no appropriate surrogate involved in the patient's care—when decisions must be based on the instruction directive alone. When a directive is so ambiguous that it fails to provide sufficient guidance, it is an ineffective and nonautonomous document. Hence, when it is set aside in favor of the patient's best interests, this action is justified precisely because there is *no violation of autonomy*. The Hopeless Ambiguity Standard marks off the boundary between an autonomous and nonautonomous directive. There is no duty to honor a nonautonomous directive; determining the action-guide for such a duty is impossible.

Because ambiguity is a fact-sensitive question of fit between prior statements and current circumstances, what makes an instruction directive ambiguous cannot be meaningfully defined in the abstract. Experience does suggest some guideposts, however. Operative language in early living wills, such as those drafted and distributed by the national advocacy organization Choice in Dying (formerly Concern for Dying and Society for the Right to Die), used terms ("heroic measures") and phrases ("no reasonable expectation of my recovery from physical or mental disability") that have proven to be especially vulnerable to ambiguity.[29] The talisman of specificity in some documents can give rise to equally important (though less obvious) concerns about ambiguity.

Future efforts to improve advance care planning would do well to avoid the pitfalls of these two extremes, while remaining mindful that there is no magic language that renders an advance directive immune to vagueness and ambiguity. As we move forward, everyone who is responsible for a patient's care should come to understand their respective obligations to confront—not shy away from—uncertainty. Physicians and other health care providers also should understand that they have essential roles as advisors, partners, and educators in the process of advance care planning, as well as in decision making at the bedside. These responsibilities include being alert to the possibility of a proxy's clearly wrong interpretation of what are in reality hopelessly ambiguous instructions of a combined directive. Health care professionals ought not arrogate the authority to declare a directive hopelessly ambiguous and ignore a prior treatment refusal, however, without first subjecting this choice to the scrutiny of others.

Radical Change in Circumstances
Treatment refusals made in anticipation of a possible future are rooted in a base of knowledge and understanding about the nature of illness, disease, and disability, as well as the nature, promise, and limitations of medicine's capacity to heal, cure, restore function, control pain, and alleviate suffering. We can think of this knowledge base as constituting a portion of the background conditions for the choices made in advance directives, at least to the extent the patient considers this information material. Hence, the current state of the medical art provides background assumptions against which a person evaluates whether a future state of illness is an acceptable or unacceptable quality of life. Suppose, however, that the background assumptions that obtained when the directive was issued are no longer valid when the directive must be implemented. What if medicine has made substantial progress in what it has to offer to the dying patient?

To illustrate the point, consider the promise of the new genetic medicine. Today, a diagnosis of Alzheimer's disease means a prognosis of inevitable, prolonged decline toward profound dementia, dependence, and often extended nursing home care. Alzheimer's is among the most feared life-threatening illnesses—a quality of life many would prefer not to endure. Suppose, looking to the not-so-distant future, that the patient's directive refuses life support in the event of severe irreversible dementia, and the patient now suffers from progressive dementia of the Alzheimer's type. Suppose further that recent breakthroughs in the search for an Alzheimer's vaccine have led to development of effective therapies to combat the effects of plaque deposits in the brain and improve mental function.[30] Should the directive be honored if the intent to refuse treatment was formed on the assumption that dementia would be irreversible, but that assumption is no longer true?

There is good reason not to honor a directive in such a case. Under the Radical Change in Circumstances Standard, holding a prior instruction directive to be nonautonomous would be justified on the ground that it failed to contemplate this new and effective therapy. Like hopeless ambiguity, a radical change in circumstances draws the line between an autonomous and nonautonomous directive. Taking a combined directive to be severable, the same may be said of the instruction part of a combined directive. In effect, holding the instruction to terminate life support to be nonautonomous removes from the proxy the authority to make this choice.

Medicine's past, present, and future offer other illustrations. Prior to development of the technical capability to perform liver transplants and of drugs such as cyclosporin to prevent rejection, diagnosis of progressive liver disease was a terminal diagnosis. Should a directive authored prior to availability of this procedure be honored if the patient is now a suitable candidate for transplant?[31] We can imagine similar scenarios for various forms of cancer, AIDS, neurological disorders such as Parkinson's and Huntington's diseases, and other targets of medical research. Since its inception in 1990, the Human Genome Project has identified more than 100 disease-linked genes; the active search for effective therapies (the "Holy Grail" of the project) is well underway.[32] Of course, the wonders of modern medicine do not literally emerge overnight. (One might even complain that the examples require some indulgence of crystal ball gazing.) Nor does medicine typically progress with great speed from treating symptoms to outright cure of terminal illness. The main point, however, is that a radical change in circumstances is more than a theoretical possibility. The intention of a prior directive must be measured against what medicine now has to offer to the patient.

A critical issue is how significant the change of circumstances must be to warrant disregard of a directive. As in the foregoing examples, the new medical intervention must offer substantial benefit for the patient—substantial reversal of symptoms, restoration of function, and extension of life, if not cure. More to the point, overriding a directive for this reason would be justified only if medicine could now alleviate the conditions of incompetence, pain, disability, dependence, and so forth that the patient considered material components of an unacceptable quality of life. A "new" ability to merely prolong life (prolong the dying process) for a while longer, with some greater measure of relief from pain and suffering than was possible years earlier, does not meet this test. Using the radical change of circumstances standard to retreat to medicine's traditional attachment to longevity alone would be an abuse. This attitude is precisely what many people reject when they refuse life support. The focus must be on quality of life, not quantity. What medicine now offers that was not available before must be *radically different*.[33]

A word of caution—or at least an admission of personal ambivalence. Many people undoubtedly would welcome the sorts of medical "miracles" identified above. If asked, when completing a directive, "If a new treatment should be developed after you become incompetent that could restore the functions you consider important, would you want that treatment to be tried despite your written refusal of treatment?" many people would say yes. For this group, a prior directive refusing treatment is rendered ineffective and nonautonomous by a radical change in critical information on which it was based. (If this sentiment has been clearly articulated in the advance directive dialogue, it would be more appropriate to say that continued treatment is consistent with the patient's intent and plan and that providing the new intervention honors patient autonomy.) This attitude will not be true for all people, however. Some people feel that "a good long life," however personally defined, is enough, and they might not desire another few years (or even 10) of quiet senescence. Any decision to continue treatment contrary to the patient's directive should always maintain sight on the person the patient has been over the course of an entire life.

Finally, we must understand what the radical change of circumstances standard is not. One can point to other circumstances that arguably may have changed, such as the patient's medical condition or the patient's interests and values. As the discussions of the *Browning* case (above) and the *Martin* case (below) show, the question of whether a patient's current medical condition was anticipated and addressed in a prior directive raises an issue of ambiguity. A choice to set aside a directive for this reason should be assessed in light of the hopeless ambiguity standard.

The suggestion that a change in the patient's interests and values may provide sufficient warrant to override a prior directive can be construed in several ways. To the extent that this suggestion posits that the now-incompetent patient has become a different person, with different interests and values, or (more modestly) that the patient's current experiential interests should predominate, these positions are fatally flawed.

Another possibility is suggested by a reversal of the case of conversion to the Jehovah's Witness faith. If the most recent set of interests and values are expressed in an intentional plan refusing treatment, the directive ought to be honored even if the patient's religious conversion is of recent origin. Suppose, however, that the patient undergoes a significant change in values (perhaps embracing a newfound religion) that strongly favors the sanctity of life but later becomes comatose before contravening a prior directive's treatment refusal.[34] The radical change in circumstances test should make room for such exceptional cases—but only in the presence of compelling evidence of the patient's commitment to longevity of life of whatever quality. Far more common are situations in which an incompetent patient's contemporaneous expressions appear to contradict a prior directive's treatment refusal. I argue below that a more constructive way to approach this problem is to construe it as an apparent change of mind and to treat the directive *as if* it has been suspended, for so long as the patient manifests a consistent desire to cling to life.

The Rebel Proxy

We commonly understand that an individual entrusted with responsibility to act on another's behalf should be deprived of the authority to do so when he or she breaches that trust. It is well-accepted in medical law that a guardian can be removed from that role for failure to fulfill his or her obligation to promote the interests of the patient. This same general rule applies to formally appointed proxies and to family members interpreting a living will. Virtually all advance directive statutes provide, either expressly or by implication, that a proxy must act within the bounds of his or her authority. When someone believes that a proxy's decisions are outside these bounds, his or her authority—like a guardian's—may be challenged in a court of law.[35] The Rebel Proxy Standard gives more targeted voice to these general principles.

In the bioethical lexicon, the term *turncoat proxy* has been used to refer to the malicious or malevolent proxy—one who says (thinks), "she deserves to suffer," "I can't wait to be rid of him," or "what will I do with all that money?" and means it. In rare instances, such as the high-profile case of Sonny von Bulow, there may even be suspicion of foul play. As the term suggests, the turncoat proxy breaches his or her fiduciary duties by contravening the patient's wishes out of ill motive. For this reason, the turncoat proxy should be removed. Of course, a proxy also may harbor malevolent feelings but not act on them. As long as the proxy does not stray from the bounds of entrusted authority, he or she cannot be called a turncoat, and there is no cause to challenge his or her role—although evidence of ill will cautions added vigilance to ensure good faith behavior.

Rebel proxy has a broader meaning. It is intended to compass as well cases in which the proxy breaches the fiduciary duty to act within the bounds of his or her authority without malevolent motive. Even granting the wide berth due the proxy's judgment, the proxy (or a family member interpreting a living will) may still misinterpret the patient's express wishes. A proxy could simply be "dead wrong." The proxy carrying the burdens of decision might press too hard to make sense of hopelessly ambiguous instructions. In some instances, a proxy might be unprepared to meet his or her responsibilities, perhaps overcome by the emotional strain of a loved one's impending death. These occurrences are real, though rare. In such cases, the proxy's specific decision (or the authority to make a decision, in the case of inaction) should be overturned. Unlike the turncoat proxy, however—who should be removed from the role of proxy altogether—the rebel proxy appropriately can continue to fill that role, assuming the ability to do so, without authority to make the particular decision in question. This resolution would facilitate the proxy's involvement in other aspects of the patient's care, including future treatment decisions. The same rule should apply to family members interpreting a living will.

Note that in nearly all cases of this sort, overturning a proxy directive also overrides prior autonomy because the vast majority of proxy directives make plain who is to fill this role and set forth sufficient markers to ascertain the fundamental bounds of the proxy's authority. (We might imagine rare exceptions in which the surrounding circumstances arguably vitiate autonomy: For example, the proxy-to-be may have disguised an evil heart in the hope of obtaining formal power over end-of-life decisions for a despised relative.) In some cases—in which the proxy's authority is annulled because he or she has clearly misinterpreted the patient's wishes—this response may protect and promote autonomy by enforcing the patient's prior expressions. The most probable scenario would involve a combined directive in which the document's treatment instructions are (reasonably) clear and a good case can be made that the proxy's judgment is wrong.

This latter possibility suggests a further question: Should the proxy's authority be limited by a standard of reasonableness? Veatch has argued that although a family member acting as surrogate decision maker in the absence of a writing (that is, exercising substituted judgment) should be given substantial deference, family surrogate decisions should not be accepted if they are based on a surrogate's unreasonable values and beliefs or on an unreasonable application of those values and beliefs. As formulated, this standard would not require a surrogate's decision to be the objectively best or most popular choice, but the treatment choice must be tolerable to the reasonable person.[36]

There is reason to be sympathetic to this position. After all, a spouse or child—perhaps but not necessarily a malevolent one—could do serious harm to the patient, including prematurely ending the patient's life, if granted unbridled discretion. This same concern is addressed by the rebel proxy standard, with an important difference. With an advance directive, the patient has committed to writing what he or she believes to be the reasonable bounds of the proxy's authority. The point of the rebel proxy test is that as long as the proxy stays within these confines, his or her authority should be recognized, however unreasonable a treatment decision may seem to others. The patient has decided what is reasonable. This judgment should not be superseded by an externally imposed standard that is based on what the average reasonable person would choose or on the basis of officially promulgated guidelines or policies embracing some version of what is reasonable or best.[37] A rebel proxy who overreaches by assigning undue importance to his or her own personal values when interpreting a directive, like the proxy who can't let go (as in the third scenario at the end of this chapter), has acted unreasonably on the patient's definition of reasonableness.

Process and Review

The Burden of Persuasion: Who Should Take the Next Step?
Suppose a cancer patient's combined directive refuses artificial nutrition and hydration in the event of terminal illness and appoints his wife as proxy to carry out his wishes. The attending physician believes that a feeding tube should be placed and cannot in good conscience abide by the patient's choice. Conversation with the wife over the course of several days fails to

resolve this impasse. As more time elapses, the attending physician is increasingly concerned for the patient's welfare and is anxious to insert the tube.

Conventional wisdom prescribes a short list of procedural rules for handling familiar conflicts such as this. Care may be transferred to another physician if the patient's welfare is not jeopardized and the new physician is prepared to honor the patient's wishes—in effect, working a brokered accommodation between patients' rights and physicians' rights of professional conscience. Another option is to ask an ethics committee or ethics consultant to become involved; the committee or consultant would clarify the issues, facilitate communication, and render advice (which might include transferring care), without usurping the traditional decisional prerogatives nested within the physician-patient-family relationship. Both approaches shelter patient care from the public eye of the courts, which remain available as the ultimate arbiter of intractable disputes.

Although these options are not recited in law in this fashion, the core features of this official mantra find ample legal and policy support. Advance directive laws uniformly provide for transfers of care.[38] Ethics committees find legal foundations in *Quinlan* and other decisions to follow its lead. Their pervasive presence in hospitals may be most strongly attributable to the nearly decade-old mandate from the Joint Commission on Accreditation of Hospital Organizations that hospitals establish and maintain mechanisms for ensuring patients' rights to be involved in consideration and resolution of ethical issues affecting their own care.[39] Physicians have long found legal shelter when claims of professional conscience are properly invoked, particularly when such claims are undertaken prudently with notice to the patient and family and without abandoning the patient's needs during the transition.[40]

Despite good moral sense and legal backing, this formula has failed to fulfill its promise. By most accounts, the dominant behavioral norm in clinical practice is that patient autonomy is respected as long as the patient's choice concurs with the physician's judgment of the patient's good. Patients' end-of-life choices are routinely ignored where the fact of patient choice matters most—when it is in conflict with the physician's view of what is best for the patient. This inattention occasionally may be excused as a by-product of the busy medical center, where simply abiding the traditional mission to preserve life sometimes is easier than engaging the family in open and timely dialogue. Nonetheless, we can reasonably infer that part and parcel of this disregard is a co-equal disdain for these widely acknowledged procedural rules. Inside the walls of the hospital, many physicians resist the felt intrusion of concurrent ethics committee participation. From the outside looking in, the comfort and carrot of legal compliance has proven to be insufficient motivation to conform, perhaps in part because the stick of potential legal liability has been so weak.

The phenomenon of passing responsibility for taking the next step to the patient, proxy, and family seems all too common. The message is that in the eyes of medicine, beneficence rather than autonomy—the physician's judgment (or the hospital's) rather than the patient's— sits atop the decisional tree. As portrayed in one of the passages that begins this chapter, patients and families, already burdened with the weight of decision, are challenged to negotiate foreign rules, processes, and cultures to show that what has been turned upside down should be reversed again.[41] For patients without family or friends involved in their care, whose control over the dying process must rely solely on the power of instruction directives, there may be no one to proclaim, with document in hand, "No—this is not what she wants."

Here, at the bedside, is where law, policy, and practice have failed to give dying patients and their loved ones the support they so much need and deserve. If autonomy is entitled to a strong presumption of respect, those who would override a directive (physician, hospital, occasionally family) should bear the burden of persuasion to overcome this presumption and justify their actions. To give true meaning to the duty to honor advance directives, the choice *not to honor* a patient's prior treatment refusal must be brought into the light, not shrouded in darkness.

The burden of justifying noncompliance must be placed squarely on the shoulders of health care providers, mending loopholes in the current scheme that have allowed physicians and others to avoid this responsibility largely without consequence. It is time to move beyond the hortatory suggestion that "if you don't want to comply with your patient's advance directive, you *should* seek the counsel of an ethics committee or consultant." This permissive approach should be supplanted by the mandate "before you choose not to comply with your patient's advance directive, you *must* subject your decision to the scrutiny of others." Physicians (and others who would choose noncompliance) also should be apprised of the nature of the task— to defend the decision to override by appeal to one of the three grounds for doing so. To borrow from the legal lexicon, the task is to rebut the presumption in favor of respect by showing that the directive is hopelessly ambiguous, there has been a radical change in circumstances, or the proxy has strayed beyond the bounds of his or her authority.

Mandating Accountability: Ethics Committees and Courts

To whom, then, should physicians or others challenging a directive's authority be held to account? Several commentators have rehearsed the comparative merits of institutional ethics committees (IECs) and courts.[42] Ethics committees have been effective in the task of resolving disagreements closer to the bedside, subjecting the private realm of the physician-patient-family relationship to a minimum of intrusion. They also offer a less formal, lower cost, and arguably more accessible resource than the courthouse. On the other hand, courts possess the publicly legitimated power to judge the patient's wishes ambiguous, order that treatment be continued, remove a rebel proxy, or bind the parties in other ways—which committees appointed by hospitals do not. Furthermore, as public officials who are not involved in the patient's care, judges can exercise more detached and objective judgment and are better suited to function as fact-finders, employing the rules of evidence and even compelling testimony.

The wisdom of the current system is that it legitimates both options: preserving the public authority of the courts while relying on local committees as facilitators of a more private solution. So too the deployment of ethics consultants, who most often function under the auspices of the IEC while offering still more flexibility and accessibility. As a general matter, current law and practice is based on an "optional/optional" model of the committee's role.[43] Participants are encouraged but not required to look to IECs (or consultants) as the forum of next resort. Recourse to the IEC creates no legal or moral obligation to follow its advice. Neither IECs nor consultants are vested with authority to impose their will on others. Decisional authority remains within the physician-patient-proxy-family relationship, with the option of adopting the IEC's recommendation(s), in whole or in part. At the same time, whatever the committee (or consultant) recommends, the door to the courthouse remains open, although only on rare occasions—such as when it becomes necessary to seek removal of a rebel proxy or surrogate decision maker—do the courts become the required venue.[44]

Alongside this reigning paradigm are some notable examples of mandated prospective review by multidisciplinary committees charged with responsibility to address ethical issues. These examples include the abortion committees of the 1960s (created by statute in several states) and the dialysis committees in Seattle and elsewhere (mandated by institutional policy) that were directed to allocate scarce dialysis machines.[45] These types of committees have since fallen out of favor and existence. On the other hand, two federal initiatives for committee review of ethical issues that arose in the 1980s remain in force today. A piece of the "Baby Doe" regulatory scheme strongly encourages (but does not actually mandate) use of infant care review committees to address proposed decisions to forgo treatment for disabled newborns.[46] Institutional review boards have become a mandated fixture nationwide since regulatory adoption in 1981 of the Federal Policy for the Protection of Human Subjects in research (now known as the "Common Rule").[47]

Closer to the idea of a limited role in end-of-life decisions, New York's do not resuscitate (DNR) law requires that disputes concerning DNR orders for incompetent patients be submitted to a dispute mediation system.[48] A growing chorus of voices, including that of the American Medical

Association, is pushing the medical futility debate toward a policy of IEC consultation when forgoing of treatment on futility grounds is contemplated, especially in cases of family-physician discord.[49] This approach to futility cases has been adopted as hospital policy in some communities,[50] and it was embraced in the 1999 revision of the Texas Advance Directives Act.[51]

The closest analogues to the scheme proposed here are in the states of Maryland and Texas. Maryland is among the very few states that has legally required establishment of hospital ethics committees (called "patient care advisory committees").[52] Under Maryland law, a health care provider who believes an incompetent patient's instruction refusing life support to be "inconsistent with generally accepted standards of patient care" must seek the advice of an IEC or petition for court review. Under Texas law (revised in 1999), an attending physician who refuses to honor an advance directive or a treatment refusal in the absence of a directive must subject that decision to review "by an ethics or medical committee."[53] Maryland and Texas are to be credited for putting the burden of going forward with physicians who would choose not to comply with treatment refusals.

A closer look, however, reveals several shortcomings in each state's law. Maryland's amorphous standard to invoke review appears to prioritize generally accepted standards of care over patients' wishes and offers an open invitation to paternalistic challenges to prior instructions. In fact, the statutory language suggests—perhaps unintentionally—that the committee's charge involves a predominantly medical rather than ethical judgment. Reliance on the phrase "generally accepted standards" also offers committees and courts no meaningful guidance in the task of assessing whether overriding the patient's wishes is ethically or legally permissible. In addition, the statute is silent on the matter of the burden of persuasion to be satisfied to override a patient's directive.

The Texas law has similar flaws. It provides no express guidance with regard to grounds for a physician's refusal to comply with a directive, nor does it allocate a burden of persuasion. Moreover, permitting review by a medical committee, not necessarily an ethics committee, suggests that a physician's decision need not be justified by appeal to ethics at all—or, at least, that it need not be subject to scrutiny from a moral standpoint.

Both states further err by conferring legal immunity on physicians who follow the committee's advice—effectively giving the physician and committee tandem authority to override the decision of the patient's proxy or one or more family members.[54] This immunity may substantially weaken any court challenge initiated by proxy or family. Texas law states that if the physician, patient, or person responsible for making decisions on the patient's behalf "[does] not agree with the decision reached during the review process . . . the physician shall make a reasonable effort to transfer the patient to a physician who is willing to comply with the directive."[55] This provision is a reasonable alternative to court intervention (it also would be an option in Maryland), but it seems to add to the committee's decisional authority. Interestingly, both states carve out additional roles in patient care for review committees. Maryland requires that in the absence of a proxy directive, disputes among surrogate decision makers of co-equal authority (for example, two adult children) must be referred to an IEC by the attending physician.[56] Texas provides that in the absence of a legally authorized surrogate, a treatment decision must be "concurred in by another physician who is not involved in the treatment of the patient or—a representative of an ethics or medical committee."[57] Another provision gives parallel authority in "futility" cases, stating that if the patient (or his or her representative) requests continued life support that "the attending physician and the review process have decided is inappropriate treatment," the patient's care should be transferred.[58]

Future efforts to manage disagreements about advance directives should follow the more specific patient-oriented guidelines I advocate here. In addition, the wiser approach is to maintain firm commitment to a purely advisory role for the committee and to insist on court intervention to resolve intractable disputes. The following section turns to the IEC's patient-centered charge and its advisory role.

Some Objections and Responses

Several sorts of objections to mandated IEC consultation can be anticipated. The idea undoubtedly will find a hostile audience among physicians and others who regard IECs as an unwarranted intrusion on professional prerogatives.[59] This attitude misses the point, however. The salutary purpose of mandatory review is that it forces physicians and other health care providers to think harder and longer about the choice not to honor a directive by putting that conviction to a simple test: persuading others of its correctness. The prod to take advance directives more seriously in the first place gives practical teeth to the normative weight of the patient's wishes.

Ideally, committee consultation would occur only when there is good reason to believe that one of the three grounds for overriding a directive applies. The outcome of this initiative ought to be that there are relatively few instances of challenge—that IEC consultation is by far the exception rather than the rule; it ought not, however, discourage physicians (or others) from acting in good conscience to promote the patient's good. If the opposite trend were to occur, overutilization of committees and associated problems (assuring the timeliness of group meetings, having adequate time for deliberation, imposing excessive demands on volunteer members, and the burdens of recordkeeping) could be addressed through greater use of ethics consultants to mediate disputes. Targeted educational initiatives could and should be developed at the institutional level to foster understanding of the rules for honoring and overriding advance directives.

Committees charged with this responsibility should be committed to a patient-centered ethic in the fulfillment of their tasks. Proponents of a fully rigorous patient-centered ethic might insist that the patient or, as appropriate, the proxy or family must consent to committee review and further that each should have the right to attend the meeting and address the committee when it deliberates. Each premise can be based on the patient's right of confidentiality, which belongs as well to the proxy or other person acting on the incompetent patient's behalf.[60] The proposed scheme should and easily can accommodate the second premise, giving patients and their chosen agents a rightful presence before the committee.

The first premise is more problematic because a proxy's (or family member's) exercise of a purported right of confidentiality here effectively blocks IEC consultation. As a general matter, this principled veto would empower patients, proxies, and families to safeguard important rights and interests; for this reason, it is worthy of serious attention. There is reason to fear, however, that in the care of incompetent dying patients this otherwise friendly amendment might well subvert the purpose and value of IEC consultation. Although many proxies undoubtedly will prefer first resort to an IEC to the prospect of a public courtroom drama, a strategizing proxy might bluntly say to physician and hospital, "Do what I say, or take me to court," hoping to coerce compliance with the proxy's judgment. Traditional disquiet over judicial intervention in patient care suggests that this gambit may be more likely than not to succeed, inducing physicians to abandon conscientious commitment to patient advocacy. This outcome is especially problematic when veto power is in the hands of a rebel proxy. For these reasons, the incompetent dying patient's interest in strict confidentiality should here yield to the patient's broader interests in more private, less cumbersome conflict resolution that is based on enhanced, shared understanding—which is what IECs have shown they can deliver. Public policy mandating review should be understood to effect a limited waiver of the patient's right—and the physician's duty—of confidentiality in deference to these broader objectives.[61]

The promise and pitfalls of IECs have generated a voluminous literature.[62] I would be remiss not to acknowledge some of the other salient general objections that might be made to the call for an expanded role for these committees, separate and apart from the narrow question of mandates. Much of the critical analysis of IECs touches on three fundamental and often interrelated themes: operating standards, the committee's mission and loyalties, and the quality of deliberations.

For the most part, IECs are unregulated participants in patient care. *Standards* governing committee operations are still found almost exclusively in institutional policy that is subject to little public scrutiny, and they can vary considerably from place to place. IECs typically are not invested in rules of procedural due process—a traditional hallmark of fairness in law. Moreover, neither committees nor consultants are accountable in meaningful ways for their actions, either within the institution or before the law. IECs and consultants have rarely been sued, and none have been found liable.[63]

The members of an IEC, most of whom are health care providers, have duties and *loyalties* to an institution, to a profession, and to colleagues that may conflict with strict fidelity to patient-centered care. Arguably, IECs cannot consistently be counted on to be strong patient advocates. In fact, the committee's *mission* remains a much-debated question: Does the committee serve—first and foremost—patients, physicians, the health care team, or the institution? Is its role to offer a collegial forum (a consultative model) or to resolve disputes (an adjudicatory model)?[64]

On the prevailing model of deliberation toward consensus, a group of mostly health care professionals who are all from the same institution may be predisposed to what has been labeled "groupthink"[65] or be unduly influenced by the forceful presence of particular members (a misgiving directed most often toward attorneys).[66] Notably, the recent report of the American Society of Bioethics and Humanities Task Force on Standards for Bioethics Consultation casts a critical eye on the core competencies of ethics consultants and committees—an important topic that bioethics as a field has only begun to seriously address.[67] In sum, there is good reason to keep a watchful eye on the *quality* of the deliberative process.

Another less commonly identified source of worry is that within the walls of a given hospital, "[t]he institutional force of some recommendations is so strong, that they are, in effect, mandatory"[68]—giving IECs *de facto* decisional authority and promoting what Agich labels "surrender of judgment."[69] Other commentators point to the absence of criteria and tools for measuring whether IECs are doing a good job.[70]

Despite persistent doubts and cautionary admonitions, IECs have continued to proliferate and evolve, gaining a stronger foothold as participants in patient care. If IECs matured from infancy to adolescence in their first two decades,[71] there is still much growing to be done. Without question, the aforementioned misgivings should continue to command our attention as IECs and consultants become increasingly integral players in the delivery of care. None of these critiques, however, points to fatal flaws in the concept or practice of IECs or the activity of ethics consultation. They offer weak foundations for objection to the modest modification of existing norms and practices endorsed here, distracting from the main point of the argument.

My essential claim is that *some* mechanism of local review is needed to hold those who would override advance directives to account for this choice. No less is called for to give advance directives their due. Investing IECs with this limited mandate adds another layer to the established institutional presence of IECs. It also builds on an important experiential base, insofar as the vast majority of case consultations involve decisions near the end of life.[72] Most important, this modest step forward calls on IECs to continue to do what they do best: to clarify issues and facilitate communication. The value and promise of the IEC lie in its contribution to the process of airing and resolving these treatment dilemmas.[73] IECs are simply the most logical—if admittedly imperfect—candidate for the task. For the rare institutions that do not have an ethics committee or similar mechanism or have failed to grant an IEC authority to provide case consultations, the choice is to look to the court as the arbiter of disputes. (Alternatively, an appropriate plan might be to collaborate with other institutions in the community to pool resources or to expand an existing committee's warrant.)

Under the scheme for which I have been arguing, a beginning sketch of an ethic of ethics committees in this limited role and a beginning, more direct response to the foregoing concerns might proceed along the following lines. The IEC's task is to adopt a patient-centered ethic that acknowledges the priority claim of prospective autonomy, not to agree on what is best for the patient.[74] The charge is to advise whether the committee believes that *not* following the directive is justified, applying the three substantive standards for overriding a directive to its own evaluation of the facts. The governing standards for overriding a directive also become standards for fulfillment of this responsibility. They shape what the committee is supposed to do, serve as guidelines for adoption of rules of process, and offer measures for assessing whether the committee has been faithful to its charge. As under the current regime, the weight of the IEC's advice may depend on its institutional status. In general, committee concurrence that the directive justifiably may be set aside should bolster health care providers' convictions that continued treatment is in the patient's best interests. On the other hand, an IEC that sides with the patient's directive (or the proxy's interpretation, as the case may be) sends a signal to those who are responsible for the patient's care to abide by the patient's wishes.[75]

Everyone involved should be mindful that helping to resolve disagreements does not mean supplanting the prerogatives of the physician-patient-proxy relationship. Those who are responsible for the patient's care should be reminded that decisional authority still resides within that relationship and that failing agreement, each retains the options of pressing their cause before a court or pursuing a transfer of care. Whatever the ultimate outcome in a particular case, the salutary contribution of IEC participation extends beyond resolution of the ethical dilemma at hand. Embraced and legitimated in policy, the command "take it to the ethics committee" issues a clarion call that advance directives are to be taken seriously.

CASE SCENARIOS AT THE EDGES

In the remainder of this chapter, I present and analyze three case scenarios. Each of these scenarios is based on actual cases (two of the three went to court). The discussion is intended to illuminate how these policy initiatives would work in practice and to bring to light some additional considerations involved in resolution of difficult cases. The analysis further demonstrates the soundness of the theory of prospective autonomy and advance directives.

Scenario One: An Ambiguous Instruction Directive?

> Tom Wirth, who is 47 years old, has been diagnosed with AIDS-Related Complex (ARC); he is a patient in the hospital's AIDS ward. Among his symptoms are multiple brain lesions that are believed to be caused by toxoplasmosis (a type of infection). According to Tom's physicians, his toxoplasmosis can be treated effectively, with a reasonable hope of recovery and return to mental function and capacity. He will continue to suffer from ARC, however—for which there is no cure and which inevitably will lead to death. Three months ago, Tom executed a living will and a durable power of attorney for health care. The latter document appointed Tom's friend John Evans to act as Tom's proxy, with authority "to make all decisions relating to [my] medical condition." The living will, executed the same day, states: "I direct that life-sustaining procedures should be withheld or withdrawn if I have illness, disease or injury or experience extreme mental deterioration, such that there is no reasonable expectation of recovering or regaining a meaningful quality of life." The living will defines life-sustaining treatments broadly to include surgery, antibiotics, feeding tubes, and other medical modalities. John insists that life-sustaining treatment (most important, antibiotics) not be provided to Tom. Tom's physicians disagree, believing that there is a reasonable likelihood that antibiotic treatment will be beneficial and that it will reverse the current bout of toxoplasmosis.

These are the facts of the case of *Evans v. Bellevue*[76]—one of only a handful of litigated cases (along with Mrs. Browning's case) in which an advance directive has been at issue. In the actual case, the court ruled that Evans did not have authority to refuse life-sustaining treatment on Wirth's behalf. The court reasoned that the living will's refusal of life-sustaining treatment if "there is no reasonable expectation of recovering or regaining a meaningful quality of life" was ambiguous as applied to the circumstances at hand because although there was no hope of recovery from ARC and AIDS, there was a reasonable prospect of recovery from the immediate threat of toxoplasmosis and restoral of Tom's ability to communicate. Significantly, this case occurred in New York—one of the states that requires clear and convincing evidence of the patient's refusal of treatment. Indicative of the role of this standard was the court's finding that the proxy's decision "did not clearly comport with the 'living will.'"[77]

The *Evans* case (also known as the Wirth case) has evoked a range of responses. Supporters of advance directives and AIDS activists have been understandably alarmed by the court's reasoning and the result. On the other hand, some commentators concur in the conclusion that the language of the living will was ambiguous and believe that the case was correctly decided.[78] Others have suggested that *Evans* illustrates the potential for conflict between the patient's past wishes and present interests and exemplifies the case for giving present interests priority.[79]

On the facts presented, the living will is ambiguous. There is a further analysis of this situation, however, that resolves the ambiguity. It is proper to hold, as the court did, that the proxy is bound to interpret and apply the express wishes of the living will, particularly when the two documents have been executed at the same time. There is no evidence that Wirth intended his living will to be strictly and literally construed—but also none that he expressly granted Evans authority to exercise his own judgment or act in his best interests. On the other hand, by charging Evans with authority to act on his behalf, Wirth has presumptively entrusted Evans with responsibility to make his best efforts to faithfully interpret the living will and to seek the objective that Wirth himself intends.

Unless the patient dictates otherwise, the proxy has the right and responsibility to interpret what a "reasonable quality of life" means.[80] Evans is best able to determine whether Wirth intended this phrase narrowly, as the court takes it, or with a longer view to the periodic bouts of opportunistic infection, illness, and inexorable decline that are characteristic of AIDS and AIDS-related illnesses. Recovery from the current illness and return to a life with ARC may not have been a reasonable quality of life for Tom Wirth. For him, continuing to live with what apparently was an advanced stage of AIDS-related illness that would bring progressive disability, dependency, and future hospitalization might have been an undignified and severely compromised quality of life—an affront to his self-image and the way he wanted to be remembered.

From this vantage point, the living will's intention is not ambiguous—or, at least, the ambiguity is resolved in a way that the patient intended. This analysis, of course, is speculation. The court apparently failed to inquire into prior conversations, personal attitudes and experiences, or other factors on which the proxy based his interpretation (at least, no such inquiry is reported in the opinion). If this were the case, however—and many activists in the AIDS community hold a view of this sort—then overriding the proxy's decision on grounds of ambiguity violated an effective exercise of prospective autonomy.

The physicians and hospital were right to seek review of their proposed decision not to comply with the proxy's request, although prior resort to an IEC is preferable to a rush to the courthouse. However, resolution of dilemmas such as this should give greater weight to the proxy's fiduciary right and responsibility to interpret the operative language of the living will in light of personal knowledge of its author. An ethic of judgment demands no less. The court's ruling seemingly ignores the fact that Wirth made an autonomous choice to rely on his proxy to interpret his living will. Had the health care professionals involved in Wirth's care shared this view, the proxy's authority and the patient's wishes could have been honored in private without the public spectacle of judicial intervention. Although there still may be room for doubt about what the patient considered a "meaningful quality of life," the proxy's interpretation rescues the directive from the charge that it is *hopelessly* ambiguous. There is no suggestion here of a lack of diligence and good faith in the proxy's behavior. John Evans clearly is not a rebel proxy—quite the opposite.

Evans raises another important issue. Is there a duty to foster opportunities for autonomous decision making—in this case, to actually restore cognitive capacity—when other patient values might be compromised? Several authorities hold that on a richer conception of respect for autonomy, physicians have a duty to promote patient autonomy and enhance opportunities for informed decision making, including efforts to restore decisional capacity. The same can be said of proxies and families. The basis for this understanding is that respect for autonomy means assisting patients to achieve their goals as autonomous agents.[81]

Here restoration of capacity was a reasonably likely outcome of treatment, according to the testimony adduced, and treatment might be justified on this basis. Thus, the judicial result might be reached on a different understanding of respect for autonomy that still honors the proxy's authority and responsibility to interpret the patient's intent in light of personal knowledge of the patient's life.

Nonetheless, it is unclear whether continuing treatment in the name of respect for autonomy would have promoted the patient's goals. A crucial factor is whether the possibility of intercurrent treatment to restore competence (and, perhaps, sufficient function to allow discharge from the hospital) was a part of the patient's prior deliberative process. This level of deliberation may reasonably be inferred in a situation of recurring illness and treatment, but it is a closer call when the issue presents itself for the first time. Nonetheless, I am persuaded that the proxy's judgment ought to control, absent substantial evidence that forgoing treatment is out of keeping with the patient's expressed wishes or that the proxy's decision is outside the bounds of his authority.

Scenario Two: Apparent Inconsistency in the Patient's Wishes

Michael Martin has suffered a traumatic brain injury in an automobile accident. He is unable to walk, is dependent on a colostomy tube and a feeding tube, and has lost several other physical abilities. He has suffered extensive and irreversible loss of cognitive functions and is unable to talk. The full extent of cognitive impairment is unknown, however, and Michael's physicians are not unanimous in their assessments. They generally agree that he retains some limited cognitive abilities but that he cannot understand the nature of his medical condition. He can engage in a very rudimentary form of communication by nodding in response to simple questions. According to one physician, Michael responded "no" with a head nod when he was asked if he was in pain. He made the same response when he was asked whether he did not want to continue living. The physicians caring for Michael all agree that he is not in PVS, nor is he terminally ill.

Michael was married 15 years ago and has three children. In numerous prior conversations over the course of approximately eight years—some of which occurred after he saw movies depicting terminal illness, infirmity, dependency, and accidental brain injuries—he stated to his wife Mary that he did not want to be maintained in a condition in which he was incapable of performing basic functions such as walking, talking, dressing, bathing, or eating and was dependent on others or machines. He elicited from Mary the promise that she would not permit it. Five years after the accident, with no signs of improvement in Michael's condition, Mary—who previously had been appointed as her husband's guardian and conservator—requested that the hospital ethics committee consider whether life-sustaining treatment should be withdrawn.

These are the basic facts of the Michigan case *In re Martin*.[82] In the actual case, the committee issued a report stating that withdrawal of the feeding tube was medically and ethically appropriate but that before the hospital would comply with the request, court approval would have to be obtained. Failure to resolve the matter at the local level led to extensive litigation, which included three appellate opinions—the last from the Michigan Supreme Court. In the legal proceedings, the patient's mother and sister opposed the wife's petition for authority to direct removal of the feeding tube.

Although this case involves substituted judgment, we can bring the scenario squarely within the current discussion by positing that Michael had appointed his wife as health care proxy, using a simple short form with no specific instructions. For all intents and purposes, this premise puts Mrs. Martin in the same legal position as she was in under court-appointed guardianship, with the caveat that a guardianship proceeding ordinarily involves the court in the specific decision about life support.

Amidst the many issues raised by this case, four important questions stand out: How specific must the patient's wishes be? What is the IEC's role? How should health care professionals respond to family discord? What moral weight is due an incompetent patient's contemporaneous expressions in favor of continued life? More extensive attention is due the last and least familiar of these questions.

Specificity of Prior Statements

As in *Browning*, a decisive question in *Martin* was whether prior statements about medical conditions that the patient considered to entail an intolerable quality of life should control when they do not fully match the current medical circumstances. Taking a different path than *Browning*, the high court of Michigan erred twice. The first error was joining the minority of courts that require clear and convincing evidence of the patient's treatment refusal. The second error was according substantial weight to the testimony of co-workers who concluded, on the basis of casual conversations, that the circumstances of the case were not the precise circumstances Michael Martin had in mind when he spoke of being allowed to die. (In these occasional conversations, Martin had spoken specifically of PVS.) The court's error is summarized in its ruling that "[o]nly when the patient's prior statements clearly illustrate a serious, well thought out, consistent decision to refuse treatment *under these exact circumstances, or circumstances highly similar to the current situation*, should treatment be refused or withdrawn."[83]

Judges in the *Martin* case may have been motivated by a well-intentioned belief that a prior refusal of life support should approximate as closely as possible contemporaneous informed refusal. Stringent interpretation of the evidentiary standard also might have been influenced by commitment to the sanctity of life (perhaps compelled in part by the shadow of Dr. Kevorkian). Whatever the underlying motivations, the case illustrates that this standard is misguided, with or without a prior written document—further attesting to the moral peril of insisting that prospective choices expressly and consistently match the circumstances of the patient's medical condition and treatment.

The Ethics Committee's Role

In this case, the IEC erroneously reversed the presumption in favor of prospective autonomy and family authority. Finding no troubling ambiguities in Mr. Martin's wishes and having concluded that withdrawal of the feeding tube was ethically permissible, the IEC should have affirmed Mrs. Martin's authority to decide. The committee might have suggested that the physician, hospital, and extended family had the right to challenge Mrs. Martin's decision, but it should have been clear that the burden of going to court was theirs, not hers. The committee's lack of courage (conviction?)

may be understood given that this was a case of first impression in Michigan; the committee apparently felt that existing legal guidance was inadequate. Nonetheless, it was wrong to shift responsibility for vindicating Mr. Martin's wishes to Mrs. Martin. A policy of mandatory review of *challenges* to prospective treatment refusals allocates this burden properly.

Handling Family Discord

The *Martin* case also presents the question of how physicians, hospitals, and courts ought to respond to family members who challenge the spouse/proxy's decision to terminate life support. Familial conflict over termination of life support is a common concern among health care professionals; along with the IEC's cowardice, it undoubtedly was a major factor in bringing Michael Martin's care before the courts. Unfortunately, there is no fully satisfactory answer to this dilemma. Families have every right to care about the welfare of loved ones, regardless of whether the patient has selected a single individual to act on his or her behalf. As long as family members act in good faith, they serve an important role as guardians (in the non-legal sense) of the patient's welfare. What the family would choose, however, does not alter the moral and legal obligation to honor the patient's advance directive or the authority of a personally selected proxy—fear of litigation notwithstanding. In fact, family-initiated legal challenges to a spouse's authority are relatively rare, and claims of bad faith and ill will have been turned away.[84] If health care professionals find that the family's allegations have merit, it is incumbent on them to explore whether the proxy (guardian) has exceeded the bounds of his or her authority and to involve an IEC or a court in this inquiry. In this case, although the court sided with the treatment choice advocated by the mother and sister, it rejected their claim that Mary Martin had rebelled against her husband's wishes in bad faith and should be removed as guardian—affirming the judgment previously reached by the IEC.

Contemporaneous Expressions in Favor of Life

Martin provides a point of departure for a fourth, more interesting, issue. How should the patient's contemporaneous expressions in favor of life be interpreted when they are contrary to a prior treatment refusal? Testimony suggesting that the patient retained some cognitive capacity and responded negatively (with a head nod) when he was asked whether he was in pain and whether he *did not want* to continue living was construed as evidence of inconsistency in the patient's wishes. The evidence here, though weak, was probative to the justices; it supported their conclusion that the clear and convincing evidence test was not satisfied. Note that Michael's response to the second query, about whether he *did not want* to go on living—the precise language attested by the physicians from the witness stand—itself is ambiguous, giving further pause with regard to the majority's conclusion.[85]

To be sure, current expressions—including responses to pain, discomfort, conversation, family, and so forth—are important clues to how the patient's prior statements should be interpreted, and such expressions may be of special significance to proxy and family whose task is to weigh the burdens and benefits of treatment in light of the patient's intentions and goals. An apparent preference for life support, like indicia that a choice is out of character, is a call to probe the question further with the patient. Respect for autonomy and beneficence counsel that physician, proxy, and family have special responsibilities to nurture capacities for choice by engaging the patient's participation in the course of his or her care.[86] Posing the question as one of inconsistency, however, avoids the harder and more meaningful issue: When, if ever, should contemporaneous expressions in favor of life supersede a prior directive refusing life support? Loosely speaking, can the incompetent patient change his mind?[87]

Two opposing responses stand out. We might hold that a prior autonomous directive always prevails over the current expressions of incompetent patients. Conversely, we might hold that the present plea for life always carries controlling moral weight. Norman Cantor holds a position close to the former response; Sanford Kadish argues for a version of the second view. Both direct our attention to problematic cases involving demented but communicative patients.

Cantor is troubled by the possibility that a patient's current desire for life will be taken to revoke a prior directive. Cantor is critical of advance directive laws that allow revocation whether the patient is competent or incompetent; he defends the moral and legal authority of a prior directive, holding that only a person's current autonomous choice should be taken to modify or invalidate the duty to respect his or her prior autonomous decision. Although Cantor notes several important reasons to engage the incompetent patient and take his or her expressions into account, he argues pointedly that "[g]iving dominion to the deranged expressions of [seriously demented] persons would make a mockery of self-determination when the expressions override a carefully considered advance directive."[88] Extrapolating slightly from the concern for revocation, the Cantor view is that we should honor the directive (though, as noted below, he seems sympathetic to a less-categorical view such as the one I develop shortly.)[89]

To support the contrary position, Kadish posits the case of a famous musician who executes a proxy directive in favor of her son, giving express instructions that if she should ever become permanently unable to appreciate music and is in need of life support, treatment should not be provided. (Kadish calls her Composer Then.) Composer Then subsequently succumbs to senile dementia, and these exact circumstances come to be. She does not appear to be uncomfortable, in pain, or unhappy (Composer Now). "When asked if she prefers to be left to die, she becomes agitated and says no, though how much she understands is unclear."[90] Kadish also holds that an incompetent patient's preference for life does not take precedence over a prior competent refusal, and he does not argue that Composer Now's response should be treated as an autonomous choice. Yet he argues that continuing life support is justified because it shows "compassion for the human being before us."[91]

When we look past the emotional and psychological pull of human compassion, we see that the attempt to shape this inchoate notion into an ethical action-guide is fatally flawed. We cannot make sense of the admonition to make the compassionate choice without simultaneously asking, What is best for the patient now? Appeal to human compassion alone as an ethical norm smuggles a current experiential best interests standard in the back door. Kadish's claim is at bottom the same as that of others who hold that a prior treatment refusal should be disregarded if the patient "would with proper care and treatment lead a life that clearly contains more pleasure and enjoyment than suffering and pain."[92] Kadish acknowledges as much, stating that he would continue treatment for Composer Now on the basis of human compassion alone, without the patient's expressed desire.[93] Furthermore, a norm of human compassion is susceptible to ready abuse. Those who believe that continued treatment serves the patient's good may find manipulating a vulnerable patient to express a desire for life an easy and inviting task. Continuing treatment for Composer Now and others like her in the name of human compassion is a gross affront to the person the patient is and has been over the course of a full life.[94]

The call to always honor a prior directive has far greater merit, but it gives too little voice to the dying patient's persistent plea for continued life. The better way to frame the inquiry is to ask whether the patient has changed his or her mind—that is, whether the patient has formed the present and persistent desire to continue living. (Note that appeal to the Radical Change of Circumstances Standard is simply inappropriate here because the "change of mind" is not that of a competent patient [person] evidencing a radical shift in values from those that informed a prior directive.)

Neither the ramblings of a demented patient nor an ambiguous response to the question "Do you want to die?" should be allowed to undermine the considered and effective exercise of prospective autonomy. Nor should an isolated statement—perhaps borne of anger, frustration, or delirium—be taken as a considered plea for life. The contradictory preferences of a patient who wants the respirator in the morning but refuses it in the afternoon show no consistency of purpose. In sum, continuation of life support for these patients on the basis of such *marginal reversals* works a serious injustice to prospective autonomy and advance directives.

On the other hand, some incompetent patients possess more significant cognitive capacity than these examples suggest and experience intermittent periods of lucidity and mental function. This pattern is characteristic of certain pathological conditions such as organic brain syndrome. For others, effective pain management or treatment of fatigue, infection, or other symptoms or conditions that impair cognition can temporarily restore abilities to appreciate important information, reason, and communicate.[95] Suppose the patient expresses a persistent and clear desire for continued life manifested at times of relative mental clarity. Should the desire for life be honored?

The answer should be that continuing life support is justified, but only as long as the patient remains consistent and persistent in this desire. Use of the term *desire* rather than the terms *choice* or *intent*—which connote autonomous action—is deliberate. As several commentators have observed, some nonautonomous dying patients regain capacity for autonomous choice.[96] In these instances, there is a duty to respect contemporaneous autonomy. Several states (e.g., New York and West Virginia) have adopted this position in their advance directive laws.[97] The most logically consistent view (apparently at work in the approaches of these two states) is that only a contemporaneous and autonomous desire (choice) takes precedence over a prior autonomous directive. Yet having and expressing a persistent desire for life does not demand the abilities to understand and reason about relevant medical information in light of personal values and goals that are the hallmarks of decisional capacity and autonomous, intentional decision making. Persistence, not just autonomy, has important moral significance here. One need not understand the nature of one's medical condition or be able to manipulate this information rationally to hold life dear. The New Jersey Bioethics Commission reached a similar conclusion—subsequently enacted into law—that commitment to respect for human life as well as "the possibility that the patient will have a change of mind as death approaches (and perhaps becomes a less abstract idea and a more real experience)" counsels respect for an incompetent patient's desire for continued life.[98]

Moreover, it is here that human compassion does important moral work. The question of whether to allow a patient to die in the face of a plea for continued life is one of the most difficult end-of-life dilemmas. The burdens of decision weigh especially heavily on loved ones who are struggling to make the "right" and "compassionate" choice. There is no "correct" choice in these circumstances. Complying with the patient's persistent entreaty (whether characterized as plea, request, or demand) is a permissible course, however. It is all the more permissible for proxy and family whose charge is to balance the patient's wishes with his or her welfare.

What, then, is the standing of the patient's directive? The advance directive should be treated *as if suspended* as long as the patient continues to manifest a desire for continued life. The contemporaneous desire for life limits but does not negate prospective autonomy. (This analysis assumes, of course, that the directive has not been revoked by the patient.)

Much of the analysis of the respective moral weight of the principles of prospective autonomy and beneficence has proceeded on the premise that a determination of incompetence (incapacity) shifts the locus of decisional authority from the patient to an advance directive—that is, to the proxy, family, or instruction directive, as the case may be. The concept of *suspension* is that the persistent desire for life support limits the weight of the directive by temporarily shifting decisional authority back to the patient. The nature of this limitation is that implementation of a prior refusal of life support is delayed. No further limitation of the proxy's role and authority is contemplated. A designated proxy should continue to be involved in the patient's care throughout, with authority to make collateral decisions on the patient's behalf.[99] If, as the patient's condition deteriorates, he or she ceases to express a desire for continued treatment, the directive should be honored and treatment should be withdrawn.[100]

It is not difficult to extrapolate from cases such as *Martin* to situations in which the incompetent patient expresses a persistent desire for continued life. The challenge to respond in an ethically appropriate fashion is likely to arise with increasing frequency as the population continues to age and health care professionals care for more and more patients with chronic and long-term illnesses who are severely debilitated and demented but have some limited capacity for interaction. In the future, we would do better to frame the issue as an inquiry into whether the patient manifests a persistent desire for life, suspending the duty to honor a prior treatment refusal as long as the patient continues to manifest the desire to live.[101]

Scenario Three: The Proxy Who Can't Let Go

> Mr. L is a 56-year-old man with a wife and two teenage children. He works as a butcher in the small Midwestern town where he was born and still lives with his family. Mr. L has diabetes, hypertension, and high cholesterol. He has been seeing the same physician, Dr. M, for the past 30 years. During the past two visits to Dr. M's office, they discussed the possibility that Mr. L's cardiovascular condition might worsen, even become critical. Mr. L clearly expressed his wish that under no circumstances would he want to be maintained on a ventilator or receive anything other than palliative care if he should have serious heart failure. Dr. M suggests that Mr. L consider putting his wishes in writing.
>
> On a return visit, Mr. L hands Dr. M a copy of his combined advance directive. The document names his wife as proxy and provides that if he should ever become terminally ill, dependent on mechanical ventilation, and unable to make his own decisions, life support should be

withheld or withdrawn. He informs his physician that he has discussed the document with Mrs. L.

Dr. M had also cared for the senior Mr. L, who died last year after a prolonged illness. Mr. L recounts that at that time, his wife had objected strongly to removal of life support from her father-in-law; she claimed that her religious convictions were strongly opposed to prematurely "ending his misery." Mr. L assures the physician that his wife has agreed to honor his wishes but points out that to make sure, he has provided that his directive is to be "strictly followed."

Eight months later, Mr. L is brought to the hospital by ambulance in severe chest pain. He has suffered acute myocardial infarction, with mild hemodynamic instability. His condition has been stabilized, but he remains confused and disoriented and is respirator-dependent. In Dr. M's opinion, Mr. L's prognosis is poor (terminal), and there is no hope of recovery. Dr. M consults Mrs. L, seeking her approval not to resuscitate should her husband undergo a critical cardiac event and to remove the respirator to allow Mr. L to die. Mrs. L insists that all aggressive measures be taken. She acknowledges her husband's prior directive, stating that it was her obligation as a dutiful wife to agree with her husband. Now that he is ill and vulnerable, however, "it is my duty to protect him in keeping with my own beliefs and values." She asserts the sincerity of her religious beliefs and asks for directions to the hospital chapel, where she can pray.

This scenario is a modified version of an actual case.[102] The patient's death shortly thereafter resolved the treatment dilemma but not the conflict. The sole issue before us is what should be done when the actions of the proxy (or family) are clearly contrary to the patient's expressed wishes. Although this particular case may be unusual, concern about the proxy's fidelity to the patient's wishes is a familiar refrain among health care professionals. Here the language of the directive is clear and unambiguous. The fact that Mr. L has anticipated his wife's struggle and directed that his treatment refusal should be strictly followed places her decision outside the scope of the otherwise broad discretion due a designated proxy.

In this scenario, advance care planning has been a model of physician-patient interaction. Physician and patient have a long-standing relationship built on mutual trust and respect. They have discussed the need for an advance care plan in the context of the patient's known health risks, and the patient has issued a directive on the basis of this discussion. As I have suggested at several points, physicians (as well as other health care professionals) have a special obligation to safeguard patient autonomy and patient well-being. Dr. M must advocate for his patient's autonomy here. As a result of his relationship with Mr. L and the prior, specific conversations about end-of-life care, there is no doubt what the patient would want at this time.

Assuming that Mrs. L cannot be persuaded to honor her husband's wishes and continues to assert her authority as proxy (that is, that she does not disqualify herself), the proper course is to seek ethics committee intervention. If this action fails to resolve the conflict, and the committee believes Mrs. L's decision is a rebellion against her husband's wishes, judicial intervention should be recommended and pursued.[103]

Note that Mrs. L harbors no ill will toward her husband, nor is there any suggestion of malevolent motive. She is not a turncoat proxy. The court order ought to be fashioned to compel Mrs. L to honor the express intent of the directive. If she accepts this ruling, her authority is set back on course, confined within its intended boundaries. If she persists in her position, she should nonetheless continue to hold authority as proxy to make collateral decisions about Mr. L's care (for example, consenting to pain relief) and should continue to be involved in the patient's care to the extent that she is willing to do so.

Suppose Mrs. L had also said, "Our children are quite upset. Our eldest graduates from school next week, and we were planning a big party." Should aggressive measures be taken for the sake of the family? Sometimes the right thing to do seems to be to keep the patient alive for a short time for the sake of the family. Without question, sensitivity to the needs of loved ones is an important factor in shaping the timing of withdrawal of life support. Modest and reasonable delay respects the patient's interests in the welfare of family members as well. In this case, however, there is no reason to believe that Mr. L has not considered his critical interests in the meaning of his decision for his family. His wishes are quite explicit in limiting his wife's discretion. She has no authority to direct aggressive measures on this basis. Nor is it permissible to impute to Mr. L an autonomy-based interest in continuing to live for the sake of his children in contravention of the clear intention of the directive. Moreover, a decision about resuscitation must be made very soon because the patient could suffer cardiac arrest at any time.

Ultimately, Mr. L's choice proved unwise because his wife was unable to fulfill her fiduciary responsibilities and would have violated her husband's autonomy. Mr. L might have fared better if he had selected another member of the family. Alternatively, he might have issued a living will, directing Dr. M to follow his wishes and specifically instructing that he intended to relieve his wife of the burdens of decision. With the benefit of hindsight, it is tempting to ask whether Mr. L's proxy designation was autonomous; we are left to wonder whether his wife at that time held and concealed her conviction that once her husband became incompetent she should base a treatment decision on her own religious beliefs—a fact that, arguably, would vitiate the autonomy of Mr. L's choice. We do not know this to be true, however, and in reality Mr. L has been more careful than most people: He has identified, discussed, and addressed his wife's reservations. Mr. L was aware of his wife's religious convictions; he believed that committing his wishes to writing and instructing that they be strictly followed would bind Mrs. L to respect his autonomy.[104]

Under the circumstances, the proposed outcome simultaneously safeguards Mr. L's prior autonomous instructions and overrides a prior autonomous proxy designation. We also might regard the resolution in this case as one that honors prior autonomy in a further limited way by confining the proxy's authority to the boundaries assigned by the patient. The result protects and honors Mr. L's interests in death with dignity, while continuing to acknowledge Mrs. L's rightful place at the bedside, as long as she abides by her husband's wishes.

CONCLUSION

Any analysis of cases is selective, of course. The three real-life scenarios above do important work in explaining how the practical and policy initiatives that follow from the theory of prospective autonomy offer concrete tools for resolving ethical dilemmas in decisions near the end of life. Explicit incorporation of an ethic of judgment as a core component of the decision-making process legitimates the wide latitude to interpret the patient's intention and plan and resolve apparent ambiguities that is the especial province of proxies and families. Giving true voice to the presumptive moral and legal weight of effective, autonomous directives demands that law and policy clearly articulate that advance directives may be justifiably overridden only when they are hopelessly ambiguous, when there has been a radical change of circumstances from those on which the directive's intentional plan was based, or when the proxy rebels against his or her fiduciary responsibilities. Giving prospective autonomy its due also requires that the burden of challenging a directive, of setting it aside on one of these three grounds, be placed squarely with those who would disregard the patient's wishes. Physicians, hospitals, and others must be held accountable for this choice. Mandatory recourse to an IEC—cast in its familiar advisory role and charged with the task of evaluating whether overriding a directive is justified in accordance with the three tests for doing so—is the logical (if not perfect) mechanism for this assignment.

NOTES

1. Joan M. Teno et al., for the SUPPORT Investigators, "Do Advance Directives Provide Instructions That Direct Care?" *Journal of the American Geriatrics Society* 45 (1997): 508–512.
2. Elisabeth Hansot, "A Letter from a Patient's Daughter," *Annals of Internal Medicine* 125, no. 2 (July 15, 1996): 149–51.
3. The law's commitment to a proxy's broad authority and discretion also is expressed in numerous health care proxy laws that are similar to New York's, which expressly grants a designated proxy authority to "make any and all health care decisions on the [incompetent patient's] behalf that the [competent] patient could make." N.Y. *Public Health Law* §2982 (Consol. 1997). As another example, standard form language for proxy directives set forth in the Iowa code states: "This document gives my agent power to make health care decisions on my behalf, including to consent, to refuse to consent, or to withdraw consent to the provision of any care, treatment, service, or procedure to maintain, diagnose, or treat a physical or mental condition." *Iowa Code Ann.* §144B.5 (West 1997). The question of whether provisions such as these, as a matter of substantive law, give a proxy virtually unfettered authority to refuse life support on the patient's behalf (assuming good faith behavior), regardless of the patient's medical condition, is an interesting issue for interpretation under state law. The point here is to further illustrate the law's strong commitment to honoring the proxy's judgment, not to parse the limits of proxy authority in these states.
4. 568 So.2d 4 (1990).
5. The medical evidence indicated that Mrs. Browning could live for up to one year with continued nasogastric tube feeding, absent infection. Ibid. at 9. In another passage, the court suggested that Mrs. Browning's condition was terminal because she would likely die within a matter of days if the feeding tube were removed. Ibid. at 17.
6. As I note in chapter one, state statutes define the term *terminal condition* in a variety of ways, all of which are centrally concerned with how close the patient is to death. The language of these statutes is imprecise; they use phrases such as "when death is imminent" or "death within a relatively short time." It is far from clear that advance directives that refuse treatment in the event of terminal illness share a common interpretation of these statutory definitions or intend them to be operative.
7. See also *Zodin v. Manor Healthcare Corp.*, No. 9010821007, slip op. (Sup.Ct., Cobb Cty. Ga., November 21, 1990). In a two-page order, the *Zodin* court upheld withdrawal of a feeding tube from a terminally ill woman at the request of her daughters on the basis of a living will that refused any life-sustaining procedures "if she were to be terminally ill with no hope of recovery." Based on the diagnosis of three physicians, the court found the patient's chronic vegetative state to be a terminal illness—thereby resolving the apparent discrepancy between the patient's condition and the terms of the directive.
8. American Bar Association (ABA) Commission on Legal Problems of the Elderly, American Medical Association (AMA), and American Association of Retired Persons (AARP), *Shape Your Health Care Future with Health Care Advance Directives* (Washington, D.C.: ABA, AMA, AARP, 1995). The quoted language appears on page 3 of the booklet's combined advance directive form.

9. See Robert M. Veatch, *The Patient-Physician Relation: The Patient as Partner, Part 2* (Bloomington: Indiana University Press, 1991), 232–35 (using the term "bonded guardian" to make a similar argument that the level of discretion and authority to act on the incompetent patient's behalf should be regarded as a function of closeness to the patient).

10. One notable exception is the New Jersey law, which prescribes a decision-making process to be followed in implementing advance directives. The statute expressly authorizes the proxy to consider personal knowledge and other reliable sources of information to determine the patient's intent. Those acting on the patient's behalf to follow an instruction directive in the absence of a proxy designation are to exercise reasonable judgment to give effect to the patient's wishes by "giving full weight to the terms, intent, and spirit of the instruction directive." New Jersey Commission on Legal and Ethical Problems in the Delivery of Health Care, *The New Jersey Advance Directives for Health Care and Declaration of Death Acts: Statutes, Commentaries and Analyses* (Princeton: N.J. Commission, 1991), 42–43.

11. SUPPORT Principal Investigators, "A Controlled Trial to Improve Care for Seriously Ill Hospitalized Patients," *Journal of the American Medical Association* 274, no. 20 (November 22/29, 1995): 1591–98.

12. Joan Teno et al., for the SUPPORT Investigators, "Advance Directives for Seriously Ill Hospitalized Patients: Effectiveness with the Patient Self-Determination Act and the SUPPORT Intervention," *Journal of the American Geriatrics Society* 45, no. 4 (April 1997): 500–507; Joan Teno et al., for the SUPPORT Investigators, "Do Advance Directives Provide Instructions That Direct Care?" *Journal of the American Geriatrics Society* 45, no. 4 (April 1997): 508–12.

13. David Orentlicher, "The Illusion of Patient Choice in End-of-Life Decisions," *Journal of the American Medical Association* 267, no. 15 (April 15, 1992): 2101–04.

14. See generally "Dying Well in the Hospital: The Lessons of SUPPORT," *Hastings Center Report* 25, no. 6, supplement (November-December 1995): S1–S36.

15. Some of these prescriptions in fact might be best effectuated through legal reform. For example, one way to truly support educational interventions would be to augment and enforce the PSDA's limited educational mandate by amending that statute and funding effective oversight of its implementation. The general tone and tenor of this literature is disdainful of law's command, however.

16. George J. Annas, "How We Lie," *Hastings Center Report* 25, no. 6 (November-December 1995): S12–S14. Annas calls for a national network of not-for-profit law firms whose mission is to educate the public and bring lawsuits, on a contingency fee basis, on behalf of hospital patients and families whose rights are violated. According to Annas, when the need for such firms ceases, we can be confident that the culture of medicine has changed. Law professor Diane Hoffmann and colleagues have a more tempered proposal for legal intervention; they advocate a legal requirement for consultation with a health care professional prior to execution of an advance directive. Diane E. Hoffmann, Sheryl Itkin Zimmerman, and Catherine J. Tompkins, "The Dangers of Directives or the False Security of Forms," *Journal of Law, Medicine & Ethics* 24, no. 4 (Spring 1996): 15. For reasons I discuss in chapter three, this requirement would be a step backward.

17. 13 Ohio App.3d 393, 469 N.E.2d 1047 (1984).
18. *Anderson v. St. Francis-St. George Hosp., Inc.*, 77 Ohio St.3d 82, 671 N.E.2d 225 (1996).
19. In brief, one approach to this type of litigation looks by analogy to "wrongful life" cases in which parents have alleged that their seriously disabled child would not have been born if the mother had had appropriate prenatal testing and diagnosis and the opportunity to make an informed decision to terminate the pregnancy. These claims, which have been unsuccessful in most states, in effect claim that "but for" the physician's negligence, the child never would have been born; they call us to compare nonexistence (the result absent professional negligence) to severely impaired existence. The assertion by analogy in the end-of-life context is that but for the wrongful continuation of life support, the patient would have died and would not continue to suffer in a severely debilitated state.
20. 671 N.E.2d 229.
21. *Allore v. Flower Hosp.*, 121 Ohio App.3d 229, 699 N.E.2d 560 (1997), offers further insights into the status of Ohio law. Applying *Anderson*, the court ruled that damage claims for "unwanted medical care, unnecessary medical bills, the unnecessary conscious pain and suffering of the [patient], and the mental anguish and severe emotional distress suffered by [the patient] prior to his death . . . all relate to the damages incurred due to the prolongation of [the patient's] life and are not recoverable." The court said that "[t]he continued viability of Leach" is "questionable." Interestingly, in *Allore* the patient had executed a living will and a durable power of attorney for health care, but the defendants claimed that they were not aware of these documents or of the patient's wishes. Lack of knowledge regarding the patient's refusal was a critical factor in the court's finding that neither the cardiologist who performed the intubation/ventilation nor the nurse committed battery.
22. *Osgood v. Genesys Regional Medical Center*, slip op., no. 94-26731-NH (Mich.Cir.Ct., Genesee Cty., Mar. 7, 1997).
23. Subsequent appeals and cross-appeals eventually resulted in a settlement of this litigation. Andrew J. Broder, "'She Don't Want No Life Support': A Summary of Osgood and Other Developments in Michigan Since Martin," *University of Detroit Mercy Law Review* 75 (spring 1998): 595–605.
24. *Grace Plaza of Great Neck, Inc. v. Elbaum*, 82 N.Y.2d 10, 603 N.Y.S.2d 386, 623 N.E.2d 513 (1993); *First Healthcare Corp. v. Rettinger*, 342 N.C. 886, 467 S.E.2d 243 (N.C. 1996), *affirming*, 118 N.C.App. 600, 456 S.E.2d 347 (1995). In each of these cases, the highest court of the state ultimately reversed a lower court ruling in favor of the family.
25. For example, see Philip G. Peters, Jr., "The Illusion of Autonomy at the End of Life: Unconsented Life Support and the Wrongful Life Analogy," *UCLA Law Review*. 45 (February 1998): 673–731; Adam M. Milani, "Better off Dead Than Disabled? Should Courts Recognize a 'Wrongful Living' Cause of Action When Doctors Fail to Honor Patients' Advance Directives?" *Washington and Lee Law Review* 54 (Winter 1997): 149–228; Maggie J. Randall Robb, "Living Wills: The Right to Refuse Life Sustaining Medical Treatment—A Right Without a Remedy?" *University of Dayton Law Review* 23 (Fall 1997): 169–88. An earlier post-*Cruzan* analysis is M. Rose Gasner, "Financial Penalties for Failing to Honor Patient Wishes to Refuse Treatment," *St. Louis University Public Law Review* 11

(1992): 499–520. These articles discuss in more depth the wrongful life and battery causes of action.

26. Another approach, untested in the courts, is to sue for violation of constitutional rights. A successful suit would supersede state law immunities but would face added hurdles in pursuit of monetary damages.

27. For specific analysis of legal enforcement of advance directives, see Norman L. Cantor, *Advance Directives and the Pursuit of Death with Dignity* (Bloomington: Indiana University Press, 1993), 130–34; "A Time to Live, a Time to Die" (note), *Akron Law Review* 24, no. 3, 4 (Spring 1991): 699–728. Arguably, a successful suit for violation of the constitutional right to refuse treatment would vitiate these statutory protections; again, however, this theory awaits judicial scrutiny.

28. I assume here, as elsewhere, the usual sorts of cases where there is some *prima facie* fit between the patient's directive and his or her medical condition. On occasion, directives are put forward in clearly inappropriate circumstances, such as when the patient suffers a sudden reversible cardiac arrest and the directive refuses life support "if I have an irreversible, terminal condition." It might be said, in such cases, that the directive simply does not apply or does not "fit." The decision to preserve life also can be justified by appeal to ambiguity or, if the proxy persists, by appeal to the rebel proxy standard (below).

29. See Stuart J. Eisendrath and Albert R. Jonsen, "The Living Will: Help or Hindrance?" *Journal of the American Medical Association* 249, no. 15 (April 15, 1983): 2054–58.

30. Laura Helmuth, "Further Progress on a B-Amyloid Vaccine," *Science* 289 (21 July 2000): 375 (reporting on animal trials with a vaccine); Jean Marx, "Drug Shows Promise for Advanced Disease," *Science* 289 (21 July 2000): 375–76 (reporting on clinical trials with the more conventional drug memantine).

31. Current work on xenografts, including genetically engineered pigs, may seem fanciful—just as human organ transplantation seemed to be a pipe dream 50 years ago. More so the prospect of genetically engineered human organ and tissue banks. Successful development of technologies such as these, however, hold the immense promise—assuming societal acceptance—of saving thousands of lives and perhaps eliminating the problem of scarcity that plagues organ transplantation. Such "wonders" probably would affect the interpretation of some prior directives refusing treatment and choosing an earlier death.

32. Francis S. Collins, "Shattuck Lecture—Medical and Societal Consequences of the Human Genome Project," *New England Journal of Medicine* 341, no. 1 (July 1, 1999): 28–37. One indicator of our vast investment in the use of genetic knowledge to develop new treatments is that by the end of 1995, 125 genetic research protocols had been approved by the Recombinant DNA Advisory Committee, and more than 40 approved protocols had been approved in other countries. Of the protocols approved in the United States, 100 involved the search for effective therapies; of those, 63 were for cancer and 12 for AIDS. W. French Anderson, "End-of-the-Year Potpourri—1995," *Human Gene Therapy* 6 (December 1995): 1505–06.

33. For a similar view, see Cantor, *Advance Directives*, 77–78.

34. David DeGrazia, "Advance Directives, Dementia, and the Someone Else Problem," *Bioethics* 13, no. 5 (1999): 375–76, posits the case of an intellectual whose directive refuses life support in the event of severe dementia but after his wife's death "finds comfort" in a religious faith that cherishes all human life. A few

years later, he becomes moderately demented; he has never expressly repudiated his prior directive, however. The time that has passed since a major sea change in life plays a critical role in the analysis of this sort of case. If incapacity comes on the heels of religious conversion, there may be reason to question the sincerity of the patient's commitment. Recall that in contrast to the Witness conversion I discuss in chapter three, here the person's new values and commitments are not committed to writing or expressly stated. If substantial time has passed, as in DeGrazia's example, one wonders why the prior directive has never been repudiated. A clear rejection of the prior directive prior to loss of capacity would count as a revocation, of course.

35. Some writers have questioned whether the legal right to challenge a proxy's decision is sufficiently clear. S. Van McCrary, William L. Allen, and Clarence L. Young, "Questionable Competency of a Surrogate Decision Maker under a Durable Power of Attorney," *Journal of Clinical Ethics* 4, no. 2 (summer 1993): 166–68. The authors propose that all states adopt the express language of New York's proxy law, which states that health care providers, family members, close friends, and state officials may initiate a legal proceeding to "have the agent removed on the ground that the agent . . . is not reasonably available, willing and competent to fulfill his or her [legal] obligations." Ibid., 167–68 (quoting *N.Y. Public Health Law*, §2992). I disagree with the authors' assessment of extant law, as well as their framing of the substantive issue as one of a proxy's decisional capacity. My purpose in recommending legal recognition of the rebel proxy standard is to make clear the proper substantive grounds for overturning a proxy's authority.

36. Veatch, *The Patient-Physician Relation*, 234–35.

37. We might regard legal limits on the right to refuse treatment as imposing a form of reasonableness standard, although we should reserve the prerogative to ask whether such limitations are reasonable, in fact, from a moral point of view.

38. A majority of states plainly make effectuating a transfer of care the responsibility of the attending physician and institution. Typically, statutes also state that transfer should be to another provider who does not have a conflict and will honor the patient's wishes. Several states admonish that physicians and facilities should not prevent or impede a transfer of care, suggesting that responsibility for arranging the transfer belongs to the proxy and family. For an illustrative comparison, see *N.J. Stat. Ann.* 26:2H-62 (West 1996) (duty to effectuate transfer belongs to attending physician); *Ohio Rev. Code Ann.* §1337.16 (Baldwin 1994) (attending physician or health care facility "shall not prevent or attempt to prevent, or unreasonably delay or attempt to unreasonably delay," a transfer.) In an unusual twist, the Iowa law—read literally—makes it the physician's responsibility to transfer care if the patient has a living will but the proxy's responsibility if there is a proxy directive. *Iowa Code Ann.* §§144A.8; 144B.9.2 (West 1997).

39. See the section on standards for "Patient Rights and Organization Ethics" in Joint Commission on Accreditation of Healthcare Organizations, Comprehensive *Accreditation Manual for Hospitals: The Official Handbook* (Chicago: Joint Commission, 2000).

40. The moral basis for a claim of professional conscience assumes that refusal to honor the patient's decision is grounded in sincerely held professional or personal convictions that continued treatment is in the patient's best interests and the belief that forcing the physician to withhold treatment would compromise

important values. In those hopefully rare instances in which the physician's behavior is motivated by prejudice, ill will, or ignorance of patients' rights, the label of *conscience* and the assertion of a right of conscience is misplaced, although transfer nonetheless might be an appropriate resolution. Extension of similar reasoning to health care institutions has led most states to recognize a right of institutional conscience, along with parallel duties of transfer in the event that conflicts prove intractable. In some states, this right has been limited to private, religiously affiliated health care facilities. For further analysis of the moral and legal basis of rights of professional and institutional conscience and the transfer of care rule, see New Jersey Commission on Legal and Ethical Problems in the Delivery of Health Care, *Problems and Approaches in Health Care Decision Making: The New Jersey Experience* (Princeton: New Jersey Commission, 1990), 113–19. For a critical view of the transfer rule as applied to institutions, see George J. Annas, "Transferring the Ethical Hot Potato," *Hastings Center Report* 17, no. 1 (February 1987): 20–21.

41. Hansot, "Letter from a Patient's Daughter"; see also Timothy Gilligan and Thomas A. Raffin, "Whose Death Is It, Anyway?" *Annals of Internal Medicine* 125 (1996): 137–41 (commenting on Hansot's case).

42. Shorter analyses include Veatch, *The Patient-Physician Relation*, 237–39; Bernard Lo, "Behind Closed Doors: Promises and Pitfalls of Ethics Committees," *New England Journal of Medicine* 317, no. 1 (July 2, 1987): 46–49. Lengthy treatments of the topic, with an emphasis on matters of due process, include Diane E. Hoffmann, "Mediating Life and Death Decisions," *Arizona Law Review* 36 (Winter 1994): 821–77; Susan M. Wolf, "Ethics Committees and Due Process: Nesting Rights in a Community of Caring," *Maryland Law Review* 50, no. 3 (1991): 798–858.

43. John A. Robertson, "Committees as Decision Makers: Alternate Structures and Responsibilities," in *Institutional Ethics Committees and Health Care Decision Making*, edited by Ronald E. Cranford and A. Edward Doudera (Ann Arbor, Mich.: Health Administration Press, 1984), 85–95.

44. To avoid repetitive references, the discussion of ethics committees should be understood to include consultants as well. Differences between the two are not pertinent to the present discussion.

45. These early examples are discussed in George J. Annas, "Legal Aspects of Ethics Committees," in Cranford and Doudera (eds.), *Institutional Ethics Committees and Health Care Decision Making*, 51–59.

46. The Department of Health and Human Services (HHS) Model Guidelines for Health Care Providers to Establish Infant Care Review Committees were originally published at 50 Fed. Reg. 14,893 (1985). These regulations, known as the "Baby Doe" regulations, implement amendments to the Child Abuse Prevention and Treatment Act of 1984, currently codified at 42 U.S.C. §5101-17 (1999). Enforcement of the HHS policy is delegated to the states through the appropriate state agency.

47. The Federal Policy for Protection of Human Subjects—known as the "Common Rule" because of its joint and widespread adoption by agencies of the federal government—is codified in 45 C.F.R. §§101 et. seq. (1999).

48. *N.Y. Public Health Law* §§2965, 2972 (Consol. 1997). The committee's charge is to mediate the dispute. Authority to decide whether a DNR order should be issued is expressly denied to the committee. The New York statute appears to impose

minimal requirements for committee membership, which are not intended to ensure a multidisciplinary review that is typical of ethics committees.
49. Report of the Council on Ethical and Judicial Affairs, "Medical Futility in End-of-Life Care," *Journal of the American Medical Association* 281, no. 10 (March 10, 1999): 937–41.
50. Amir Halevy and Baruch A. Brody, "A Multi-Institution Collaborative Policy on Medical Futility," *Journal of the American Medical Association* 276, no. 7 (August 21, 1996): 571–74; Lawrence J. Schneiderman and Alexander Morgan Copron, "How Can Hospital Futility Policies Contribute to Establishing Standards of Practice?" *Cambridge Quarterly of Healthcare Ethics* 9 (2000): 524–31 (a review of 26 hospital policies showed that all described a role for an ethics committee in dealing with futility cases).
51. *Tex. Health and Safety Code,* §166.046 (West Supp. 2001).
52. *Md. Code Ann., Health–Gen.* §§19-370 *et seq.* (Michie 1996). As I note in chapter one, other state mandates appear in health facilities regulations in New Jersey and Texas. As I have noted, New York mandates a hospital-based dispute resolution system for DNR orders.
53. *Tex. Code Ann.* §166.046 (West Supp. 2001).
54. *Md. Code Ann., Health-Gen.* §§5-605(b); 5-609; 5-612 (Michie 2000); *Tex. Health and Safety Code* §166.045(d).
55. Ibid., §166.046(d).
56. *Md. Code Ann., Health-Gen.* §5-605(b).
57. *Tex. Health and Safety Code* §166.039.
58. Ibid., §166.046.
59. See, e.g., Mark Siegler, "Ethics Committees: Decisions by Bureaucracy," *Hastings Center Report* 16, no. 3 (June 1986): 22–24.
60. Veatch, *The Patient-Physician Relation,* 255; Wolf, "Ethics Committees and Due Process," 812–13.
61. This position might be argued on a theory of implied consent to the limited disclosure that is necessary to fulfill the purposes of committee consultation, but the point need not be pressed further here. Note that there are two ways in which a waiver of confidentiality would be limited: First, it would apply only in the circumstances I set forth; second, as participants in patient care, the committee members themselves would have duties of confidentiality.
62. Among the more comprehensive treatments of the subject are Judith Wilson Ross, *Handbook for Hospital Ethics Committees* (Chicago: American Hospital Publishing, 1986); Judith Wilson Ross, John W. Glaser, Dorothy Rasinski-Gregory et al., *Health Care Ethics Committees: The Next Generation* (Chicago: American Hospital Publishing, 1993); Cranford and Doudera, *Institutional Ethics Committees;* and *Maryland Law Review* 50, no. 3 (Symposium issue, 1991). The most extensive analysis of the accountability and liability of ethics committees is Sigrid Fry-Revere, *The Accountability of Bioethics Committees and Consultants* (Frederick, Md.: University Publishing Group, 1992). The *Journal of Clinical Ethics,* established in 1990, is devoted to issues of interest to ethics committees and consultants.
63. Comprehensive analysis of regulating ethics committees appears in Diane E. Hoffmann, "Regulating Ethics Committees in Health Care Institutions— Is It Time?" *Maryland Law Review* 50, no. 3 (1991): 746–97. Extensive critical

analysis of IECs and due process appears in Wolf, "Ethics Committees and Due Process."

The only known case in which an IEC was named as a defendant is *Bouvia v. Superior Court*, 179 Cal. App. 3d 1127, 225 Cal.Rptr. 297 (1986); claims against the committee were voluntarily dropped. The rare lawsuits that have named ethics consultants as defendants have never reached the merits of liability; they offer no judicial signposts of proper conduct for IECs engaged in case consultation. For discussion of these cases, see John C. Fletcher, Paul A. Lombardo, Mary Faith Marshall, and Franklin G. Miller, eds., *Introduction to Clinical Ethics*, 2nd ed. (Frederick, Md.: University Publishing Group, 1997), 271–75; John C. Fletcher, Robert J. Boyle, and Edward M. Spencer, "Errors in Healthcare Ethics Consultation," in *Margin of Error: The Ethics of Mistakes in the Practice of Medicine*, edited by Susan B. Rubin and Laurie Zoloth (Hagerstown, Md.: University Publishing Group, 2000), 357–60. I explore how a legal standard of care in ethics consultation might evolve in "Ethics Consultation and the Law: What's the Standard of Care?" in *Margin of Error,* 287–303. An early exploration of *potential* legal pitfalls for IECs is Andrew L. Merritt, "The Tort Liability of Hospital Ethics Committees," *Southern California Law Review* 60, no. 5 (1987): 1239–97.

64. Wolf, "Ethics Committees and Due Process"; Veatch, *The Patient-Physician Relation,* 237–39.

65. Lo, "Behind Closed Doors."

66. The attorney's role as a member of the IEC is discussed in Ross, *Health Care Ethics Committees,* chapter 9; Bruce White and Lawrence E. Gottlieb, "Point and Counterpoint: Should an Institution's Risk Manager/Lawyer Serve as HEC members?" *HEC Forum* 3, no. 2 (1991): 87–93; and Suzanne M. Mitchell and Martha S. Swartz, "Is There a Place for Lawyers on Ethics Committees? A View from the Inside," *Hastings Center Report* 20, no. 2 (March/April 1990): 32–33.

67. American Society for Bioethics and Humanities (ASBH), *Core Competencies for Health Care Ethics Consultation* (Glenview, Ill.: ASBH, 1998). See also Mark P. Ausilio, Robert M. Arnold, and Stuart J. Youngner, for the Society for Health and Human Values—Society for Bioethics Consultation Task Force on Standards for Bioethics Consultation, "Health Care Ethics Consultation: Nature, Goals, and Competencies," *Annals of Internal Medicine* 133, no. 1 (July 4, 2000): 59–69.

68. Karen Ritchie, "When It's Not Really Optional," *Hastings Center Report* 18, no. 4 (August-September 1988): 25.

69. George Agich, "Authority in Ethics Consultation," *Journal of Law, Medicine & Ethics* 23 (1995): 273–83. Courts have attached varying degrees of importance to the IEC's role and recommendations. No court has taken the committee's judgment to be dispositive. Uncertainty and lack of uniformity regarding the legal status of IEC advice may contribute to a perception that following the IEC's advice is a legally safe course. Compare *In re Conservatorship of Torres,* 357 N.W.2d 332, 335 n.2 (Minn., 1984) ("these committees are uniquely suited to provide guidance to physicians, families and guardians when ethical dilemmas arise"); *Spahn v. Eisenberg,* 563 N.W.2d 485 (Wis., 1997) (Abrahamson, C.J., concurring) (reciting the lower court's criticism of the IEC and discounting its recommendations because of its failures of process and its understanding "that its function was to reach a determination that would insulate the facility from legal liability"); *In re L.H.R.,* 253 Ga. 439, 321 S.E.2d 716 (1984) (noting and

apparently ignoring the infant care review committee); *Conservatorship of Wendland*, 78 Cal.App.4th 517, 93 Cal.Rptr.2d 550 (2000) (mentioning the IEC's recommendation only in a recitation of the facts). For an early review, see Susan M. Wolf, "Ethics Committees in the Courts," *Hastings Center Report* 16, no. 3 (June 1986): 12–15.

70. Gail J. Povar, "Evaluating Ethics Committees: What Do We Mean by Success?" *Maryland Law Review* 50, no. 3 (1991): 904–19.

71. Cynthia B. Cohen, "The Adolescence of Ethics Committees," *Hastings Center Report* 20, no. 2 (March/April 1990): 29; Wolf, "Ethics Committees and Due Process," 807.

72. James A. Tulsky and Ellen Fox, "Evaluating Ethics Consultation: Framing the Questions," *Journal of Clinical Ethics* 7, no. 2 (Summer 1996): 110–11.

73. Janet E. Fleetwood, Robert M. Arnold, and Richard J. Baron, "Giving Answers or Raising Questions? The Problematic Role of Institutional Ethics Committees," *Journal of Medical Ethics* 15 (1989): 137–42 (noting many of the concerns about ethics committees identified here and concluding that the major strength of IECs is their contribution to the process of examining bioethical conflicts).

74. Veatch, *The Patient-Physician Relation*, 250–60 (arguing that an ethic for ethics committees must be patient-centered and suggesting what such an ethic would look like).

75. Of course there is always the theoretical possibility that the outcome of IEC consultation may be that all concerned—proxy, physician, and committee—come to agreement that a directive's treatment refusal should be set aside; yet the shared judgment that the directive is nonautonomous is incorrect, in fact: They are all wrong.

76. Index no. 16536/87, *New York Law Journal* (Sup. Ct. N.Y.Cty. July 28, 1987), 11.

77. Ibid.

78. Tom L. Beauchamp and James F. Childress, *Principles of Biomedical Ethics*, 4th ed. (New York: Oxford University Press, 1994), 177.

79. Rebecca S. Dresser and John A. Robertson, "Quality of Life and Non-Treatment Decisions for Incompetent Patients: A Critique of the Orthodox Approach," *Law, Medicine & Health Care* 17, no. 3 (Fall 1989): 237–38. The authors state, however, that we cannot determine from the facts of the case whether there was a genuine conflict between Wirth's current interests and his past statements.

80. This case arose several years prior to enactment of New York's health care proxy law, which establishes the proxy's best interests authority, subject to the limitations stated in the document.

81. Beauchamp and Childress, *Biomedical Ethics*, 127; New Jersey Commission, *Problems and Approaches*, 99. The New Jersey advance directive statute makes the obligation to foster opportunities for autonomy explicit and extends this rule to the patient's health care proxy. N.J. Stat. Ann. 26-2H-63b.

82. 538 N.W.2d 399 (Mich. 1995).

83. Ibid. at 411 (emphasis added). The evidentiary finding ignored the substantial weight of the evidence, which included testimony from Michael's mother and sister—who acknowledged, although they were opposed to removal of life support, that he would not have wanted to continue living in this condition. For a contrary reading of this case, see Rebecca Dresser, "Still Troubled: *In re Martin*," *Hastings Center Report* 26, no. 4 (July-August 1996): 21–22. For a response

to Dresser, see Robert S. Olick, "In re Martin" (letter), *Hastings Center Report* 27, no. 3 (May-June 1997): 4.
84. *In re Donlan*, no. A-3103-89t5F, slip op. (N.J. App. Div. Oct. 24, 1990); *In re Smerdon*, no. A-6031-89T1, slip op. (N.J. App. Div. Apr. 8, 1991).
85. The relevant passage in the opinion reads as follows: "According to Dr. Kreitsch, Michael seemed content with his environment and indicated 'no' with a head nod when asked whether he has been in any pain and discomfort, and also when asked if there were ever any times when he felt he did not want to go on living." 538 N.W.2d at 403.
86. Of course, there are other reasons to continue to involve the incapacitated but communicative patient in the shaping of his or her treatment plan. Actively involving the patient in his or her own care, including gaining the patient's assent (as opposed to consent), displays basic human compassion and shows respect for personal dignity.
87. The mother and sister also contended that Michael had changed his mind, but this way of framing the issue was largely ignored by the majority. See the dissenting opinion of Justice Levin, 538 N.W.2d at 416, note 23.
88. Cantor, *Advance Directives*, 85.
89. I share the concern that contemporaneous expressions will be misconstrued as valid revocations of a prior directive and am inclined to agree that statutes that freely allow revocation by an incompetent patient have fallen into error. Proper recognition of an incompetent patient's revocation must distinguish apparent rejection of an instruction directive or dismissal of a proxy or family member out of anger, frustration, or depression. These occurrences should not simply be accepted as valid; they should occasion further inquiry into the patient's meaning and intention. The issue before us—namely, what weight is due contemporaneous expressions in favor of life—is different, although factual circumstances may be quite similar to those that raise the revocation question. A current preference for life is not in itself a revocation of prior instructions unless the patient intends to invalidate the prior document—nor does a plea for life speak to the legitimacy of the proxy's role.
90. Sanford H. Kadish, "Letting Patients Die: Legal and Moral Reflections," *California Law Review* 80 (1992): 871-72.
91. Ibid., 876.
92. Allen E. Buchanan and Dan W. Brock, *Deciding for Others: The Ethics of Surrogate Decision Making* (Cambridge: Cambridge University Press, 1989), 111.
93. Kadish, "Letting Patients Die," 878.
94. I am not prepared to completely rule out the possibility that there may be exceptional situations in which honoring an advance directive and discontinuing life support would be horribly inhumane and the choice not to do so would be justifiable. Ignoring an opportunity to take advantage of a cutting-edge therapy—a radical change of circumstances—would be one such possibility. Human compassion alone does not provide the justificatory ground for doing so, however.
95. Paul S. Appelbaum and Thomas Grisso, "Assessing Patients' Capacities to Consent to Treatment," *New England Journal of Medicine* 319, no. 25 (December 22, 1988): 1635-38; President's Commission for the Study of Ethical Problems in Medicine and Biomedical and Behavioral Research, *Making Health Care Decisions*,

Vol. 1 (Washington, D.C.: G.P.O., 1982), 56–62; New Jersey Commission, *New Jersey Advance Directives*, 92–98. The Presidential and New Jersey commissions recommend a decision-specific approach to assessing a patient's capacity for autonomous choice which would allow that patients with diminished or fluctuating capacity might be able to make some decisions but not others.

96. Appelbaum and Grisso, "Assessing Patients' Capacities to Consent to Treatment"; President's Commission, *Making Health Care Decisions*; New Jersey Commission, *New Jersey Advance Directives*; David L. Jackson and Stuart J. Youngner, "Patient Autonomy and 'Death with Dignity': Some Clinical Caveats," *New England Journal of Medicine* 301 (August 1979): 404-08.
97. N.Y. *Public Health Law* §2983 (5-7); W.Va. *Code* §16-30-6(d) (2000).
98. New Jersey Commission, *New Jersey Advance Directives*, 106. The commission did not reach the question of whether only a persistent—as opposed to occasional—desire for life is worthy of respect when such a desire is in conflict with a prior treatment refusal.
99. The origins of this approach can be found in the work of the New Jersey Bioethics Commission and the state's advance directive law developed by the commission. The New Jersey statute contemplates the possibility that a patient with impaired capacity may express what appears to constitute a revocation of a directive out of anger or depression and later reverse this desire (but not be competent to issue a new document). In such cases, the directive should be treated as if it were suspended, allowing the patient the opportunity to reinstate his or her prior competently expressed wishes. Another provision states that a clear, contemporaneous expression in favor of life should take precedence over a directive that refuses life support. New Jersey Commission, *New Jersey Advance Directives*, 18–19. The approach I recommend here differs from that of the commission when the patient expresses a desire for life support: I call for automatic reinstatement of the directive when the patient no longer maintains this desire.
100. Cantor appears sympathetic to this position: "At most, an understanding (even if not deliberately considered) expression by an incompetent patient ought to suspend implementation of an advance directive which conflicts with the expression." He goes on to say that to have moral weight, the patient's life-affirming expression ought to be minimally based on an understanding of the concept of death. "Even then, the force of such an expression probably ought to continue only so long as the position is being communicated by the patient." Cantor, *Advance Directives*, 85–86.
101. We also can easily imagine the reverse scenario, in which an incompetent patient with a prior protreatment directive now manifests an apparent desire to forgo treatment, perhaps uttering vague complaints about pain or pulling out a feeding tube. Those who would honor contemporaneous expressions in favor of life are unlikely to advocate simply honoring an incompetent patient's contemporaneous treatment refusal here—nor does that seem to be an appropriate course. It also is not clear that a proxy with best interests discretion should be permitted to make this judgment—at least not without further examination of the patient's best interests. Furthermore, the strategy of suspending the directive in such cases is inappropriate because death would quickly follow, making a temporary suspension permanent. Cases such as these illustrate one of the more subtle ways in which this approach to prior treatment refusals cannot be enlisted wholesale to handle dilemmas involving protreatment directives.

102. I thank Richard Dobyns, M.D., for his assistance in the preparation of this scenario.
103. Suppose Mrs. L were to assert a legally recognized right to veto committee consultation by refusing to consent to disclosure of her husband's medical records and other pertinent information before the committee. The result might well be that Dr. M would soften, even abandon, his advocacy for Mr. L's autonomous treatment refusal, perhaps hoping for a change in Mr. L's condition or in his wife's attitude. It is hard to see why we should favor a mechanism that shields the judgment of a rebel proxy at the expense of patient autonomy in cases such as this one. Alternatively, Dr. M (or the hospital) would petition a court for a more public airing of the dispute, seeking to remove Mrs. L as proxy and thereby escalating existing tensions among physician, proxy, and hospital (and more than likely children and other family members as well). Of course, this escalation might occur anyway if Mrs. L were to reject the committee's advice, but the committee's recommendations would make a powerful statement about the appropriate outcome.
104. Standard language in the recommended form for advance directives contained in the recently revamped West Virginia Health Care Decisions Act states that it is the author's (patient's) intent that decisions made by a health care representative "not be the subject of review by any health care provider or administrative agency." *W.Va. Code,* §16-30-4. The intent of this provision is to insulate the proxy from challenge. The story of Mr. L shows why this protection may not always be a wise course.

CONCLUSION

Over the past quarter-century, an ethical, legal, and societal consensus surrounding decisions near the end of life for incompetent patients has taken its place as a cornerstone of the bioethical landscape. The clarion call of the consensus is that deciding how we die—variously described as the right to die; the pursuit of "death with dignity"; and, more precisely, the right to refuse treatment—is the special province of patients and families. A patient's prior autonomous refusal of life support trumps others' views of the patient's best interests.

Nonetheless, there is considerable and lively debate about the theoretical underpinnings of the consensus, the nature and limits of the principle of prospective autonomy, and the moral and legal weight of advance directives. The preeminence of autonomy remains contested terrain, and a substantial body of empirical data suggests that ethical and legal norms have not been translated effectively into practical clinical norms. Many physicians (and health care facilities) routinely ignore dying patients' wishes. Too often, advance directives—which are widely regarded as the best mechanism for making future-oriented treatment decisions—do not control care near the end of life.

The central themes and goals of this book have been to develop a theory of prospective autonomy and advance directives that reaffirms and strengthens the core tenets of the consensus; to clarify widespread confusion about the moral and legal weight of advance directives; and to point to practical policy initiatives that are designed to ensure that prospective autonomy and advance directives are taken seriously in the care of dying patients.

Pivotal to the theory of prospective autonomy is the distinction between autonomous persons and autonomous actions. The position for which I argue is that we ought to understand what it means to be an autonomous person on the model of autonomy as integrity. We ought to understand what it means to act autonomously in particular instances—to make autonomous (or other choices) is what the patient intended. An effective, autonomous proxy directive provides sufficient guidance to determine the intended boundaries of the proxy's authority. The morally licit response to the inevitable uncertainties and ambiguities that are endemic to future-oriented choice is to straightforwardly embrace an ethic of judgment that reposes broad authority in proxies and families to interpret the intent of a directive and to implement the patient's wishes or to act in the patient's best interests on the basis of what is known about his or her wishes, remaining faithful to the bounds of the authority established by the document. An effective, autonomous directive imposes on proxies, families, physicians, and other members of the health care team duties to honor its intentions. It functions as a shield and as a constraint against interventions that others think best.

To be sure, advance care planning ought to aspire to be a process of informed consent in consultation with one's physician, proxy, family members, religious advisors, or others. Intentional plans that are formed through discussion with others may be more informed and perhaps all the more effective. Holding advance directives to standards of contemporaneous informed consent shaped by meaningful dialogue between patient and physician, however, erroneously transforms an ideal into a requirement. Elevating specific matching of clinical conditions with a series of treatment options to a benchmark of autonomy misconstrues the essentially outcome-oriented nature of prospectively intentional plans. At bottom, both views fail to appreciate the natural limitations of future-oriented choice under conditions of uncertainty and seemingly embrace an almost irrational (or at least highly idealistic) belief in the powers of anticipatory reason.

One result of understanding advance directives in the way I describe in this book should be that more directives are regarded as autonomous and worthy of respect, and fewer should be considered ambiguous, unclear, and unhelpful. This paradigm for understanding advance directives is not a panacea, however, for the natural limits of human foresight or efforts to capture even carefully considered anticipations on paper. The task at the bedside is to distinguish autonomous directives from those that are not autonomous.

Instruction directives (or the instruction directive part of a combined directive) may fail to provide sufficient guidance when they are hopelessly ambiguous or when what medicine has to offer has changed radically from the circumstances contemplated by the directive. In these sorts of cases, holding that the directive may be justifiably overridden because it is nonautonomous is proper. A proxy directive also may be overridden justifiably when the proxy rebels against the bounds of his or her authority. It will most often be proper to understand removal of a rebel proxy as an instance of justified overriding of an autonomous proxy directive. In some cases—

such as those in which the patient has issued a combined directive with otherwise effective and autonomous instructions—overturning the proxy's authority but not the patient's instructions simultaneously safeguards and honors patient autonomy.

It follows from the presumptive weight of a prospectively autonomous advance directive that the burden of showing why the document should not be followed properly rests with those who would set it aside. Unfortunately, this simple premise runs counter to the prevailing medical culture, which commonly shifts to families the burden of navigating unfamiliar institutions, rules, and conventions to vindicate their loved ones' wishes. This is where patients and families most need the kind of support and assistance that law and policy can offer.

To right the course—to give advance directives their due—we should embrace three practical policy initiatives. First, law and policy should clearly enunciate the three—and only three—grounds on which an advance directive may justifiably be overridden by embracing the Hopeless Ambiguity, Radical Change of Circumstances, and Rebel Proxy standards for setting a directive aside. Second, the burden of showing why a directive should be overridden for one of these three reasons should be placed squarely on physicians, hospitals, and families who challenge the directive's authority. Third, challenges to directives should be subject to mandatory review before an ethics committee or court, with an expectation that the path to the courthouse is likely to be the road less traveled. A mandated role for IECs here compels those who would override a directive to put that conviction to the test, to measure their reasons against the three standards on which this decision may be justified, and to have others do the same. These amendments to the existing consensus would give true voice to the moral weight of advance directives. They also hold the salutary promise of reversing prevailing norms and practices that improperly force proxies and families to persuade physicians, hospitals, and others that they are ethically and legally bound to honor the intentional plans of their patients.

The time has come for a new and more probing dialogue about the nature and limits of prospective autonomy and advance directives and our approach to decisions near the end of life for incompetent, dying patients. Revision of theory, policy, and practice as set forth in these pages would do important work in cementing the place of prospective autonomy and respect for advance directives in the care of dying patients. As champions of individual rights, law and policy should once again enter the arena to amend the rules for dying, right the balance of power, and ensure that advance directives are taken seriously. Our commitment to the legacy of Karen Ann, Joseph, and Julia Quinlan; to Nancy Beth Cruzan and her family; and to all those who have been and will be fellow travelers in their struggle requires no less.

INDEX

A
accident victims, 93–97
actions, 90–91, 211–12. *See also* intentional actions
  autonomy of, 77–78, 87, 88–89, 111–12, 211–12
  hierarchical theory of, 88–89
  integrity and, 79, 85–87, 88–89, 212
  motivation for, 82, 89
  understanding and, 78, 113–14n7
  values and, 51, 86
advance directives. *See also* living wills; proxy directives
  ambiguous. *See* ambiguous directives
  challenging, 167–84
  combined, 108, 110, 172, 194, 215
  disease-specific, 106
  effectiveness of, 80–81, 97–111, 213–14
  forms for, 101, 209n104
  implementing, 161–215
  institutional policies on, 29
  next generation, 165
  outcome-oriented, 98, 99–103, 107, 110
  overriding. *See* noncompliance with directives
  practical problems of, 102
  protreatment, xv, 73n48, 208n101
  respect for, xviii, 64–65
  statistics on, xv–xvi
  suspension of, 193–94, 208n99
  writing, 78–79
advocacy, 183
agency, unity of, 140–41, 157n43
agents, moral, 140, 141–42, 212
Agich, George, 183, 205–6n69
AIDS patients, 62, 185–86
Alabama legislation, on treatment refusal, 22
Alaska legislation, on living wills, 22
Allore v. Flower Hosp., 200n21
Alzheimer's patients, 58, 128, 137–38

ambiguous directives, 163, 166, 214
  case studies of, 185–87
  noncompliance with, 170–72, 197
American Association of Retired Persons, 165
American Bar Association, 165
American Medical Association, 165, 179–80
American Society of Bioethics and Humanities Task Force on Standards for Bioethics Consultation, 183
amnesia, 159n68
Anderson v. St. Francis-St. George Hosp., Inc., 168–69
Annas, George, 13, 31n3, 168, 169, 199n16
anticipatory judgment, 78, 100, 102, 104
artificial feeding, 12, 19, 101
  case studies of, 176–78, 188–94
  state legislation on, 23–24, 41n127
assisted suicide, 20–21, 40n114
attitudes, 86–87
Austin, J. L., 83
authenticity, 50–51, 92. *See also* integrity
authority
  decisional, 90, 179, 184
  of ethics committees, 180–81
  identity and, 128
  proxy, 109–10, 174–76
authorship, 78–79, 81, 213
autonomy, xiii, 2, 27, 85. *See also* prospective autonomy
  of actions, 77–78, 87, 88–89, 111–12, 211–12
  vs. beneficence, 92, 94, 178
  vs. best interests standard, xiv, 59–60
  vs. competence, 113n4
  contemporaneous, 105, 193
  criteria for, 90
  vs. current interests, 47, 61
  decisional, 57, 58
  definition of, 46
  degrees of, 80
  future-oriented, 46

autonomy—*continued*
  hierarchical theory of, 88–89
  identity and, 50–51
  incompetent patients and, xvi, 14
  as integrity, xvii, 46–47, 54, 60–61, 68,
    85–87
  intentional actions and, 78, 79, 81–85
  interests and, 46, 47–50
  precedent, 56–57, 112
  respect for, 53, 55–57, 81
  sufficient, 80–81

B
Baby Doe regulations, 203n46
bad-faith behavior, 169
battery, 169
Beauchamp, Tom L., 78, 115n14
beneficence, 63, 92, 94, 178
best interests standard, 9, 13–16, 45
  ambiguous directives and, 166
  vs. autonomy-based interests, xiv, 59–60
  connectedness and, 155n25
  current experiences and, 192
  vs. current interests, 57–59, 72n45, 192
  guardianship and, 3, 7
  individual interests and, 67
  new persons and, 148
  proxy directives and, 109
  substituted judgment and, 14–15, 16
bioethics, autonomy and, 2
blood transfusions, 60, 91, 93–94,
  119–20n59, 119n56
bodily continuity, 139, 143–44, 151, 153n14,
  156n39, 156n40
bodily death, 129, 136, 139–40, 142–45,
  156n39
brain death, 32n9, 60, 74n53, 160n74
Brennan, William, 39–40n106
Brock, Dan
  on psychological continuity, 128–29, 131,
    134, 142
  on surviving interests, 145, 146
Browning case. *See In re Guardianship of
  Browning v. Herbert*
Buchanan, Allen
  on psychological continuity, 128–29, 131,
    134, 142
  on surviving interests, 145, 146
Buñuel, Luis, 127
burden of persuasion, 176–78, 197
burden of proof, 15, 16
burials, 67–68, 136, 143–44

C
California courts
  on assisted suicide, 40n114
  on life-sustaining treatment refusal, 11–12

California legislation, on advance
  directives, 22
cancer patients, 90–91, 176–78
Cantor, Norman
  on contemporaneous expressions, 191,
    208n100
  on current interests, 72n38
  on image, 55
  on living wills, 56, 77
  on quality of life, 101–2
  on values, 62, 71n33
Cardozo, Benjamin, 29
careers, 51–52
case law
  on artificial feeding, 188–94
  on assisted suicide, 20–21, 40n114
  ethics committees and, 205n63
  on feeding tubes, 12, 18–19
  on guardianship, 164–65
  on life-sustaining treatment refusal, 12,
    18–20, 185–87
  on living wills, 17–18, 164–65
  monetary damages and, 168–69
  on proxy directives, 17, 169
  on substituted judgment, 12, 36n56
  on treatment refusal, 2–8
case studies
  of ambiguous directives, 185–87
  of artificial feeding, 176–78, 188–94
  of identity, 136–38
  of inconsistent patient wishes, 188–94
  of intentional plans, 94–97
  of life-sustaining treatment refusal,
    137–38, 185–87, 188–97
  of living wills, 93–97, 137–38
  of noncompliance with directives, 194–97
  of prospective decisional autonomy,
    93–97
  of proxy directives, 137–38, 185–87,
    188–94, 194–97
  of psychological discontinuity, 136–38
  of religious beliefs, 93–97
  of treatment refusal, 93–97
causal agents, 82
change of mind, 193
character
  acting in, 48, 85, 96
  acting out of, 70n25, 117–18n39
Childress, James F., 78
choices, 51, 63, 85, 88. *See also* decisions
  compassionate, 192
  inauthentic, 96
  treatment, 90–91, 92, 93, 146–47
chronic diseases, xiii, xviiin3
circumstances
  radical change in, 172–74, 192, 201n31, 214
  specificity of, 189

Index

clear and convincing evidence, 11–12, 15, 16–17, 19, 24
clinical behavior, 167–70, 177
coercion, 26
cognitive impairment
   continuity and, 133, 159n68
   degree of, 135, 193
   restoration of capacity, 187, 190
Colorado legislation, on treatment refusal, 22
coma, irreversible, 136, 149, 160n70
combined directives, 108, 110, 172, 194, 215
commitment
   decisive, 88, 118n41
   first-order vs. second order, 85–86, 87
   harm and, 64
   identity and, 50–51, 70n25
   integrity and, 52
   intentional plans and, 83
common law, 9, 10, 35n45
Common Rule, 179
commonsense view of directives, 98–103, 107
communication, 108, 123n86, 184, 191, 207n85
compassion, 192, 207n94
Compassion in Dying, 20
competence vs. autonomy, 113n4
competent patients, xiii, 12–14, 20–21, 30, 76n70
confidentiality, 182, 204n61, 209n103
conflicts, case studies in, 176–78
connectedness, psychological, 132–33, 154n23, 155n25, 213
In re Conroy, 12
constitutional rights, 24–25
consultation
   with ethics committees, 178–84
   with health care professionals, 171–72, 214
   informed decisions and, 110–11
   legislation on, 199n16
   with physicians, 103, 105–6, 123n86, 171–72
contemporaneous autonomy, 105, 193
contemporaneous expressions, 190–94, 208n100
continuity. *See* psychological continuity
controlling influences, 78, 114n7
Coordinating Council on Life-Sustaining Medical Treatment Decision Making, 17
core values
   actions and, 86, 87, 88
   integrity and, 51, 52
   treatment choices and, 92, 93
costs, 25, 169
courts, 178–84, 215. *See also* case law; legal consensus

critical interests, 50–53, 56–57
   autonomy and, 68
   vs. dignity interests, 71–72n34
   vs. experiential interests, 48–49, 50, 56–57
   future-oriented decision and, 49–50
   intentional actions and, 81–82
   of new persons, 146–49
   patient wishes and, 60–61
critically ill patients, 97
Cruzan, Nancy Beth, 11, 18–20, 127
Cruzan v. Director, Missouri Dept. of Health, 18–20, 21, 43n143
current experiences, 58, 165, 192
current interests, xvii, 57–59, 61–62, 72n38, 73n48
   vs. autonomy-based interests, 47, 61–62
   vs. best interests standard, 57–59, 72n45, 192
   connectedness and, 155n25
   continued life and, 63
   of new persons, 148–49
   proxy directives and, 73n46

D

damages, monetary, 28, 168–69, 200n21
Danforth, John, 25
death. *See also* dying
   of the body, 129, 136, 139–40, 142–45, 156n39
   brain, 32n9, 60, 74n53, 160n74
   dignity after, 64
   vs. dying, 53
   interests after, 63–65
   legal, 32n9, 142, 143–44, 148–49, 158n57
   of permanently unconscious patients, 160n74
   of the person, 129, 136, 138, 139–40, 142, 156n39
   premature, 58
   right to, 1–2
   statistics on, xiii, xviiin3
death rituals, 67–68, 136
   bodily continuity and, 139, 143–44, 151, 156n39
death with dignity, 46–47, 53–55, 96, 211
   intentional plans and, 84–85, 111
debilitating illness. *See* progressive illness
decision making, xiii, 30. *See also* end-of-life decisions
   future-oriented, 49–50, 55, 99
   by incompetent patients, xiii–xiv, xvi, 187, 207n89
decisions
   attitudes toward, 86–87
   authentic, 92
   autonomous, 57, 58, 90

decisions—*continued*
  core values and, 88
  respect for, 90–91
Defining Death, 144
dementia patients
  continuity and, 128–29, 134, 135, 155n33
  identity and, 128
  memories of, 132–33
  as new persons, 130, 135, 138, 149
  personhood and, 158n63
  surviving interests of, 59–62, 129
dependence, 54, 59
desires
  first-order, 85–86, 88–89, 118n41
  vs. intention, 193
  for life, 190–94
  second order, 85–86, 88–89, 118n41
  third-order, 88
diagnosis, incorrect, 159n68
dignity, xvii, 13, 53–54, 60–64. *See also* death with dignity
  after death, 64
  familial, 71–72n34
  integrity and, 52–53
  intentional plans and, 84–85, 111, 212
  interests, 71–72n34
  intrinsic, 71n27
disclosure, 120n66
discontinuity theories, 129, 134–35, 142, 145, 213. *See also* psychological continuity
  case study of, 136–38
  identity and, 131–39
  new persons and, 148–49
  nonpersons and, 150
disease-specific directives, 106
diseases. *See* illness
disposal, right of, 146–47, 159n65, 159n66
disrespect, 53
do-not-resuscitate orders, 179
Dresser, Rebecca
  on best interests, 45, 72n45
  on current interests, 57–58, 61–62, 73n46
  on evidence, 15, 16
  on identity, 128, 134, 152n5, 155n25
durable power of attorney, xiv, 22, 105
duty, 27, 214
Dworkin, Gerald, 85–86
Dworkin, Ronald, 45, 46, 48, 55–56, 72n38
dying. *See also* death
  control over, 46–47, 54, 84, 112
  current experience of, 165
  vs. death, 53
  family welfare and, 54
  natural, 30
  quality of, 100
  social relationships and, 141

E

education, 167
effectiveness
  of advance directives, 80–81, 97–111, 213–14
  of intentional plans, 97–98, 111, 214
  of living wills, 98–107, 110–11, 214
  outcome-oriented, 99–103
  of proxy directives, 107–10, 123–24n88
  treatment specificity and, 103–7
elderly, death rate of, xiii
Emanuel, Linda, 103, 104–5, 108
end-of-life decisions, 5, 7–8, 18, 19–20, 118n40
  legislation on, 19–20, 21–26
  monetary damages and, 168–70
  Patient Self-Determination Act and, 25
  rights and, 2
  standards for, 108
  uncertainty in, 162
ends, 50
equality, 13–14
Estate of Leach v. Shapiro, 168–69
ethic of judgment, 162, 164, 187, 197
ethics committees, 7–8, 183
  authority of, 180–81
  confidentiality and, 182
  consultation with, 178–84
  legal consensus on, 18, 205–6n69
  liability and, 34n37, 205n63
  in the *Martin* case, 189–90
  noncompliance and, 178–84
  in nursing homes, 39n99
  patient-centered, 184
  role of, 8, 29, 34n39, 215
  standards for, 182–83
  state legislation on, 39n98, 180
euthanasia, 3–4
evaluational system, 82
Evans, John, 185–87
Evans v. Bellevue Hosp., 17, 185–87
evidence, 14–18, 19, 24, 29
  clear and convincing, 11–12, 15, 16–17, 19, 24
  written documentation as, 17–18, 22, 27
experiences
  connections between, 131–32
  current, 58, 165, 192
  of incompetent patients, 59
  subjects of, 131–32, 141–42, 151
experiential interests
  vs. critical interests, 48–49, 50, 56–57
  identity and, 134
  of incompetent patients, 58, 62, 73n46, 212
  of new persons, 146
  vs. prospective autonomy, 78

F

Faden, Ruth R., 78, 115n14
family
  authority of, 162, 163–64
  Cruzan case and, 18–19
  disagreement in, 190
  ethics committees and, 8
  of permanently unconscious patients, 150–51
  proxy directives and, 108, 110
  role of, 5, 16, 58, 211
  unity of life and, 141
family welfare, xvii, 46–47, 54
  fiscal, 71n31
  future-oriented interest in, 60–61, 62, 64
  noncompliance and, 196
In re Farrell, 35n45
federal legislation, 25–26
Federal Policy for the Protection of Human Subjects in Research, 179
feeding tubes, 11–12, 18–19, 23–24. *See also* artificial feeding
Feinberg, Joel, 47, 50, 64, 69n7
Final Exit (Humphrey), 83
flexibility, of proxy directives, 109
Florida courts
  on assisted suicide, 40n114
  on living wills, 17, 164–65
Florida legislation, 23, 121n71
focal aims, 69n7
foresight, 111
forms, for advance directives, 101, 209n104
Frankfurt, Harry, 85–86
funerals, 67–68, 136, 143–44
futile treatment, xv, 150, 180, 181
future-oriented interests, 46, 60–61, 62, 64, 141
future-oriented rights, 46, 68
future persons, 140–41

G

genetic therapy, 173
Georgia courts, on living wills, 17
Glantz, Leonard, 13
good faith behavior, 28, 169, 190
groupthink, 183
guardianship. *See also* proxy directives
  ad litem, 3
  best interests standard and, 3, 7
  bonded, 165, 199n9
  case law on, 164–65
  of new persons, 136, 142, 148, 151
  of nonpersons, 136, 142, 150
  obligations of, 174–75
  Quinlan case and, 3, 4, 6, 7, 34n32
  self-determination and, 10–11

In re Guardianship of Browning v. Herbert, 164–65, 174, 198n4

H

Halachic Living Will, 124–25n100
Hardwig, John, 125n104
harm, 47, 50, 60, 65–66
  posthumous, 63–65, 75–76n67
health care institutions
  death in, xiii
  immunity for, 28
  noncompliance and, 167
health care professionals, xvi, 25, 26, 108, 167, 183. *See also* physicians
  consultation with, 171–72, 214
health care representatives. *See* proxy directives
Hippocratic tradition, xvi
history, subjects of, 141, 151
Hoffmann, Diane, 199n16
homicide, 3, 30
hopeless ambiguity standard, 170–72
hospitals. *See* health care institutions
Hughes, Richard J., 1, 5
human animals, vs. persons, 157n50
humiliation, 59
Humphrey, Derek, *Final Exit*, 83

I

identity, 127–60, 212–13
  autonomy and, 50–51
  bodily continuity and, 139, 143–44, 151, 153n14, 156n39, 156n40
  case study of, 136–38
  continuity of, 131–39, 154n23, 155n25, 213
  critical interests and, 50–51
  experiential interests and, 134
  of incompetent patients, xviii, 127–60
  integrity and, 46–47
  loss of, 127–30, 135
  of new persons, 128–29, 145–49
  newly dead and, 142–45
  of nonpersons, 128–29, 149–51
  over time, 152n9, 157n49
  of permanently unconscious patients, 149–51
  unity of life and, 139–42
illness. *See also* terminal illness
  chronic, xiii, xviiin3
  possible, 100
  progressive, 23, 36n55, 54, 121n71
immunity, legal. *See* legal immunity
implied consent, 204n61
incompetence, suspension of, 194
incompetent patients, 1–43. *See also* new persons; nonpersons

incompetent patients—*continued*
  autonomy and, xvi, 14
  best interests standard and, 13–14, 45
  cognitive capacity of, 190, 193
  communication by, 191, 207n85
  vs. competent patients, 13–14, 30
  confidentiality for, 182
  continued life and, 58
  decision making by, xiii–xiv, xvi, 30, 207n89
  desires of, 191–94
  experiences of, 59
  experiential interests of, 58, 62, 73n46, 212
  guardianship for. *See* guardianship
  identity of, xviii, 127–60
  interests of, 56–58, 59
  as objects, 63, 73n47
  as organ donors, 14, 148–49
  past of, 61, 62
  person life stages and, 131
  privacy rights and, 6
  prognosis and, 12
  self-determination for, 13–14, 191
  state legislation on, 22–23
indignity, 53, 54, 59
individuals, 143–44, 156n39, 158n64. *See also* persons
infant care review committees, 179
infinite regress, 88–89
information, 98, 120n66
informed consent, 9, 80, 103, 104–7, 110–11
  legislation on, 120n66
  real-time, 99, 104–5, 110–11
injury. *See* harm
innocent parties, 10
institutional ethics committees. *See* ethics committees
institutional policies, 29
institutional review boards, 179
instruction directives. *See* living wills
integrity, 50–53, 93, 97, 118n40
  actions and, 79, 85–87, 88–89, 212
  authorship and, 79
  autonomous actions and, 77–78, 88–89, 111–12
  autonomy as, xvii, 46–47, 54, 60–61, 68, 85–87
  definition of, 51, 70n19, 70n21
  dignity and, 52–53
  identity and, 46–47
  intentional plans and, 84–85, 91
  paternalism and, 91–92
  personal vs. moral, 70n19
  preferences and, 119n53
  reflective acceptance and, 93, 95–96
intentional actions, 212
  autonomous, 78, 79, 81–85
  motivation and, 91

vs. plans, 115n17
values and, 89
intentional plans, 81–85, 90, 111, 213
  vs. actions, 115n17
  case study of, 94–97
  vs. desires, 193
  dignity and, 84–85, 111, 212
  effectiveness of, 97–98, 111, 214
  outcomes and, 116n21
interests. *See also* best interests standard; critical interests
  after death, 63–65
  appreciation of, 59–62
  autonomy-based, 46, 47–50
  dignity, 54
  experiential. *See* experiential interests
  familial, 54
  future-oriented, 46, 60–61, 62, 64, 141
  harm to, 47, 59–62
  of incompetent patients, 56–58
  quality of life and, 48–50
  respect for, 48
  surviving, 59–62, 67–68, 128–29, 145–49, 151
  ulterior, 69n7
  ultimate, 50
interpretation, 166
interventions, definition of, 24
intestate succession, 66
intrinsic value, 13, 45, 71n27
Iowa legislation, on proxy directives, 198n3
irreversible coma, 136, 149, 160n70

J

Jackson, David, 97
Jacobson v. Massachusetts, 35–36n49
Jehovah's Witnesses, 60, 91, 93–94, 119n56
Jewish law, 66, 124–25n100, 143–44
John F. Kennedy Hosp. v. Bludworth, 17
Joint Commission on Accreditation of Healthcare Organizations, 18, 177
Judeo-Christian tradition, 139, 143–44
judgment
  anticipatory, 78, 100, 102, 104
  ethic of, 162, 164, 187, 197
  evaluative, 90
  normative, 80
  by physicians, 93, 177–78
  reflective acceptance and, 93
  substituted. *See* substituted judgment
  surrender of, 183
  uncertainty and, 78
judicial consensus. *See* legal consensus

K

Kadish, Sanford, 191–92
Korsgaard, Christine M., 140
Kuhse, Helga, 158n63

Index

L

laws. *See also* case law; legislation
   common, 9, 10, 35n45
lawsuits. *See* case law
Leach case. *See Estate of Leach v. Shapiro*
legal consensus
   development of, 31n4
   on ethics committees, 18, 205–6n69
   on evidence, 14–18
   on life-sustaining treatment refusal, 9–18, 29–30
   on substituted judgment, 9, 14–18
legal death, 32n9, 142, 143–44, 148–49, 158n57
legal immunity
   for health care institutions, 28
   for physicians, 8, 28, 33–34n30, 43n142, 169, 180–81
legislation, xiv, 1–2, 21–26, 120n66. *See also* state legislation
   on consultation, 199n16
   federal, 35–36
liability
   bad-faith behavior and, 169
   ethics committees and, 34n37, 205n63
   immunity from, 8, 33–34n30
   in noncompliance cases, 177
   in treatment refusal cases, 28
life
   continued, 58, 63, 190, 191
   control over, 61
   longevity of, 173, 174
   memories of, 64
   preference for, 190–94, 208n100
   preservation of, 10, 11, 19
   stages of, 131
   unity of, 139–42, 151
   wrongful, 200n19
life-sustaining treatment refusal, xvi, 1–43. *See also* artificial feeding
   best interests standard and, 3, 7, 9
   case law on, 12, 18–20, 185–87
   case studies of, 137–38, 185–87, 188–97
   common law and, 10
   definition of, 101
   dignity and, 53–54
   vs. euthanasia, 3–4
   legal consensus on, 9–18, 29–30
   medical standards and, 5, 10–11
   physicians on, 3–4, 5
   privacy and, 4, 6, 9, 20
   right of, 4, 9–12
   specific treatments and, 100–101
   state legislation on, 41n123, 101, 121n71
   statistics on, xiii, 160n70
   vs. suicide, 4, 10
Lifton, Robert Jay, 70–71n25
litigation. *See* case law

living wills
   case law on, 17–18, 164–65
   case studies of, 93–97, 137–38
   commonsense view of, 98–103, 107
   condition-specific, 98, 99
   definition of, xiv
   disease-specific, 106
   effectiveness of, 98–107, 110–11, 214
   as evidence, 17
   language of, 171
   noncompliance with. *See* noncompliance with directives
   outcome-oriented, 98, 99–103, 107, 110
   physician-patient relationship and, 103, 105–6
   reactionary view of, 99, 103–7
   state legislation on, 21–25, 41n125, 43n142
   vs. testamentary wills, 65
   treatment-specific, 98–99, 103–7
living, wrongful, 168–69
Locke, John, 132, 156n40
longevity, 173, 174
loyalty, 183
Lynn, Joanne, 77

M

MacIntyre, Alasdair, 141
marriage, 143
In re Martin, 188–94, 206–7n83, 207n85
Martin, Michael, 174, 188–94, 206–7n83, 207n85
Maryland legislation, on ethics committees, 39n98, 180
Massachusetts courts
   on ethics committees, 18
   on substituted judgment, 36n56
materiality, 98, 120n66
May, William, 139, 158n56
medical culture, xvi, 167–68, 178, 215
Medical Directive, 103, 105
medical ethics, 5, 10–11
medical futility. *See* futile treatment
medical profession. *See* health care professionals; physicians
medical standards, 5, 10–11
Meisel, Alan, 38n91
memories, 127, 132–33
Michigan courts, on monetary damages, 169
Miller, Bruce, 92, 93
minimally conscious states, 11
misdiagnosis, 159n68
misinterpretation, 175, 176
Missouri courts, on life-sustaining treatment refusal, 18–20
monetary damages, 28, 168–69, 200n21
moral agents, 51, 140, 141–42, 212
moral weight, 112, 128, 191

motivation, 82, 89, 90, 91, 116n24
Moynihan, Daniel Patrick, 25
Muir, Robert, 3–4
multidisciplinary committees, 179

N
narratives, 141
Natural Death Act, 22
Nelson, Hilde Lindemann, 77, 108
Nelson, James Lindemann, 108
neurological death. *See* brain death
New Jersey Bioethics Commission, 193, 208n99
New Jersey legislation
    on advance directives, 23
    on contemporaneous autonomy, 193
    on directive revocation, 208n99
    on ethics committees, 39n98
    on life-sustaining treatment refusal, 41n123, 101, 121n71
    on proxy directives, 199n10
New Jersey Supreme Court
    on *Conroy*, 12, 35n45
    on *Quinlan*, 4–8, 34n39
new persons, xviii, 73n45, 145–49, 213
    best interests standard and, 148
    continuity threshold and, 130, 135, 136
    current interests of, 148–49
    dementia patients as, 130, 135, 138, 149
    guardianship of, 136, 142, 148, 151
    identity and, 128–29, 145–49
    interests of, 145–49
    judgment of, 134
    vs. nonpersons, 130
    as property, 148, 151, 159n65
    rights of, 146–47, 148
New York courts
    on assisted suicide, 20–21
    on life-sustaining treatment refusal, 185–87
    on living wills, 17
    on monetary damages, 169
New York legislation
    on artificial feeding, 41n127
    on contemporaneous autonomy, 193
    on DNR orders, 179
    on proxy directives, 198n3, 202n35
New York University Medical Center, policies, 29
newly dead persons, 142–45
next generation directives, 165
noncompliance with directives, xviii, 68, 197
    accountability for, 178–84, 215
    ambiguous directives and, 170–72, 197
    autonomy and, 72n38, 112

case studies of, 94, 194–97
circumstances and, 172–74, 192, 214
ethics committees and, 178–84
grounds for, 161–63, 170–76, 181, 184, 197, 215
by hospitals, 167
justifying, 176–78
legal context for, 26–29, 169, 177, 178–84, 208n99
by physicians, 27–29, 112, 167–69, 177, 211
procedure for, 167–84
proxy directives and, 125n104, 162, 174–76, 194–97, 214–15
responsibility for, 162–63, 176–78
nonpersons, xviii, 139, 150
    continuity threshold and, 135, 136
    guardianship of, 136, 142, 150
    identity and, 128–29, 149–51
    judgment of, 134
    vs. new persons, 130
North Carolina courts, on monetary damages, 169
nurses, predictions by, 108
nursing homes, ethics committees in, 39n99
nutritional therapy. *See* artificial feeding

O
objective standards, 75n62
objects, incompetent patients as, 63, 73n47
obligations, 2, 10, 27–39, 66
    of guardianship, 174–75
    surviving, 145–49, 151
O'Connor, Sandra Day, 19, 20, 43n143
Ohio courts, on monetary damages, 168–69
Ohio legislation, on monetary damages, 200n21
oral expression, vs. written, xiv–xv
Oregon legislation
    on advance directives, 23, 41n125, 121n71
    on assisted suicide, 40n114
organ donor cards, 74n52
organ donors
    discontinuity theory and, 148–49
    incompetent patients as, 14
    nonpersons as, 150
    policies on, 158n56
    Uniform Anatomical Gift Act on, 60
organ transplantation, 173, 201n31
organic brain syndrome, 193
Orthodox Jewish law, 124–25n100
Osgood v. Genesys Regional Medical Center, 169
outcome-oriented directives, 98, 99–103, 107, 110
outcomes, 81, 116n21
overriding directives. *See* noncompliance with directives

Index 225

P
Parfit, Derek, 131–33, 134, 154n23
past preferences, 61, 62
paternalism, 91–93, 96, 111, 115n16, 180
patient care
  standards of, 180
  transfer of, 177, 202n38
patient-centered approach, 75n62
Patient Self-Determination Act, 25–26, 42n137
patients. *See also* incompetent patients
  competent, xiii, 12–14, 20–21, 30, 76n70
  critically ill, 97
  dementia. *See* dementia patients
  inconsistent wishes of, 188–94
  permanently unconscious. *See* permanently unconscious patients
  wishes of. *See* wishes (patient)
patients' rights, 38n83, 167, 177
permanently unconscious patients
  case law on, 164–65
  continuity threshold and, 134, 135, 213
  death of, 160n74
  family of, 150–51
  identity of, 149–51
  as nonpersons, 130, 139
persistence, 193
persistent vegetative state, 32n9, 136, 149, 153n10
  Browning case and, 164–65
  Cruzan case and, 11, 18–20
  Quinlan case and, 2–3, 4
personal identity. *See* identity
personhood, 128–29, 130, 158n63
persons. *See also* new persons; nonpersons
  of action, 211–12
  death of, 129, 136, 138, 139–40, 142, 156n39
  future, 140–41
  vs. human animals, 157n50
  vs. individuals, 158n64
  life stages of, 131
  new persons as, 147–49
  newly dead, 142–45
  respect for, 62–63, 68, 74n59
physician-assisted suicide, 20–21, 40n114
physician-patient relationship, 2, 92, 103, 105–6, 184
physicians. *See also* health care professionals
  ambiguous directives and, 166
  attitudes of, xvi, 3–4, 5, 27–29, 42n140
  consultation with, 103, 105–6, 123n86, 171–72
  on ethics committees, 8, 181
  judgment by, 93, 177–78
  legal immunity for, 8, 28, 33–34n30, 43n142, 169, 180–81
  noncompliance by, 27–29, 112, 167–69, 177, 211
  paternalism of, 91–93, 96, 111, 115n16, 180
  patient self-determination and, 10–11
  predictions by, 108
  professional conscience of, 177, 202–3n40
  Quinlan case and, 3–4, 5, 10–11, 33–34n30
  as surrogates, 165–66
  transfer of care and, 177, 202n38
policies, institutional, 29
posthumous harm, 63–65, 75–76n67
precedent autonomy, 56–57, 112
predictions, 107–8
preferences, 85, 107–8, 119n53
  first-order, 86
  for life, 190–94
  past, 61, 62
  predictions of, 107–8
pregnancy
  advance directives and, 24, 35–36n49
  terminal illness in, 36n49
President's Commission for the Study of Ethical Problems in Medicine and Biomedical and Behavioral Research, 144
presumptive weight, 162
prior expressions, 14, 15–16, 190–91
privacy, 4, 6, 9, 18
  Cruzan case and, 17, 20, 39–30n106
probative value, 15
professional conscience, 177, 202–3n40
professional organizations, 10–11
professional success, 51–52
prognosis, 8, 12, 23
progressive illness, 23, 36n55, 54, 121n71
projects, 69n7. *See also* critical interests
proof, burden of, 15, 16
property, new persons as, 148, 151, 159n65
prospective autonomy, xiv, xvii, 1–43, 45–76, 211–12
  vs. contemporaneous autonomy, 105
  current interests approach and, 47, 61–62
  definition of, xv
  ethical foundation of, 45–76
  exercise of, 102
  vs. experiential interests, 78
  incompetent patients and, 1–43
  intentional actions and, 81–85
  legislation and, 22
  proxy directives and, 108
  respect for, 55–57
  testamentary wills and, 65
  unity of life and, 140

prospective decisional autonomy, 57, 77–125
  case study of, 93–97
  integrity and, 85–87
  intentionality and, 81–85
prospective review, 179
protreatment directives, xv, 73n48, 208n101
proxy directives. *See also* guardianship
  alternates in, 125n101
  authority of, 109–10, 174–76
  best interests standard and, 109
  case law on, 17, 169
  case studies of, 137–38, 185–87, 188–97
  current interests approach and, 58, 73n46
  effectiveness of, 107–10, 123–24n88
  family and, 108, 110
  noncompliance with, 125n104, 162, 174–76, 194–97, 214–15
  O'Connor on, 43n143
  Quinlan case and, 6–7
  rebel proxy and, 174–76, 182, 214–15
  religious beliefs and, 124–25n100, 195–97
  respect for, 163–64
  role of, xiv, 30, 80, 84
  state legislation on, 22, 198n3, 199n10, 202n35, 209n104
  trust and, 108, 109, 110
  turncoat proxy and, 175
psychological continuity, 128–29, 142, 212–13
  case study of, 136–38
  identity and, 131–39, 154n23, 155n25, 213
  new persons and, 130, 135, 136
  normal cause of, 154n23
  recovery of, 159n68
  threshold of, 134–35, 149, 154n24, 155n32, 155n33, 213
PVS. *See* persistent vegetative state

Q

quality of life
  interests and, 48–50
  intolerable, 101–2, 103, 189
  legislation and, 24
  vs. preservation of life, 10, 11, 19
  prospective autonomy and, 45
  Quinlan case and, 3–4
  radical change standard and, 173
  reasonable, 186
  substituted judgment and, 16
In re Quinlan, 1, 2–9, 33–34n30, 34n39
Quinlan, Joseph, 4, 6
Quinlan, Karen Ann, 2–9, 32n8

R

radical change in circumstances standard, 172–74, 192, 201n31, 214
Raleigh Fitkin-Paul Morgan Memorial Hosp. v. Anderson, 35–36n49

reactionary view, 99, 103–7
rebel proxy standard, 174–76, 182, 214–15
recovery, 159n68
reflective acceptance, 85–87, 92–93, 95–96, 119n53, 213
refusal of treatment. *See* treatment refusal
Rehnquist, William, 1, 19, 21
reliability, 15
religious beliefs
  bodily continuity and, 139
  bodily death and, 143–44
  brain death and, 74n53
  case study of, 93–97
  conversion to, 93–94, 174, 201–2n34
  death rituals and, 67–68
  death with dignity and, 96
  proxy directives and, 124–25n100
  violation of, 60
reputation, 48
respect
  for actions, 90–91
  for advance directives, xviii, 64–65
  for autonomy, 53, 55–57, 81
  for choices, 63, 90–91
  for interests, 48
  for persons, 62–63, 68, 74n59
responsibility, 55, 176–78
Rhoden, Nancy, 15–16
rights
  constitutional, 24–25
  death and, 1–2
  of disposal, 146–47, 159n65, 159n66
  future-oriented, 46, 68
  harm to, 47
  legal, 2
  of new persons, 146–47, 148
  obligations and, 2, 10
  of patients, 38n83, 167, 177
  to privacy, 4, 6, 9, 20
  of professional conscience, 177, 202–3n40
Robertson, John
  on best interests, 45, 72n45
  on current interests, 57–58, 61–62, 73n46
  on identity, 128, 152n5

S

Saikewicz case. *See Superintendent of Belchertown State School v. Saikewicz*
Saunders v. State, 17
Scalia, Antonin, 19
Scrooge, Ebenezer, 52
self-authorship, 50–51
self-destruction, 4
self-determination, xiii, 4, 6
  common law right to, 9, 10, 35n45
  death with dignity and, 54
  for incompetent patients, 13–14, 191
  Patient Self-Determination Act on, 25–26

self-determination—*continued*
  physicians and, 10
  state legislation on, 22–23
  substituted judgment and, 16
  surviving interests and, 146
self-esteem, 59
self-identification, 50–51, 87
self, loss of, 128
self-study, 87
shape-shifters, 70–71n25
social relationships, 141
social workers, predictions by, 108
standards
  for ethics committees, 182–83
  medical, 5, 10–11
  objective, 75n62
  for patient care, 180
  subjective, 75n62, 98
state courts. *See also* case law; *specific states*
  on assisted suicide, 20–21
  on life-sustaining treatment refusal, 11–12
  on living wills, 17, 164–65
  on monetary damages, 168–69
  on proxy directives, 169
state interests, in preservation of life, 10, 11, 19
state legislation, 21–25. *See also specific states*
  on advance directives, 21–25, 41n125, 43n142
  on artificial feeding, 23–24, 41n127
  on assisted suicide, 40n114
  on contemporaneous autonomy, 193
  on directive revocation, 208n99
  on DNR orders, 179
  on durable power of attorney, 22
  on ethics committees, 39n98, 180
  on immunity, 169
  on incompetent patients, 22–23
  on life-sustaining treatment refusal, 41n123, 101, 121n71
  on living wills, 22
  on monetary damages, 200n21
  patients' rights and, 38n83
  on prognosis, 23
  on progressive illness, 23, 36n55, 121n71
  on proxy directives, 22, 198n3, 199n10, 202n35, 209n104
  on self-determination, 22–23
  testamentary wills and, 65
Stevenson, C. L., 69n7
Strunk v. Strunk, 14
Study to Understand Prognoses and Preferences for Outcomes and Risks of Treatment. *See* SUPPORT
subjective standards, 75n62, 98
substituted judgment, 5–7, 14, 16, 30
  best interests standard and, 14–15, 16
  case law on, 36n56

  legal consensus on, 9, 14–18
  uncertainty and, 166
success, professional, 51–52
suicide, 20–21, 40n113
  vs. dying, 30
  intentional, 83
  vs. life-sustaining treatment refusal, 4, 10
  preventing, 10
Superintendent of Belchertown State School v. Saikewicz, 13
SUPPORT, xvi, 167
Supreme Court
  on assisted suicide, 20–21, 40n114
  on *Cruzan*, 11, 19–20
  on end-of-life decisions, 19–20
  on privacy, 39–30n106
  on treatment refusal, 19–20
surrogates. *See also* proxy directives
  bonded, 166, 199n9
  disputes between, 181
  physicians as, 165–66
surviving interests, 59–62, 67–68, 128–29, 145–49, 151
suspension of directives, 193–94

T

Taylor, Gabriele, 86, 117–18n39
technology, 5, 173, 201n31
Teel, Karen, 34n37
Teno, Joan, 77, 161
terminal illness
  assisted suicide for, 20–21
  costs of, 25
  definition of, 23, 165, 198n5
  language of, 100
  in pregnancy, 36n49
  social relationships and, 141
  state legislation and, 23
testamentary wills, 65–67, 76n70
Texas Advance Directives Act, 180
Texas legislation, on ethics committees, 39n98, 180
theory of the will, 85–86, 88
third party judgment. *See* substituted judgment
transfer of care, 177, 202n38
treatment
  costs of, 169
  definition of, 24
  futile, xv, 150, 180, 181
  for nonpersons, 150
  protreatment directives and, xv, 73n48, 208n101
  radical change in, 172–73, 201n31
  without advance directives, 66–67
  wrongful continuation of, 169
treatment choices, 90–91, 92, 93
  of new persons, 146–47

treatment refusal, xv, 1–43. *See also* life-sustaining treatment refusal
  autonomy and, xiii
  case study of, 93–97
  common law right to, 9, 10
  legal consensus on, 9–18, 29–30
  legislation on, 21–26
  liability and, 28
  motivation for, 91, 97
  noncompliance with. *See* noncompliance with directives
  Quinlan case and, 2–8
  specific treatments and, 100–101, 103–7
  statistics on, xiii
  substituted judgment and, 5–7
  Supreme Court on, 19–20
  treatment, thent-specific documents, 98–99, 100–101, 103–7
trust, 80, 105, 108–9, 110, 174, 186
turncoat proxy, 175

U

ultimate interests, 50
uncertainty, 78, 104, 162, 163, 166
unconscious patients. *See* permanently unconscious patients
understanding, actions and, 78, 113–14n7
Uniform Anatomical Gift Act, 60
uninsured persons, 105
unity of agency, 157n43
unity of life, 139–42, 151
unity relation, 131, 133
U.S. Supreme Court. *See* Supreme Court

V

Vacco v. Quill, 21
values. *See also* core values
  actions and, 51, 86
  changes in, 174, 202n34
  first-order vs. second order, 85–86
  intentional plans and, 83
  intrinsic, 13, 45, 71n27
  vs. motivations, 116n24
  proxy, 176
Values History, 55
Values Profile, 71n33
Veatch, Robert M., 109, 139, 156n39, 176
Virginia legislation, on advance directives, 43n142
volitions, second-order, 85–86, 87, 118n41

von Bulow, Sonny, 175
vulnerable patients, 24

W

wanting, vs. willing, 116n21
wards. *See* guardianship
Washington courts, on assisted suicide, 20–21
Washington v. Glucksberg, 1, 21
Watson, Gary, 116n24
well-being, 16
West Virginia Health Care Decisions Act, 209n104
West Virginia legislation
  on contemporaneous autonomy, 193
  on proxy directives, 209n104
will, theory of the, 85–86, 88
willful disregard, 28
Williams, Bernard, 69n7, 140–41
willing, vs. wanting, 116n21
wills
  living. *See* living wills
  testamentary, 65–67, 76n70
Winter, Edward, 168–69
Wirth, Tom, 185–87
Wisconsin courts, on life-sustaining treatment refusal, 11–12
wishes (patient)
  best interests standard and, 13
  clear and convincing evidence for, 11–12
  critical interests and, 60–61
  ignored, 167
  inconsistent, 188–94
  prior expressions of, 15–16
  proxy directives and, 125n104
  specificity of, 189
written documentation, xiv–xv, 23, 27
  as evidence, 17–18, 22, 27
wrongful life, 200n19
wrongful living, 168–69

X

xenografts, 201n31

Y

Youngner, Stuart, 97

Z

Zodin v. Manor Healthcare Corp., 17, 198n7